GENOSYS–Exam Preparatory Manual for Undergraduates

Biochemistry

GENOSYS–Exam Preparatory Manual for Undergraduates

Biochemistry

(A Simplified Approach)

Neethu Lakshmi N
MBBS Final Year (Part-I) Student
Kannur Medical College
Kannur, Kerala, India

Aiswarya S Lal
MBBS Final Year (Part-I) Student
Kannur Medical College
Kannur, Kerala, India

Nikhila K
MBBS Final Year (Part-I) Student
Kannur Medical College
Kannur, Kerala, India

Divya JS
MBBS Final Year (Part-I) Student
Kannur Medical College
Kannur, Kerala, India

Nimisha PM
MBBS Final Year (Part-I) Student
Kannur Medical College
Kannur, Kerala, India

JAYPEE The Health Sciences Publisher

New Delhi | London | Philadelphia | Panama

Jaypee Brothers Medical Publishers (P) Ltd

Headquarters

Jaypee Brothers Medical Publishers (P) Ltd
4838/24, Ansari Road, Daryaganj
New Delhi 110 002, India
Phone: +91-11-43574357
Fax: +91-11-43574314
Email: jaypee@jaypeebrothers.com

Overseas Offices

J.P. Medical Ltd
83 Victoria Street, London
SW1H 0HW (UK)
Phone: +44 20 3170 8910
Fax: +44 (0)20 3008 6180
Email: info@jpmedpub.com

Jaypee-Highlights Medical Publishers Inc
City of Knowledge, Bld. 237, Clayton
Panama City, Panama
Phone: +1 507-301-0496
Fax: +1 507-301-0499
Email: cservice@jphmedical.com

Jaypee Medical Inc
The Bourse
111 South Independence Mall East
Suite 835, Philadelphia, PA 19106, USA
Phone: +1 267-519-9789
Email: jpmed.us@gmail.com

Jaypee Brothers Medical Publishers (P) Ltd
17/1-B Babar Road, Block-B, Shaymali
Mohammadpur, Dhaka-1207
Bangladesh
Mobile: +08801912003485
Email: jaypeedhaka@gmail.com

Jaypee Brothers Medical Publishers (P) Ltd
Bhotahity, Kathmandu, Nepal
Phone +977-9741283608
Email: kathmandu@jaypeebrothers.com

Website: www.jaypeebrothers.com
Website: www.jaypeedigital.com

Inquiries for bulk sales may be solicited at: jaypee@jaypeebrothers.com

GENOSYS–Exam Preparatory Manual for Undergraduates—Biochemistry

First Edition: **2015**

ISBN: 978-93-5152-636-0

Printed at Rajkamal Electric Press, Plot No. 2, Phase-IV, Kundli, Haryana.

Dedicated to

Our Parents and Teachers

Preface

The first year of MBBS has become an increasingly tough year. As we experienced ourselves with anatomy, physiology and biochemistry covered during first year, biochemistry tends to receive the least attention by most of the students. At that point of time, we always felt a need for a comprehensive and examination-oriented preparatory manual for biochemistry. It is with great pleasure and satisfaction we are presenting *GENOSYS-Exam Preparatory Manual for Undergraduates—Biochemistry*. This book is a yield of notes with the information gathered from various standard textbooks.

Biochemistry is a highly volatile subject. Most of the standard textbooks available are too vast and inconclusive to study. It becomes a herculean task for most of them to study the entire syllabus or even revise the same just before the examination and what matters more than hard work is smart work. This is when GENOSYS comes to the rescue of the students. We hope that this book will help the students to perfect their examination preparation. It is something we wished to be available for us when we were in the MBBS first year.

For any subject, there is no easy way out; it has to be learnt in depth to understand. A concerted effort has been made to make this process an easy affair with lucid language, illustrations, flow charts and tables. Clinical correlations are incorporated at the end of appropriate topics. This will be extremely useful in developing interest of the students in the subject. Practicals are covered in a systematic manner. We have also included viva voce, important topics, multiple choice questions and a separate chapter on biochemical pathways for better understanding.

We have put all our efforts in creating this meticulous handbook, pretty simple, and at the same time, covering all the essentials of biochemistry. But we would like to clearly emphasize that this is not a textbook, but rather a supplement to recommended texts. So, we kindly request prospective students to read their prescribed textbooks first before reading this book.

Although this book has been written primarily for undergraduate MBBS students, it should also prove to be useful to alternative medicine students like BDS, BAMS, BHMS, Unani and Siddha, etc.

Sincere attempts have been made to maintain the accuracy and correctness of the subject. But we solicit your valuable comments and criticism to improve this book and make it more useful.

In conclusion, we acknowledge the Almighty with whose blessings, this book has become a reality. Wishing all the best to all the students in forthcoming examinations.

Neethu Lakshmi N
Aiswarya S Lal
Divya JS
Nikhila K
Nimisha PM

Preface

Acknowledgments

We thank God first for giving us this opportunity and for helping us complete the book successfully. We thank our parents for giving us support and encouragement we needed.

We wish to express the deepest gratitude to Dr Sanoop KS of 2007 batch (Kannur Medical College, Kannur, Kerala, India) who guided us with valuable inputs and corrected our mistakes. He gave us selfless support for preparing the manuscript of this book. He cleared our doubts and helped us to make this book as close to perfect as possible. Without his guidance and help, the completion of this book could never have been realized.

We also extend our gratitude to Dr Seetha, Head of the Department of Biochemistry, Kannur Medical College and all the faculty members for their valuable advices.

Last but not least, we thank Dr Nishanth PS (Kannur Medical College), Mohammed Ashkar (2011 MBBS, Kannur Medical College), Mashhood VP (2011 MBBS, Kannur Medical College), Nandita Ranjit (2011 MBBS, Kannur Medical College) and all our batchmates (2011 MBBS) for their support throughout this venture.

We also thank Shri Jitendar P Vij (Group Chairman), Mr Ankit Vij (Group President), Mr Tarun Duneja (Director-Publishing) of M/s Jaypee Brothers Medical Publishers (P) Ltd, New Delhi, India and all other staff of Bengaluru branch, for their encouragement and support, which made this book possible.

Contents

Section I: Theories

Section II: Practicals

Viva Voce

Appendix 1

Appendix 2

Section 1

Theories

Chapter 1

Cell and Subcellular Organelles

Biochemistry can be defined as the science concerned with the chemical basis of life (Greek bios means 'life'). The cell is the structural unit of living systems. Thus, biochemistry can also be described as the science concerned with chemical constituents of living cells and with the reactions and processes they undergo. By this definition, biochemistry encompasses large areas of cell biology, of molecular biology and of molecular genetics.

CELL

The cell is the structural and functional unit of life. It is also known as the basic unit of biological activity.

Prokaryotic and Eukaryotic Cell

Present-day living organisms can be divided into two large groups, i.e the prokaryotes and eukaryotes. The prokaryotes are represented by bacteria (eubacteria and archaebacteria). These organisms do not possess a well-defined nucleus.

The eukaryotes include fungi, plants and animals, and comprise both unicellular and multicellular organisms. Multicellular eukaryotes are made up of a wide variety of cell types that are specialized for different tasks. A comparison of characteristics between prokaryotes and eukaryotes are listed in Table 1.1.

Table 1.1: Comparison between prokaryotic and eukaryotic cell

Characteristics	Prokaryote	Eukaryote
Organisms	Eubacteria Archaebacteria	Fungi Plants Animals
Form and size	Singlecelled; 1–10 μm	Single or multicellular; 10–100 μm
Organelles, cytoskeleton, cell division apparatus	Missing	Present, complicated, specialized
Nucleus	Not well-defined	Well-defined
Deoxyribonucleic acid (DNA)	Small, circular, no introns, plasmids	Large, in nucleus, many introns
Cell membrane	Cell is enveloped by a rigid cell wall	Cell is enveloped by a flexible plasma membrane
Ribonucleic acid (RNA): Synthesis and maturation	Simple, in cytoplasm	Complicated, in nucleus
Protein: Synthesis and maturation	Simple, coupled with RNA synthesis	Complicated, in the cytoplasm and the rough endoplasmic reticulum
Metabolism	Anaerobic or aerobic very flexible	Mostly aerobic, compartmented
Endocytosis and exocytosis	No	Yes

Structure of an Animal Cell

In the human body alone, there are at least 200 different cell types. The basic structures of an animal cell are as shown in the Figure 1.1.

The eukaryotic cell is subdivided by membranes. On the outside, it is enclosed by a plasma membrane. Inside the cell, there is a large space containing numerous components in solution—the cytoplasm. Different organelles are distributed in the cytoplasm.

The largest organelle is the nucleus. It is surrounded by a double membrane nuclear envelope. The endoplasmic reticulum (ER) is a closed network of shallow sacs and tubules, and is linked with the outer membrane of the nucleus. Another membrane bound organelle is the Golgi apparatus, which resembles a bundle of layered slices. The endosomes and exosomes are bubble-shaped compartments (vesicles) that are involved in the exchange of substances between the cell and its surroundings. Probably the most important organelles in the cell's metabolism are the mitochondria, which are around the same size as bacteria. The lysosomes and peroxisomes are small, globular organelles that carry out specific tasks. The whole cell is traversed by a framework of proteins known as the cytoskeleton.

Functions of Cellular Organelles

1. Centrioles: Help to organize the assembly of microtubules.
2. Chromosomes: House cellular deoxyribonucleic acid (DNA).
3. Cilia and flagella: Aid in cellular locomotion.
4. Endoplasmic reticulum: Synthesizes carbohydrates and lipids.
5. Golgi complex: Manufactures, stores and ships certain cellular products.
6. Lysosomes: Digest cellular macromolecules (hence they are called suicidal bags).

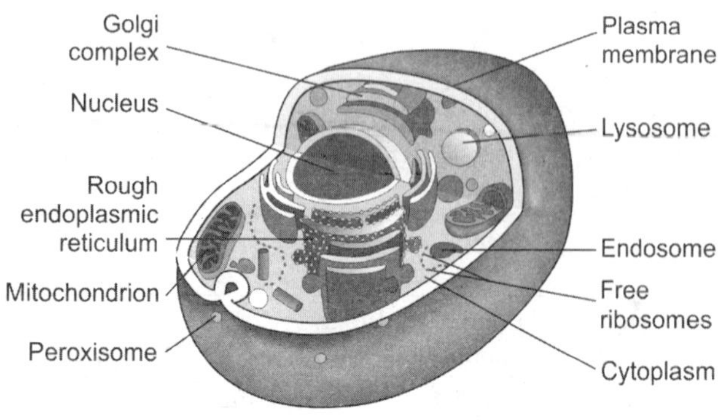

Fig. 1.1: Structure of animal cell

7. Mitochondria: Provide energy for the cell.
8. Nucleus: Controls cell growth and reproduction.
9. Peroxisomes: Detoxify alcohol, form bile acid and use oxygen to breakdown fats.
10. Ribosomes: Responsible for protein production via translation.

Cell Membrane

The plasma membrane is an envelope covering the cell. It separates and protects the cell from external environment. Besides being the protective barrier, it also provides a connecting system between the cell and environment.

Structure of Cell Membrane

The membrane is composed of lipids, proteins and carbohydrates. A lipid bilayer model for biological membrane was originally proposed in 1935 by Davson and Danielli. Later, the structure of the cell membrane was described as a ***fluid mosaic model*** by Singer and Nicolson in 1972 (Fig. 1.2).

The membrane consists of a bimolecular lipid layer with proteins inserted in it or bound to either surface. Integral membrane proteins are firmly embedded in the lipid layers. Some of these proteins completely span the bilayer called transmembrane proteins, while others are embedded in either the outer or inner leaflet of the lipid bilayer.

Loosely bound to the outer or inner surface of the membrane are the peripheral proteins. Many of the proteins and lipids have externally exposed oligosaccharide chains:

1. Extrinsic (peripheral) membrane proteins are loosely held to the surface of the membrane and they can be easily separated, e.g. cytochrome of mitochondria.
2. Intrinsic (integral) membrane proteins are tightly bound to lipid bilayer and they can be separated only by the use of detergents or organic solvents, e.g. hormone receptors and cytochrome P450.

LYSOSOMES

Lysosomes are tiny enzymes, which are considered as the bag of enzymes.

Enzymes Present

1. Polysaccharide hydrolyzing enzymes (α-glucosidase, α-fucoside, β-galactosidase and hyaluronidase).
2. Protein hydrolyzing enzymes (cathepsins, collagenase, elastase).
3. Nucleic acid hydrolyzing enzymes (ribonuclease and deoxyribonuclease).
4. Lipid hydrolyzing enzymes (fatty acyl esterase and phosphor lipases).

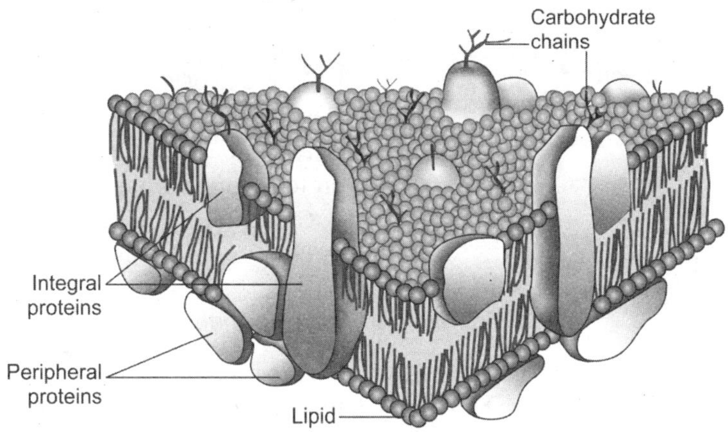

Fig. 1.2: Fluid mosaic model

Clinical Correlation of Lysosomes

1. In gout, urate crystals are deposited around knee joints. These crystals are easily phagocytosed, causing physical damage to lysosomes and release of enzymes.
2. Following cell death, lysosomes rupture releasing the hydrolytic enzymes.
3. Lysosomal proteases, cathepsins are implicated in tumor metastasis. Cathepsins, which are normally restricted to interior of lysosomes degrade basal lamina by hydrolyzing collagen and elastin so that other tumor cells can travel to form distant metastasis.

PEROXISOMES

Peroxisomes are also called microbodies, are single membrane cellular organelles.

Enzymes Present

Catalases and peroxidases are the enzymes present in peroxisomes, which will destroy the unwanted peroxides and radicals.

Clinical Correlation of Peroxisomes

1. Deficiency of peroxisomal proteins can lead to adrenoleukodystrophy (ALD) or Brown-Schilder's disease characterized by progressive degeneration of liver, kidneys and brain.
2. In Zellweger syndrome, proteins are not transported into peroxisomes leading to formation of empty peroxisomes or peroxisomal ghosts.

MITOCHONDRIA

Mitochondria are enclosed by two membranes—a smooth outer membrane and a markedly folded or tubular inner mitochondrial membrane, which has a large surface and encloses the matrix space. The folds of the inner membrane are known as cristae and tube-like protrusions are called tubules. The intermembrane space is located between the inner and the outer membranes.

Functions

1. Mitochondria are also described as being the cell's biochemical powerhouse, since through oxidative phosphorylation (refer page 69), they produce the majority of cellular adenosine triphosphate (ATP).
2. Pyruvate dehydrogenase (PDH), the tricarboxylic acid cycle, β-oxidation of fatty acids and parts of the urea cycle are located in the matrix. The respiratory chain, ATP synthesis and enzymes involved in heme biosynthesis are associated with the inner membrane.
3. In addition to the endoplasmic reticulum, the mitochondria also function as an intracellular calcium reservoir. The mitochondria also plays an important role in 'programmed cell death'—apoptosis.

MARKER MOLECULES

Marker molecules are molecules that occur exclusively or predominantly in one type of organelle (Table 1.2). The activity of organelle-specific enzymes (marker enzymes) is often assessed. The distribution of marker enzymes in the cell reflects the compartmentation of the processes they catalyze.

TRANSPORT MECHANISMS

Many small uncharged molecules pass freely through the lipid bilayer. Charged molecules, larger uncharged molecules and some small uncharged molecules are transferred through channels or pores, or by specific carrier proteins.

The transport mechanisms (Fig. 1.3) are classified into:

1. Passive transport: Transport of molecules in accordance with concentration gradient:
   a. Simple diffusion.
   b. Facilitated diffusion.
   c. Ion channels.
2. Active transport.

Table 1.2: Marker enzymes

Subcellular organelle	Marker enzyme
Nucleus	–
Mitochondria	Adenosine triphosphate (ATP) synthase
Lysosome	Cathepsin
Golgi complex	Galactosyltransferase
Microsomes	Glucose-6-phosphatase
Cytoplasm	Lactate dehydrogenase

Passive Transport

Simple Diffusion

In order for molecules to simply diffuse across a membrane, they must either be quite small so as to enter membrane pores, go via the paracellular route or be soluble in the lipid membrane. No energy is required.

Facilitated Diffusion

Transport is facilitated by a transport protein therefore this is a carrier-mediated transport. The driving force is the concentration gradient. Glucose and amino acids use this mechanism.

Aquaporins

1. Water channels that serve as selective pores through which water crosses plasma membrane of cells.

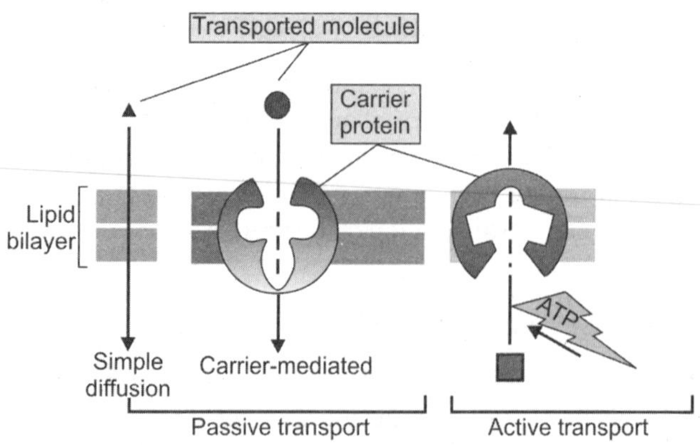

Fig. 1.3: Transport mechanism (ATP, adenosine triphosphate)

2. Form tetramers in cell membrane.
3. Facilitate transport of water and hence, control water content of cells.

Clinical correlation

Channelopathies are disorders due to abnormalities in proteins forming ion pores or channels. For example:

- Cystic fibrosis (chloride channels)
- Liddle's syndrome (sodium channels).

Ion Channels

Ion channels are transmembrane proteins that allow the selective entry of various ions. Selective ion-conductive pores are selective for one particular ion. Channels generally remain closed and they open in response to stimuli. The regulation is done by gated channels such as ligand-gated ion channel and calcium channel. For example:

- Nerve impulse propagation
- Synaptic transmission
- Secretion of active substances from cell.

Ionophores

Ionophores are membrane shuttles for specific ions, which transport certain ions. There are two types of ionophores:

- Mobile ion carriers (e.g. valinomycin)
- Channel formers (e.g. gramicidin).

Clinical correlation

Valinomycin allows potassium to permeate mitochondria and so it dissipates the proton gradient. Hence, it acts as an uncoupler of electron transport chain.

Active Transport

- Require 40% of total energy used
- Unidirectional
- Need special integral protein, called transporter protein
- System is saturated at high concentration of solutes
- Susceptible for inhibition by specific organic or inorganic compounds. For example, sodium-potassium pump (Na^+ -K^+ ATPase) cell has less concentration of sodium and high concentration of potassium (K). This is maintained by pump and the pump is activated by ATPase enzyme. They have binding sites for ATP and Na^+ on inner side and K^+ on outer side.

TRANSPORT SYSTEMS

Carrier is a transport protein that binds ions and other molecules and then changes their configuration, thus moving the bound molecule from one side of cell membrane to other.

Table 1.3: Comparison between symport and antiport

Symport	Antiport
Simultaneously two molecules are carried across membrane in same direction	Simultaneously two molecules are carried across membrane in opposite direction
For example, sodium-dependent glucose transporter	For example, sodium pump or chloride-bicarbonate exchange in red blood cell (RBC)

Types

There are two types of transport system.

Uniport

Uniport-carries single solute across the membrane (e.g. glucose transporter in most cells).

Cotransport

Cotransport is of two types—symport and antiport (Table 1.3).

Chapter 2

Enzymology

ENZYMES

Characteristics of enzymes are:
- Biological catalysts
- Not consumed during a chemical reaction
- Speed up reactions from 10^3 to 10^{17}
- Exhibit stereospecificity
- Exhibit reaction specificity.

NOMENCLATURE

Trivial Names

Typically add '-ase' to the name of substrate, e.g. lactase breaks down lactose (disaccharide of glucose and galactose).

IUBMB System of Classification

The International Union of Biochemistry and Molecular Biology (IUBMB) classifies enzymes based upon the class of organic chemical reaction catalyzed (Table 2.1).

Table 2.1: Enzyme classification

Enzyme class	Example for enzyme	Reaction catalyzed
Oxidoreductase	Alcohol dehydrogenase Cytochrome oxidase	Oxidation → Reduction
Transferase	Hexokinase Transaminase	Group transfer
Hydrolase	Lipase Cholinesterase	Hydrolysis
Isomerase	Triose phosphate isomerase Retinol isomerase	Interconversion of isomers
Lyases	Aldolase Fumarase	Addition → Elimination
Ligases	Glutamine synthetase Acetyl-coA carboxylase	Condensation [usually dependent on adenosine triphosphate (ATP)]

PROSTHETIC GROUPS, COFACTORS AND COENZYMES

Many enzymes contain small non-protein molecules and metal ions that participate directly in substrate binding or catalysis. These are termed as prosthetic groups, cofactors and coenzymes.

Prosthetic Groups

Prosthetic groups are tightly integrated into an enzyme's structure. These are distinguished by their tight, stable incorporation into a protein's structure by covalent or non-covalent forces. Examples include pyridoxal phosphate, flavin mononucleotide (FMN), flavin dinucleotide (FAD), thiamin pyrophosphate, biotin; and the metal ions of cobalt (Co), copper (Cu), magnesium (Mg), manganese (Mn), selenium (Se) and zinc (Zn). Metals are the most common prosthetic groups. Roughly, one third of all enzymes that contain tightly bound metal ions are termed metalloenzymes. Metal ions that participate in redox reactions generally are complexed to prosthetic groups such as heme or iron-sulfur clusters. Important metalloenzymes are:
- Carbonic anhydrase, alcohol dehydrogenase, carboxypeptidase: Zinc
- Hexokinase, phosphofructokinase, enolase: Magnesium
- Tyrosinase, cytochrome oxidase, superoxide dismutase: Copper

Mnemonic:
'**O**ver **T**he **HILL**':

- ***O***xidoreductases
- ***T***ransferases
- ***H***ydrolases
- ***I***somerases
- ***L***igases
- ***L***yases

Enzymes get reaction over the hill

- Cytochrome oxidase, catalase, peroxidase: Iron
- Lecithinase, Lipase: Calcium
- Xanthine oxidase: Molybdenum.

Cofactors

Cofactors associate reversibly with enzymes or substrates. Cofactors serve functions similar to those of prosthetic groups, but bind in a transient, dissociable manner either to the enzyme or to a substrate such as adenosine triphosphate (ATP). Unlike the stably associated prosthetic groups, cofactors therefore must be present in the medium surrounding the enzyme for catalysis to occur. The most common cofactors also are metal ions. Enzymes that require a metal ion cofactor are termed metal-activated enzymes to distinguish them from the metalloenzymes for which metal ions serve as prosthetic groups.

Coenzymes

Coenzymes serve as recyclable shuttles or group transfer reagents that transport many substrates from their point of generation to their point of utilization. Association with the coenzyme also stabilizes substrates such as hydrogen atoms or hydride ions that are unstable in the aqueous environment of the cell. Other chemical moieties transported by coenzymes include methyl groups (folates), acyl groups (coenzyme A) and oligosaccharides (dolichol).

ENZYME KINETICS

Mathematical and graphical study of the rates of enzyme-catalyzed reactions are detailed below:

$$S \xrightarrow{k} P$$

$$A + B \xrightarrow{k} C$$

The velocity of this reaction can be summarized by the following equation:

$$V = k\,[S] \text{ or } V = k\,[A][B]$$

This reaction is considered a first order reaction, determined by the sum of the exponents in the rate equation, i.e. the number of molecules reacting.

There are also bimolecular reactions, which involve two substrates:

$$S_1 + S_2 \longrightarrow P_1 + P_2$$

$V = k\,[S_1][S_2]$, first order for each reactant.

For enzyme-catalyzed reactions:

$$E + S \longrightarrow ES \longrightarrow E + P$$

The rate or velocity is dependent upon both the enzyme and substrate.

In reactions:

$$E + S \underset{k_{-1}}{\overset{k_1}{\rightleftharpoons}} ES \xrightarrow{k_{cat}} E + P$$

where,
k_1 and k-1 govern the rates of association and dissociation of ES; k_{cat} is the turnover number or catalytic constant:

$$V_{ES} = k_1\,[E][S]$$

$$V_{E+S} = k_{-1}\,[ES]$$

$$V_{E+P} = k_{cat}\,[ES]$$

Usually an enzyme's velocity (V_o) is measured under initial conditions of [S] and [P].

These same reactions can be described graphically:

- At low [S], V_o increases as [S] increases
- At high [S], enzymes become saturated with substrates and the reaction is independent of [S].

$$V_{max} = k_{cat}\,[ES]$$

or because the [S] is irrelevant at high [S],

$$V_{max} = k_{cat}\,[E]$$

The graph is a hyperbola and the equation for a hyperbola is:

$$y = \frac{ax}{b + x}$$

where,
a is the asymptote
b is the value at a/2

Substituting equation parameters:

$$V_o = \frac{V_{max}[S]}{K_m + [S]}$$

MICHAELIS-MENTEN THEORY

According to this enzyme-substrate complex theory put forward by Michaelis and Menten, the enzyme (E) combines with the substrate (S), to form an enzyme-substrate (ES) complex, which immediately breaks down to the enzyme and the product (P).

$$E + P \rightleftharpoons ES \text{ complex} \longrightarrow E + P$$

Different enzymes reach V_{max} at different [S], because enzymes differ in their affinity for the substrate or K_m:

1. The greater the tendency for an enzyme and substrate to form an ES, the higher the enzyme's affinity for the substrate, i.e. lower K_m.
2. The greater the affinity of enzymes, the lower the [S] needed to saturate the enzyme or to reach V_{max}.

Enzyme-substrate affinity and reaction kinetics are closely associated:

[S] at which $V_o = 1/2$

$V_{max} = K_m$

Here,

K_m is a measure of enzyme affinity

So,

$$K_m = \frac{k_{-1}}{k_1}$$

Where,

K_1 and K_1 are reaction constants of association and dissociation of ES:

- A small K_m (high affinity) favors E + S ⟶ ES
- A large K_m (low affinity) favors ES ⟶ E + S
- Meaning that the lower the K_m, the less substrate is needed to saturate the enzyme.

These two parameters K_m and V_{max} are used to describe the efficiency of enzymes.

These are graphically done by taking the reciprocal of both sides of the equation, i.e. double reciprocal plot or Lineweaver-Burk plot (Fig. 2.1).

$$V_o = \frac{V_{max}[S]}{K_m + [S]}$$

$$\frac{1}{V_o} = \frac{K_m}{V_{max}} \frac{1}{[S]} + \frac{1}{V_{max}}$$

FACTORS AFFECTING ENZYME ACTIVITY

Substrate Concentration

Maximal velocity: The rate or velocity of a reaction (V) is the number of substrate molecules converted to product per unit time; velocity is usually expressed as µmol of product formed per minute. The rate of an enzyme-catalyzed reaction increases with substrate concentration until a maximal velocity (V_{max}) is reached (Fig. 2.2).

Hyperbolic shape of the enzyme kinetics curve: Most enzymes show Michaelis-Menten kinetics in which the plot of initial reaction velocity (V_o) against substrate concentration [S], is hyperbolic. In contrast, allosteric enzymes do not follow Michaelis-Menten kinetics and show a sigmoidal curve.

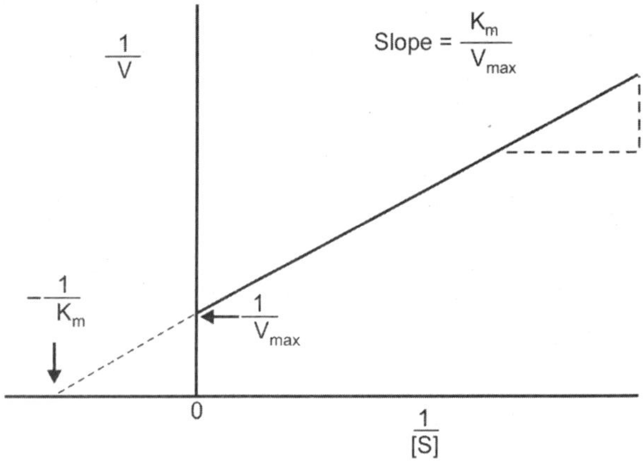

Fig. 2.1: Relation between K_m and V_{max} (Lineweaver-Burk plot)

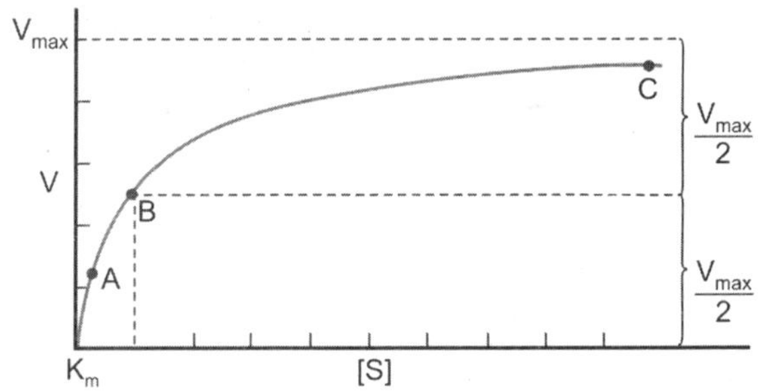

Fig. 2.2: Effect of enzyme concentration on initial velocity

Temperature

Increase of velocity with temperature: The reaction velocity increases with temperature until a peak velocity is reached. This increase is the result of the increased number of molecules having sufficient energy to pass over the energy barrier and form the products of the reaction.

Decrease of velocity with higher temperature: Further elevation of the temperature results in a decrease in reaction velocity as a result of temperature-induced denaturation of the enzyme.

The optimum temperature for most human enzymes is between 35°C and 40°C. Human enzymes start to denature at temperatures above 40°C, but thermophilic bacteria found in the hot springs have optimum temperatures of 70°C.

Effect of pH

Effect of pH on the ionization of the active site: The concentration of H^+ affects reaction velocity in several ways. First, the catalytic process usually requires that the enzyme and substrate have specific chemical groups in either an ionized or unionized state in order to interact. For example, catalytic activity may require that an amino group of the enzyme be in the protonated form ($-NH_3^+$). At alkaline pH, this group is deprotonated and the rate of the reaction, therefore declines.

Effect of pH on enzyme denaturation: Extremes of pH can also lead to denaturation of the enzyme, because the structure of the catalytically active protein molecule depends on the ionic character of the amino acid side chains.

Covalent Modification

Enzyme activity may be increased or decreased either by addition of a group by covalent bond or by removal of a group by cleaving covalent bond. For example, zymogen activation by partial proteolysis, adenosine diphosphate (ADP) ribosylation and reversible protein ribosylation (commonest type).

INHIBITION OF ENZYME ACTIVITY

Any substance that can diminish the velocity of an enzyme-catalyzed reaction is called inhibitor. In general, irreversible inhibitors bind to enzymes through covalent bonds.

General Types of Inhibitors

Competitive Inhibitor

1. Competes with substrate for active site of enzyme.
2. Both substrate and competitive inhibitor bind to active site.
3. These inhibitors are often substrate analogs (similar in structure substrate), but still no product is formed.
4. Can be overcome by addition of more substrate (overwhelm inhibitor; a numbers game).

   For example, malonate inhibition of succinate dehydrogenase

   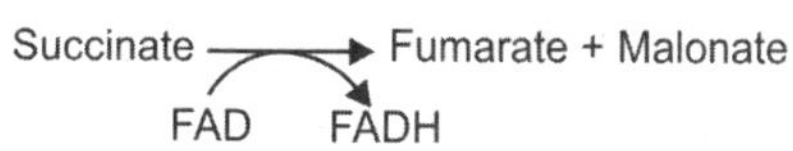

   For example, azidothymidine (AZT) inhibition of human immunodeficiency virus (HIV) reverse transcriptase actual substrate is deoxythymidine triphosphate (dTTP).
5. It can be represented by the following equation:

$$E + S \rightleftharpoons ES \longrightarrow E + P$$
$$I \rightleftharpoons EI$$

   Graphical representation of competitive inhibitors is shown in Figure 2.3.
6. Affects K_m (increases K_m, decreases affinity; need more substrate to reach half-saturation of enzyme).
7. V_{max} unaffected.

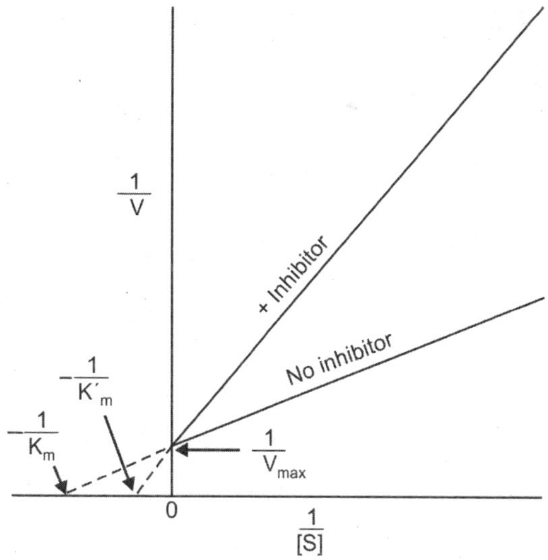

Fig. 2.3: Competitive inhibition

Note: Mnemonics: Competition is hard because we have to travel more kilometers (K_m) with the same velocity. With competitive inhibitors, velocity remains same, but K_m increases.

Uncompetitive Inhibitor

1. Typically seen in multisubstrate reactions (here, there is a decrease in product formation, because the second substrate cannot bind).
2. Inhibitor binds to ES, but not enzyme.

$$E + S \rightleftharpoons ES \longrightarrow E + P$$
$$ES + I \rightleftharpoons ESI$$

   Graphical representation of uncompetitive inhibitors is shown in Figure 2.4.
3. Both K_m and V_{max} are lowered, usually by the same amount
4. Ratio K_m/V_{max} unchanged and hence no change in slope.

Pure Non-competitive Inhibitor

1. Can bind to enzyme and ES complex equally.
2. Does not bind to same site as substrate and is not a substrate analog.
3. Cannot be overcome by increases in substrate. For example, lead, mercury, silver, heavy metals.
4. Lineweaver-Burk plot of showing:

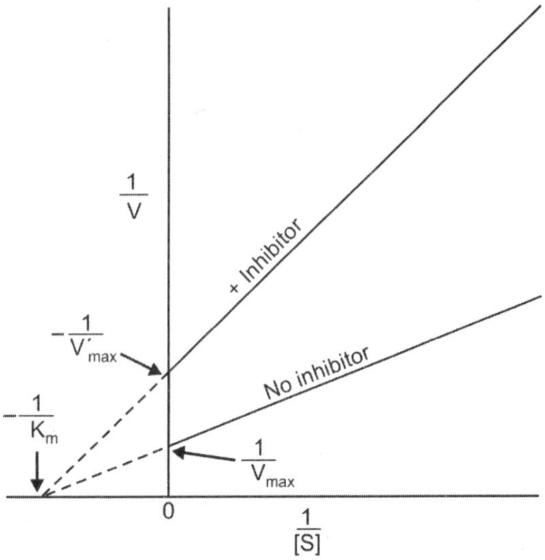

Fig. 2.4: Lineweaver-Burk plot for uncompetitive inhibition

a. No effect on K_m, because those enzyme molecules that are unaffected have normal affinity.
b. V_{max} is lowered.

REGULATION OF ENZYME ACTIVITY

There are many ways to regulate enzyme activity at different levels.

Regulation of Rate of Synthesis or Degradation

1. Is fairly slow (several hours), so is really too slow to be effective in eukaryotic cells.
2. Need something that can occur in seconds or less.
3. Usually done through regulatory enzymes and occur in metabolic pathways early or at first committed step:

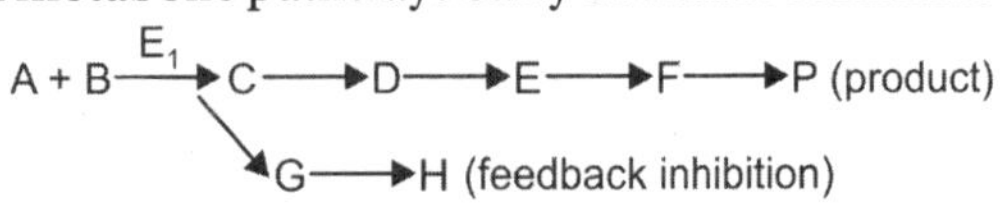

4. Result is to conserve material and energy by preventing accumulation of intermediates.

Allosteric Regulation

1. Done through allosteric sites or regulatory sites on enzymes—site other than active site where inhibitor or activator can bind.
2. Properties of allosteric enzymes:
   a. Sensitive to metabolic inhibitors and activators.
   b. Binding is noncovalent; not chemically altered by enzyme.
   c. Regulatory enzymes possess quaternary structure; individual polypeptide chains may or may not be identical.
   d. Enzyme has at least one substrate that gives sigmoidal curve due to positive cooperativity because of multiple substrate binding sites.

SPECIFICITY OF ENZYMES

Specificity is a characteristic property of active site.

1. Stereospecificity: Enzymes act only on one monomer and thus show stereospecificity. But isomerases do not show this property, as they are specialized in interconversion of isomers. For example:
   - Hexokinase acts on D-hexoses
   - Glucokinase acts on D-glucose
   - Cellulase cleaves β-glycosidic bonds.
2. Reaction specificity: The same substrate can undergo different types of reactions, each catalyzed by a separate enzyme. For example, enzymes are different for reactions such as transamination, oxidative deamination, decarboxylation and racemization, etc.
3. Substrate specificity: It varies from enzyme to enzyme. It is divided into:
   a. Absolute substrate specificity. Certain enzymes act only on one substrate. For example:
      - Glucokinase acts on glucose to give glucose-6-phosphate
      - Urease acts only on urea and not on thiourea.
   b. Relative substrate specificity: Some enzymes act on structurally related compounds that may be dependent upon the specific group or bond present. For example:
      - Action of trypsin (for group specificity)
      - Glycosidases acting on glycosidic bond of carbohydrates (for bond specificity).
   c. Broad specificity: Some enzymes act on closely related substrates. For example:
      - Hexokinase acts on glucose, fructose, mannose, glucosamine and not on galactose.

CLINICAL ENZYMOLOGY

The quantitative determination of the activities of certain enzymes in serum has been found to be of great value in clinical diagnosis of diseases. In general, clinical laboratories are principally concerned with changes in the activity in serum or plasma of such enzymes, which are predominantly intracellular and that are normally present in the serum at low activities only. Such enzymes therefore have a diagnostic significance.

Cardiac Biomarkers

A biomarker is a clinical laboratory test, which is useful in detecting dysfunction of an organ. Cardiac biomarkers are used to detect cardiac diseases such as:

- Acute coronary syndrome resulting from myocardial ischemia
- Congestive cardiac failure (CCF) due to ventricular dysfunction.

Isoenzymes

Isoenzymes are the physically distinct forms of an enzyme, which have the same specificity, but may be present in different tissues of the same organism, in different cell type or subcellular compartments. Besides the source, they also differ from each other with respect to their structure, electrophoretic mobility and immunological properties.

Isoenzymes that have wide clinical applications include lactate dehydrogenase, creatine phosphokinase and alkaline phosphatase.

Creatine Phosphokinase

Normal serum value of creatine phosphokinase (CPK) or creatine kinase (CK) are:

- Males = 15–100 U/L
- Females = 10–80 U/L.

The CPK exists in three forms. Each isoenzyme is a dimer composed of two subunits, i.e. muscle (M) type and brain (B) type. The three isoenzymes are (Table 2.2):

- CPK1 (BB) found in brain
- CPK2 (MB) in myocardium
- CPK3 (MM) in skeletal muscle.

The CPK-MB isoenzyme is present in very small amount in serum.

Table 2.2: Characteristics of isoenzymes of creatine kinase (CK)

Isoenzyme	Electrophoretic mobility	Tissue of origin	Mean percentage in blood
MM (CK3)	Least	Skeletal muscle	80%
MB (CK2)	Intermediate	Heart	5%
BB (CK1)	Maximum	Brain	1%

Heart disorder

The CK level rises within 4–6 hours in acute myocardial infarction (AMI) and reaches to a maximum within 1 day of the infarction.

Muscle diseases

- The level of CK in serum is very much elevated in muscular dystrophies (500–1,500 IU/L)
- The CK level is highly elevated in crush injury, fracture and acute cerebrovascular accidents
- Estimation of total CK is employed in muscular dystrophies and MB isoenzyme is estimated in myocardial infarction.

Lactate Dehydrogenase

Normal value of lactate dehydrogenase (LDH) in serum is 100-200 U/L. The LDH is a tetramer, i.e. it has four polypeptide subunits. Each subunit may be one of the two types, known as the H-type (heart type) and the M-type (muscle type).

Lactate dehydrogenase exists in serum in five distinct forms (isoenzymes), which have different proportions of the H- and the M-subunits (Table 2.3):

- LDH_1 has 4 H type of polypeptide chains (H_4) and is predominantly found in myocardium and red blood cell (RBC)
- LDH_5 has 4 M subunits (M_4) and is the predominant form in the hepatic tissue and the skeletal muscle
- The other forms are LDH_2 (H_3M), LDH_3 (H_2M_2) and LDH_4 (HM_3).

LDH_1 becomes greater than LDH_2 (known as a flipped ratio) between 12 and 24 hours following an AMI. Raised LDH_4 and LDH_5 are diagnostic of secondary congestive liver involvement.

Table 2.3: Characteristic features of LDH isoenzyme

Isoenzyme		Tissue	Mean percentage
LDH_1*	H_4†	Heart muscle	30%
LDH_2	H_3M_1‡	RBC§	35%
LDH_3	H_2M_2	Brain	20%
LDH_4	H_1M_3	Liver	10%
LDH_5	M_4	Skeletal muscle	5%

*LDH, lactate dehydrogenase; †H, heart type; ‡M, muscle type; §RBC, red blood cell.

Troponin

Troponins are not enzymes. However, they are now accepted as reliable markers for myocardial infarction. The troponin complex consists of three components:

- Troponin C (calcium-binding subunit)
- Troponin I (actomyosin ATPase inhibitory subunit)
- Troponin T (tropomyosin-binding subunit).

Troponin I is released into the blood within 4 hours after the onset of symptoms of myocardial ischemia; peaks at 14–24 hours and remains elevated for 3–5 days post-infarction.

Serum level of troponin T (TnT) increases within 6 hours of myocardial infarction, peaks at 72 hours and then remains elevated up to 7–14 days.

Alkaline Phosphatase

Different tissues contain different forms of alkaline phosphatase. A major portion of alkaline phosphatase in serum is derived from liver and its level rises in posthepatic jaundice. In growing children, the major isoenzyme is from the bone, which is related to its increased osteoblastic activity. During the last trimester of pregnancy, there is an increase in alkaline phosphatase, which is of placental origin. This isoenzyme is heat stable and is called heat-stable alkaline phosphatase.

ENZYME PATTERN (ENZYME PROFILE) IN DISEASES

Hepatic Diseases

1. Alanine amino transferase (ALT): Marked increase in parenchymal liver diseases.
2. Aspartate amino transferase (AST): Elevated in parenchymal liver disease.
3. Alkaline phosphatase (ALP): Marked increase in obstructive liver disease.
4. Gamma glutamyl transferase (GGT): Increase in obstructive and alcoholic liver.

Myocardial Infarction

Following are serum enzyme profile in AMI (Fig. 2.5):

1. Creatine kinase (CK-MB): First enzyme to rise following infarction CK-MB isoenzyme is specific.
2. Aspartate amino transferase: Rises after the rise in CK and returns to normal in 4–5 days.
3. Lactate dehydrogenase: LDH_1 becomes more than two (flipped pattern).

Muscle Diseases

1. Creatine kinase (CK-MM): Marked increase in muscle diseases; CK-MM fraction is elevated.

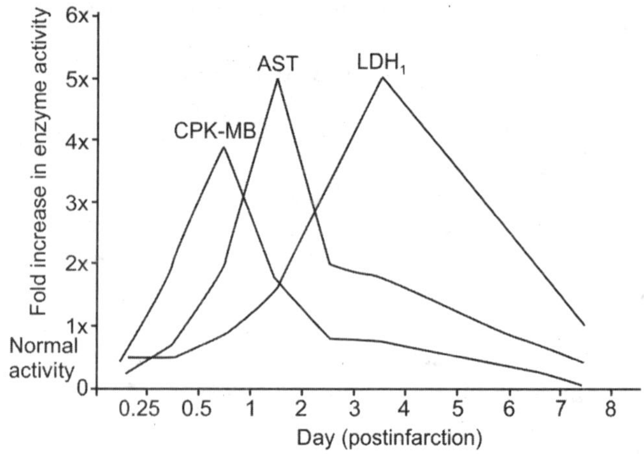

Fig. 2.5: Serum enzyme profile in acute myocardial infarction (AST, aspartate aminotransferase; CPK-MB, creatine phosphokinase-muscle and brain type; LDH, lactate dehydrogenase).

2. Aspartate amino transferase (AST): Increase in muscle disease; not specific.
3. Aldolase (ALD): Earliest enzyme to rise, but not specific.

Bone Diseases

1. Alkaline phosphatase: Marked elevation in rickets and Paget's disease; heat labile bone isoenzyme (BAP) is elevated.

Prostate Cancer

1. Prostate-specific antigen (PSA): Marker for prostate cancer. Mild increase in benign prostate enlargement.
2. Acid phosphatase (ACP): Marker for prostate cancer. Metastatic bone disease especially from a primary from prostate. Inhibited by L-tartrate.

Chapter 3

Carbohydrates

Carbohydrates may be defined as polyhydroxy aldehydes or ketones or compounds, which produce them on hydrolysis.

FUNCTIONS OF CARBOHYDRATES

1. Carbohydrates are the most abundant dietary source of energy (4 kcal/g) for all organisms.
2. Carbohydrates are precursors for many organic compounds (fats and amino acids).
3. Carbohydrates participate in the structure of cell membrane.
4. Storage form of energy (starch and glycogen).
5. Structural basis of many organisms: Cellulose of plants; exoskeleton of insects, cell wall of microorganisms, mucopolysaccharides as ground substance in higher organisms.

CLASSIFICATION OF CARBOHYDRATES

1. Monosaccharides: It cannot be further hydrolyzed (glucose, fructose, galactose).
2. Disaccharides: On hydrolysis, they yield two monosac charide units (maltose, lactose, sucrose).
3. Oligosaccharides: It include trisaccharides, tetrasaccharides (raffinose), etc.
4. Polysaccharides: On hydrolysis, they yield more than 10 monosaccharides (starch, glycogen, cellulose).

Monosaccharides

Epimers: If two monosaccharides differ from each other in their configuration around a single specific carbon (other than anomeric) atom, they are referred to as epimers to each other:

- Glucose and galactose are C4 epimers
- Glucose and mannose are C2 epimers (Fig. 3.1).

Anomer: The alpha- and beta-cyclic forms of D-glucose are, known as anomers. They differ from each other in the configuration only around C1 known as anomeric carbon. The anomers differ in certain physical and chemical properties.

Mutarotation: Is defined as the change in the specific optical rotation representing the interconversion of alpha and beta forms of D-glucose to an equilibrium mixture.

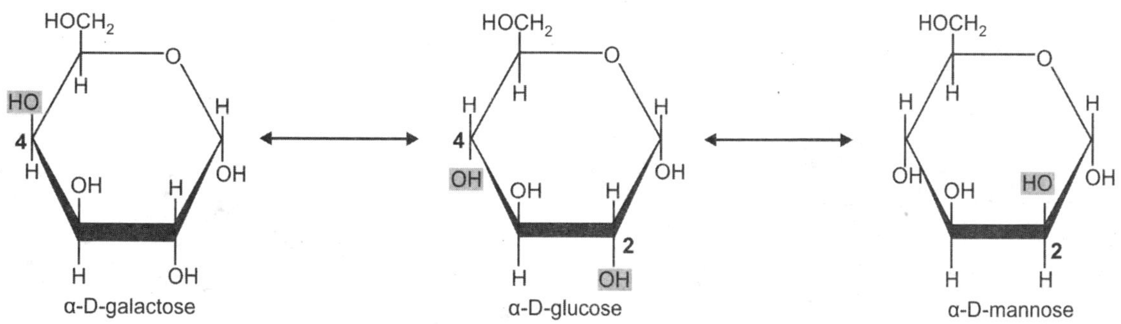

Fig. 3.1: Epimers of glucose

In case of fructose, pyranose ring is converted to furanose ring.

Reactions of Monosaccharides

Enediol formation: In mild alkaline solutions, carbohydrates containing a free sugar group will tautomerise to form enediols, where two hydroxyl groups are attached to the double-bonded carbon atoms.

In mild alkaline conditions, glucose is converted into fructose and mannose. The interconversion of sugars through a common enediol form is called Lobry de Bruyn-van Ekenstein transformation.

Enediols are highly reactive, so sugars are powerful reducing agents in alkaline medium.

Benedict's reaction: It is very commonly employed to detect the presence of glucose in urine (glucosuria). It is a standard laboratory test employed to diagnose diabetes mellitus. Benedict's reagent contains sodium carbonate, copper sulfate and sodium citrate. In alkaline medium, sugars form enediol, cupric ions are reduced, correspondingly sugar is oxidized.

Osazone formation: All reducing sugars will form osazones with excess of phenylhydrazine when kept at boiling temperature. Osazones are insoluble. Each sugar will have characteristic crystal form of osazones. Glucose, fructose and mannose produce same ozasone (Figs 3.2 to 3.4).

Oxidation: Under mild oxidation conditions (Br_2/H_2O), aldehyde group is oxidized to carboxyl group to produce aldonic acid (glucose oxidized to gluconic acid). When aldehyde group is protected and molecule is oxidized, uronic acid is produced (glucose oxidized to glucuronic acid). Under strong oxidation conditions (HNO_3), dicarboxylic acid, saccharic acids are formed.

Dehydration: When treated with H_2SO_4, monosaccharides undergo dehydration to form a furfural derivative. These furfurals can condense with phenolic compounds to form colored products. This is the basis of molisch test.

Reduction: When treated with reducing agents (sodium amalgam) aldehyde or keto group is reduced to alcohol.

D-glucose → D-sorbitol
D-galactose → D-dulcitol
D-mannose → D-mannitol
D-fructose → D-mannitol + D-sorbitol
D-ribose → D-ribitol

Clinical correlation: Sorbitol and dulcitol accumulate in tissues cause strong osmotic effects leading to swelling of cells and cataract. Mannitol is useful to reduce intracranial tension by forced diuresis.

Formation of esters: The hydroxyl (OH) group of sugars can be esterified to form acetates, benzoates, phosphates, etc. Glucose-6-phosphate and glucose-1-phosphate are important intermediates of glucose metabolism.

Glycosides

When the hemi-acetal group (hydroxyl group of the anomeric carbon) of a monosaccharide is condensed with an alcohol or phenol group, it is called glycoside. The non-carbohydrate group is called aglycone. Glycosides do not reduce Benedict's reagent, because the sugar group is masked. Physiologically important glycosides are:

- Glucovanillin is a natural substance that imparts vanilla flavor
- Cardiac glycosides (steroidal glycosides): Digoxin and digitoxin contain the aglycone steroid and they stimulate muscle contraction
- Streptomycin, an antibiotic used in the treatment of tuberculosis is a glycoside
- Ouabain inhibits Na^+- K^+ ATPase.

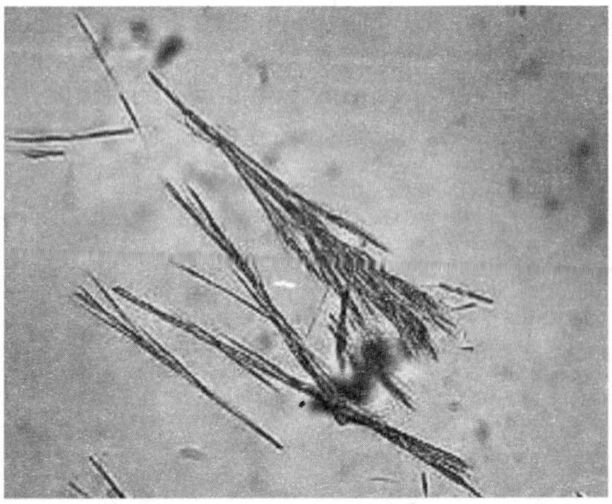

Fig. 3.2: Glucosazone—needle-shaped crystals appearance

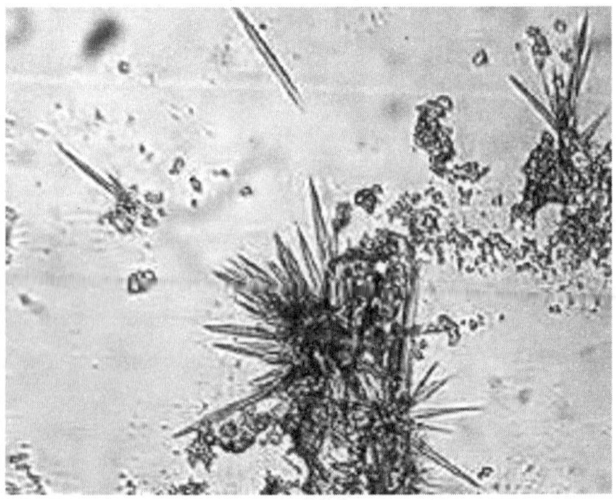

Fig. 3.3: Lactosazone—hedgehog or pin cushion with pins appearance

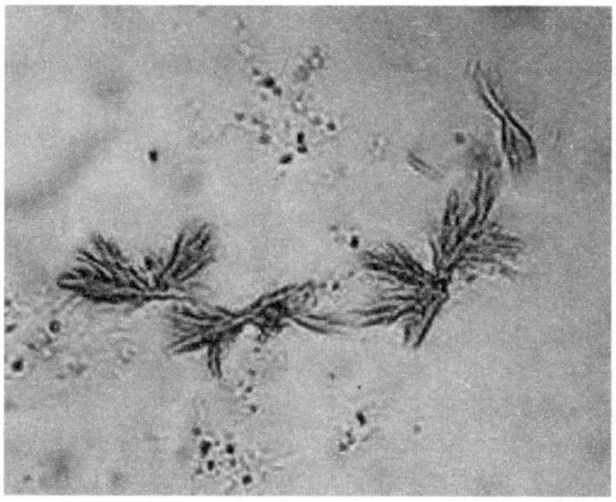

Fig. 3.4: Maltosazone (sunflower- or petal-shaped crystals)

Amino sugars

Amino groups may be substituted for hydroxyl groups of sugars to give rise to amino sugars. Amino sugars will not show reducing property. They will not produce osazones. For examples, galactosamine, glucosamine, mannosamine. The amino group in the sugar may be further acetylated to produce N-acetylated sugars such as N-acetyl-glucosamine (GluNAc or NAG), N-acetylgalactosamine (GalNAc).

Deoxy sugars

These are the sugars that contain one oxygen less than that present in the parent molecule:

- Deoxy sugars will not reduce and will not form osazones
- Deoxyribose is an important part of nucleic acid.

Disaccharides

When two monosaccharides are combined together by glycosidic linkage, a disaccharide is formed:

1. Reducing disaccharides with free aldehyde or keto group (maltose, lactose).
2. Non-reducing disaccharides with no free group (sucrose).

Sucrose

1. Sucrose is the sweetening agent known as cane sugar. It is present in sugarcane and various fruits.
2. Sucrose contains glucose and fructose. It is not a reducing sugar; and it will not form osazone (Fig. 3.5).
3. When sucrose is hydrolyzed, the products have reducing action. A sugar solution, which is originally non-reducing, but becomes reducing after hydrolysis, is identified as sucrose (specific sucrose test).
4. Hydrolysis of sucrose (optical rotation +66.5°) will produce one molecule of glucose (+52.5°) and one molecule of fructose (-92°). Therefore, the products will change the dextrorotation to levorotation, or the plane of rotation is inverted. Equimolecular mixture of glucose and fructose thus formed is called invert sugar. The enzyme producing hydrolysis of sucrose is called sucrase or invertase.

Lactose

1. Lactose is the sugar present in milk. It is a reducing disaccharide. On hydrolysis lactose yields glucose and galactose. Beta-1,4-glycosidic linkage is present in lactose (Fig. 3.6).
2. Lactose exhibits reducing properties and form osazones.

Maltose

- Maltose contains two glucose residues. There is alpha-1, 4 linkage (Fig. 3.7)
- It is a reducing disaccharide
- It forms petal-shaped crystals of maltose-osazone.

Polysaccharide

They are polymerized products of many monosaccharide units. It is of two types:

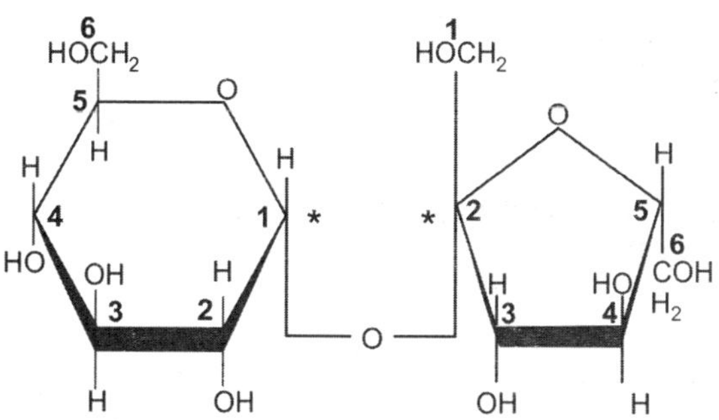

Fig. 3.5: Sucrose

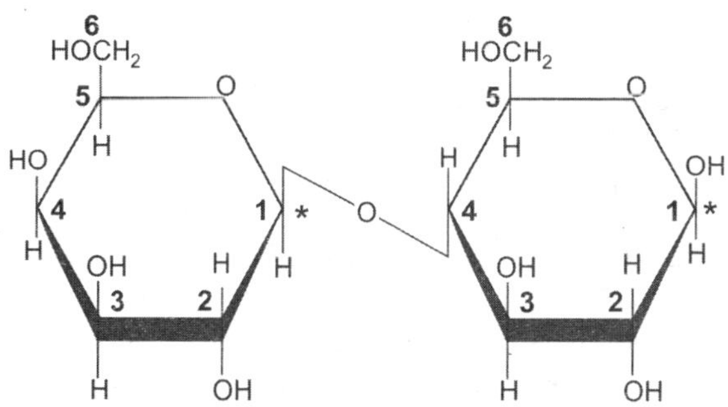

Fig. 3.6: Lactose

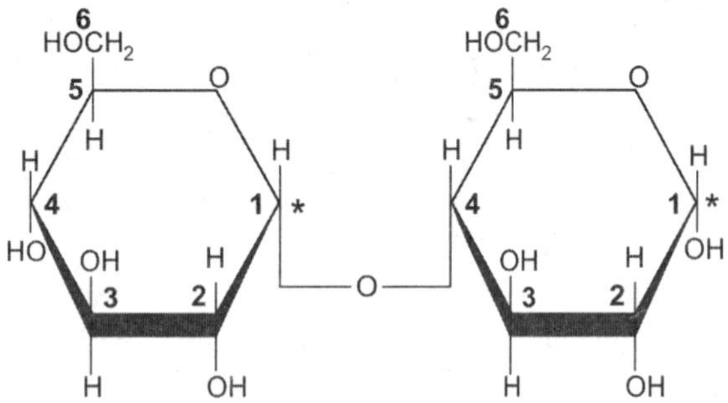

Fig. 3.7: Maltose

1. Homopolysaccharides, which on hydrolysis yield only a single type of monosaccharide, e.g. starch, glycogen and cellulose. Inulin, dextrans, chitin, etc. are homopolysaccharides.
2. Heteropolysaccharides on hydrolysis yield a mixture of a few monosaccharides or their derivatives, e.g. hyaluronic acid.

Starch

1. Starch is the reserve carbohydrate of plants.
2. High content of starch is found in cereals, roots, tubers and vegetables.
3. Starch is composed of amylose and amylopectin.
4. Amylose (soluble) is made up of glucose units with alpha-1,4 glycosidic linkages.
5. The insoluble part absorbs water and forms paste like gel and this is called amylopectin. Amylopectin is also made up of glucose units, but is highly branched. Branching points are made by alpha-1,6 linkage.
6. Starches are hydrolyzed by amylase (pancreatic or salivary) to liberate dextrins, and finally maltose and glucose units. Amylase acts specifically on alpha-1,4 glycosidic bonds.
7. Hydrolysis for a short time produces amylodextrin, which gives violet color with iodine and is non-reducing. Further hydrolysis produces erythrodextrin, which gives red color with iodine and mild reduction of Benedict's solution. Later achrodextrins (no color with iodine, but reducing) and further on, maltose (no color with iodine, but powerfully reducing) are formed on continued hydrolysis.

Glycogen

1. Glycogen is the reserve carbohydrate in animals. It is stored in liver and muscle.
2. Glycogen is composed of glucose units joined by alpha-1,4 links in the straight chains.
3. Has alpha-1,6 glycosidic linkages at the branching points.
4. Innermost core of glycogen contains a primer protein, glycogenin. Glycogen is more branched and more compact than amylopectin.

Cellulose

1. Cellulose occurs exclusively in plants and it is the most abundant organic substance in plants.
2. Constituent of plant cell wall.
3. Cellulose is made up of glucose units combined with beta-1,4 linkages. It has a straight line structure, with no branching points.
4. Beta-1,4 bridges are hydrolyzed by the enzyme cellobiase. But this enzyme is absent in animal and human digestive system, and hence cellulose cannot be digested.

Heteropolysaccharide

When the polysaccharides are composed of different types of sugars or their derivatives, they are referred to as heteropolysaccharides or heteroglycans.

Mucopolysaccharides

Mucopolysaccharides or glycosaminoglycans (GAG) are heteropolysaccharides, containing uronic acid and amino sugars.

Hyaluronic Acid

- Present in connective tissues, tendons, synovial fluid and vitreous humor
- It serves as a lubricant and shock absorbant in joint cavities.

Heparin

- Heparin is an anticoagulant widely used
- It is present in liver, lungs, spleen and monocytes.

Chondroitin Sulfate

Chondroitin sulfate is present in ground substance of connective tissues widely distributed in cartilage, bone, tendons, cornea and skin.

Keratan Sulfate

- Keratan sulfate is the only GAG, which does not contain any uronic acid
- It is found in cornea and tendons.

Dermatan Sulfate

Dermatan sulfate is found in skin, blood vessels and heart valves.

Glycoproteins

Proteins, which are covalently bound to carbohydrates are referred to as glycoproteins. The carbohydrate content of glycoprotein varies from 1% to 90% by weight. Mucoprotein is glycoprotein with carbohydrate concentration more than 4%.They perform many functions—role as enzymes, hormones, transport proteins and receptors. Glycophorin is the major membrane glycoprotein of RBC.

METABOLISM OF CARBOHYDRATES

In the diet carbohydrates are present as complex polysaccharides (starch, glycogen) and to a minor extent, as disaccharides (sucrose and lactose). They are hydrolyzed to monosaccharide units in the gastrointestinal tract.

The process of digestion starts in the mouth. Steps are given in Table 3.1.

Table 3.1: Digestion of carbohydrate

Enzyme	Site of action	Function
Salivary amylase	Mouth	Starch/Glycogen → Maltose, oligosaccharides, isomaltose
Pancreatic amylase	Small intestine	Oligosaccharides → Maltose, isomaltose
Disaccharidases	Small intestine	
Sucrase Lactase Maltase Isomaltase		Sucrose → Glucose + Fructose Lactose → Glucose + Galactose Maltose → Glucose Isomaltose → Glucose

After digestion by the action of various enzymes, dietary carbohydrates are released and absorbed as monosaccharides, which are almost completely absorbed from the small intestine.

Amongst the various monosaccharides, galactose and glucose are absorbed from the small intestine very rapidly, by the active process, which is linked to the transport of sodium and requires energy, in the form of hydrolysis of a high energy phosphate bond of adenosine triphosphate (ATP). A sodium-dependent glucose transporter, called sodium glucose transporter or SGLT-1 (Table 3.2), binds both glucose and sodium at separate sites and transports them through the plasma membrane of the intestinal cells.

Clinical Correlation: Lactose Intolerance

It is a condition resulting from a deficiency of intestinal lactase so that the individual is unable to digest the milk sugar.

Table 3.2: Glucose transporters (GLT)

Transporter	Locations	Properties
Glu T1	RBC, kidney, brain, retina, placenta	Glucose uptake in most of cells
Glu T2	Intestine, liver, pancreas	Glucose uptake in liver (low affinity)
Glu T3	Neurons, brain	High affinity, glucose uptake in brain
Glu T4	Skeletal, heart muscles, adipose tissue	Insulin-mediated glucose uptake
Glu T5	Small intestine, sperms, kidney	Fructose transporter
Glu T7	Liver endoplasmic reticulum	Glucose from ER to cytoplasm
SGLT	Intestine, kidney	Cotransport from lumen to cell

Lactase deficiency results in the accumulation of undigested lactose. Lactose moves to the colon where its bacterial fermentation generates CO_2 and organic acids. The symptoms include abdominal cramps, diarrhea and flatulence. Secondary lactase deficiency may result from damage to villi caused by drugs, prolonged diarrhea and malnutrition. Cheese is well tolerated since lactose gets removed during manufacturing. The management strategy is to gradually increase the intake of milk products, to take them with other foods and to spread their intake over the day. 'Acidophilus milk', i.e. milk pretreated with the bacteria *Lactobacillus acidophilus* is commercially available.

GLYCOLYSIS (EMBDEN-MEYERHOF-PARNAS PATHWAY)

Oxidation of glucose is known as glycolysis. Glucose is oxidized to either lactate or pyruvate. Under aerobic conditions, the dominant product in most tissues is pyruvate and the pathway is known as aerobic glycolysis. When oxygen is depleted, as for instance during prolonged vigorous exercise, the dominant glycolytic product in many tissues is lactate and the process is known as anaerobic glycolysis (Tables 3.3 and 3.4).

The pathway of glycolysis can be seen as consisting of two separate phases. The first is the chemical priming phase requiring energy in the form of ATP, and the second is considered the energy-yielding phase. In the first phase, two equivalents of ATP are used to convert glucose to fructose-1,6-bisphosphate (F1,6BP) (Fig. 3.8). In the second phase F1,6BP is degraded to pyruvate, with the production of four equivalents of ATP and two equivalents of nicotinamide adenine dinucleotide (NADH) (refer Fig. 3.8).

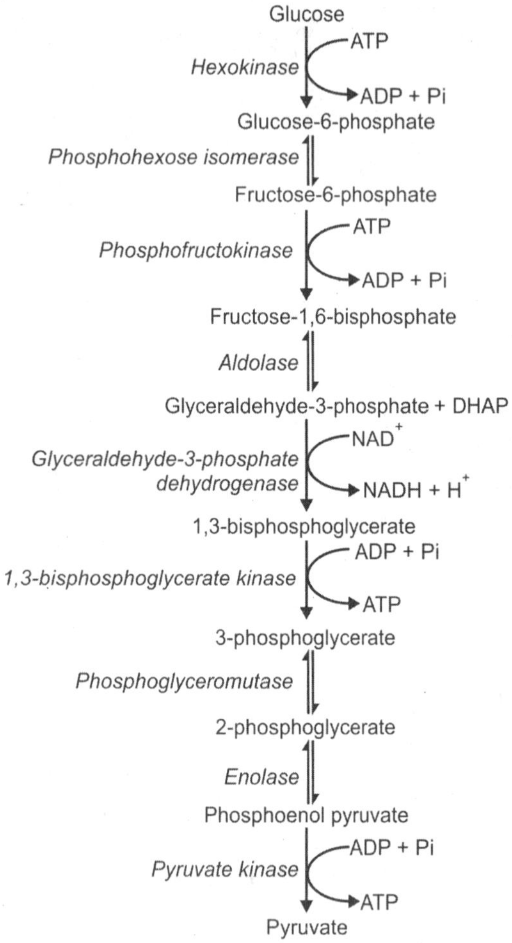

Fig. 3.8: Glycolysis (ADP, adenosine diphosphate; ATP, adenosine triphosphate; Pi, inorganic phosphate; DHAP, dihydroxyacetone phosphate; NAD, nicotinamide adenine dinucleotide).

Table 3.3: Energetics of aerobic glycolysis

Step	ATP (used –) (produced +)
1	–1
3	–1
5—NADH to ETC to FAD = 2 step 5 (twice)	2 × 2 = +4
6 (twice)	1 × 2 = +2
9 (twice)	1 × 2 = +2
Net	6 ATP

Table 3.4: Energetics of anaerobic glycolysis

Step	ATP (used –) (produced +)
1	–1
3	–1
5—NADH to pyruvic acid to lactic acid ETC not used	0
6 (twice)	1 × 2 = +2
9 (twice)	1 × 2 = +2
Net	2 ATP

Glycolysis step mnemonic

"**G**oodness **G**racious **F**ather **F**ranklin **D**id **G**o **B**y **P**icking **P**umpkins (to) **P**r**EP**are **P**ies":
- ***G***lucose
- ***G***lucose-6-P
- ***F***ructose-6-P
- ***F***ructose-1,6-diP
- ***D***ihydroxyacetone-P
- ***G***lyceraldehyde-P
- 1,3-***B***iphosphoglycerate
- 3-***P***hosphoglycerate
- 2-***P***hosphoglycerate
- ***P***hosphoenolpyruvate (**PEP**)
- ***P***yruvate

Glycolytic enzymes mnemonic

"**H**igh **P**rofile **P**eople **A**ct **T**oo **G**lamorous, **P**osing **E**very **P**lace":
- ***H***exokinase
- ***P***hosphoglucose isomerase
- ***P***hosphofructokinase (PFK)
- ***A***ldolase
- ***T***riose phosphate isomerase
- ***G***lyceraldehyde-3-phosphate dehydrogenase
- ***P***hosphoglycerate mutase
- ***E***nolase
- ***P***yruvate kinase

Irreversible Enzymes of Glycolysis

The 'irreversible' enzymes of glycolysis are those that involve ATP.

Hexokinase

- Irreversible
- Uses 1 ATP per glucose
- Low km (high affinity for glucose)
- Hexokinase is in all cells, and its isozyme glucokinase (aka hexokinase IV) is found in the liver. Glucokinase has a higher Km
- Active after meals (high glucose concentration in liver)
- Allosteric inhibition by product (glucose-6-phosphate).

Phosphofructokinase-1

- Irreversible
- Uses 1 ATP per glucose
- Major rate regulator: At this point, the product has to continue in glycolysis (glucose and glucose-6-phosphate

can have other fats until this point, i.e. glycogen synthesis or pentose phosphate pathway)
- Allosteric regulation
- Negative—ATP, citrate
- Positive—AMP, ADP, fructose-2,6-bisphosphate.

Pyruvate Kinase

1. Irreversible.
2. Makes 2 ATP per glucose (1 per PEP): Transfers phosphoryl group from PEP to ADP, producing ATP.
3. Allosteric regulation:
   a. Negative:
      - ATP
      - Acetyl-CoA
      - Fatty acids
      - Alanine 2.
   b. Positive:
      - Fructose-1,6-bisphosphate.

Energy Yield from Glycolysis

Net reaction: As given below:

$$\text{Glucose} + 2\text{NAD}^+ + 2\text{ Pi} + 2\text{ ADP} \longrightarrow 2\text{ pyruvate} + 2\text{ATP} + 2\text{ NADH} + 2H_2O$$

Regulation of Glycolysis

Regulatory mechanisms controlling glycolysis include allosteric and covalent modification mechanisms.

Glycolysis is regulated reciprocally from gluconeogenesis. Molecules, such as F2, 6BP, that turn on glycolysis, turn off gluconeogenesis. Conversely, acetyl-CoA turns on gluconeogenesis, but turns off glycolysis.

The principle enzymes of glycolysis involved in regulation are hexokinase (reaction 1), phosphofructokinase (reaction 3) and pyruvate kinase (reaction 10):

1. Hexokinase is allosterically inhibited by glucose-6-phosphate. That is, the enzyme for first reaction of glycolysis is inhibited by the product of first reaction. As a result, glucose and ATP (in reactions 1 and 3) are not committed to glycolysis unless necessary.
2. Phosphofructokinase (PFK) is a major control point for glycolysis. The PFK is allosterically inhibited by ATP and citrate, allosterically activated by AMP, ADP and F2, 6BP. Thus, carbon movement through glycolysis is inhibited at PFK when the cell contains ample stores of ATP and oxidizible substrates. Additionally, PFK is activated by AMP and ADP because they indicate low levels of ATP in the cell. The F2,6BP is the major activator, though, because it reciprocally inhibits F1,6BP bisphosphatase, which is the gluconeogenic enzyme that catalyzes the reversal of this step.
3. Pyruvate kinase is allosterically inhibited by acetyl-CoA, ATP and alanine, allosterically activated by F1,6BP.

CORI CYCLE (LACTIC ACID CYCLE)

1. Lactate is formed in the active muscle to regenerate NAD^+ from NADH so that glycolysis can continue.
2. The muscle cannot spare NAD^+ for reconversion of lactate back to pyruvate.
3. Thus, lactate is transported to the liver, where, in the presence of oxygen, it undergoes gluconeogenesis to form glucose.
4. The glucose is supplied by the liver to various tissues including muscle.
5. This interorgan cooperation during high-muscular activity is called 'Cori cycle' (Fig. 3.9).

Significance

The cycle's importance is based on the prevention of lactic acidosis in the muscle under anaerobic conditions. However, normally before this happens the lactic acid is moved out of the muscles and into the liver.

The cycle is also important in producing ATP, an energy source, during muscle activity. The Cori cycle functions more efficiently when muscle activity has ceased. This allows the oxygen debt to be repaid such that the Krebs cycle and electron transport chain can produce energy at peak efficiency.

RAPOPORT-LUEBERING REACTION

Rapoport-luebering reaction (BPG shunt) is the part of glycolytic pathway characteristic of human erythrocytes in which 2,3-bisphosphoglycerate (2,3-BPG) is formed as an intermediate between 1,3-bisphosphoglycerate and 3-phosphoglycerate by the enzyme bisphosphoglycerate mutase enzyme.

Significance

The 2,3-BPG is an important regulator of the affinity of hemoglobin (HB) for oxygen. It combines with Hb and

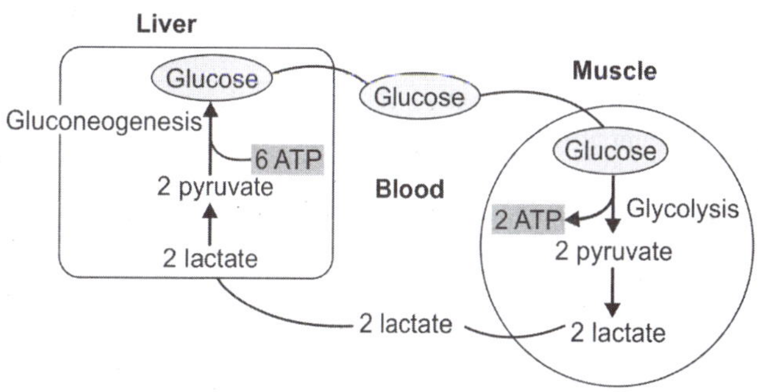

Fig. 3.9: Cori cycle

decreases the affinity of Hb to oxygen, thus it helps in unloading O_2 from oxyhemoglobin in the tissues. An increase in 2,3-BPG is observed in hypoxia, high altitude, fetal tissues and in anemia.

$$HbO_2 + 2,3\text{-BPG} \longrightarrow Hb2,3\text{-BPG} + O_2$$

Energetics

No ATP is generated.

GLUCONEOGENESIS

The synthesis of glucose from non-carbohydrate compounds is known as gluconeogenesis. The major substrates/precursors for gluconeogenesis are lactate, pyruvate, glucogenic amino acids, propionate and glycerol. Gluconeogenesis occurs mainly in the liver. The pathway is partly mitochondrial and partly cytoplasmic. Gluconeogenetic pathway is shown in Figure 3.10.

Key Gluconeogenic Enzymes

- Pyruvate carboxylase
- Phosphoenolpyruvate carboxykinase (PEPCK)
- Fructose-1,6-bisphosphatase
- Glucose-6-phosphatase.

Pyruvate Carboxylase Reaction

Pyruvate in the cytoplasm enters the mitochondria. Then, carboxylation of pyruvate to oxaloacetate is catalyzed by a mitochondrial enzyme and pyruvate carboxylase. It needs the coenzymes biotin and ATP.

The carboxylation of pyruvate takes place in mitochondria. So, oxaloacetate is generated inside the mitochondria. This oxaloacetate has to be transported from mitochondria to cytosol, because further reactions of gluconeogenesis are taking place in cytosol. This is achieved by the malate aspartate shuttle.

Phosphoenolpyruvate Carboxykinase

In the cytoplasm, PEPCK enzyme then converts oxaloacetate to phosphoenolpyruvate by removing a molecule of CO_2. The guanosine triphosphate (GTP) or inositol triphosphate (ITP) donates the phosphate. The net effect of these two reactions is the conversion of pyruvate to phosphoenol pyruvate.

Fructose 1,6-bisphosphatase

Fructose 1,6-bisphosphate is then acted upon by fructose 1,6-bisphosphatase to form fructose-6-phosphate. Then fructose-6-phosphate is isomerized to glucose-6-phosphate by the freely reversible reaction catalyzed by hexosephosphate isomerase.

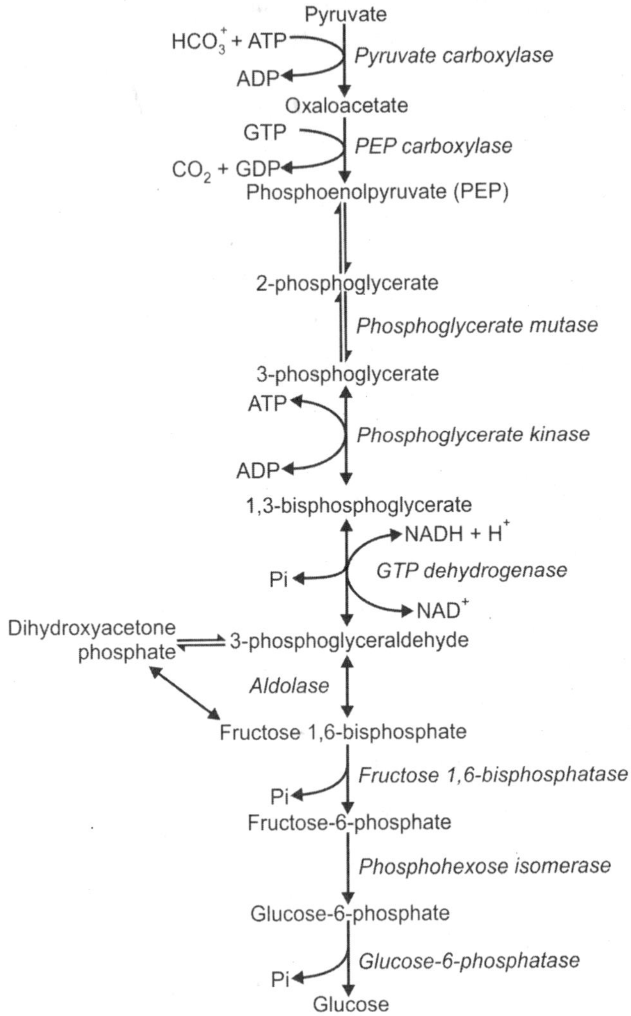

Fig. 3.10: Gluconeogenesis (ADP, adenosin diphosphate; ATP, adenosin triphosphate; CO_2, Carbon dioxide; GDP, guanosine diphosphate; GTP, guanosine triphosphate; HCO_3, bicarbonate; NADH, nicotinamide adenine dinucleotide Pi, inorganic phosphate).

Glucose-6-phosphatase Reaction

The glucose 6-phosphate is hydrolyzed to free glucose by glucose-6-phosphatase. Gluconeogenesis utilizes 6 ATPs. The overall summary of gluconeogenesis is given below:

$$2\text{ pyruvate} + 4\text{ ATP} + 2\text{ GTP} + 2\text{ NADH} + 2\text{ H}^+ + 6\text{ H}_2\text{O} \longrightarrow \text{glucose} + 2\text{ NAD} + 4\text{ ADP} + 2\text{ GDP} + 6\text{ Pi} + 6\text{ H}^+.$$

Glucose-alanine Cycle

Alanine is transported to liver and used for gluconeogenesis. This glucose may again enter the glycolytic pathway to form alanine. This cycle is known as glucose-alanine cycle.

It is important in starvation. Net transfer of amino acids from muscle to liver and corresponding transfer of glucose from liver to muscle is affected (Fig. 3.11).

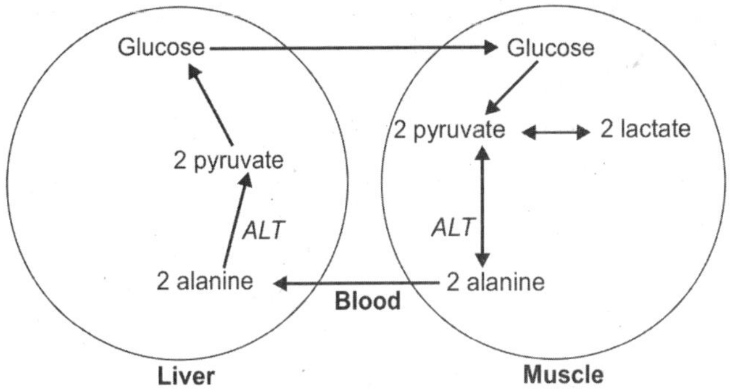

Fig. 3.11: Glucose-alanine cycle (ALT, alanine transaminase)

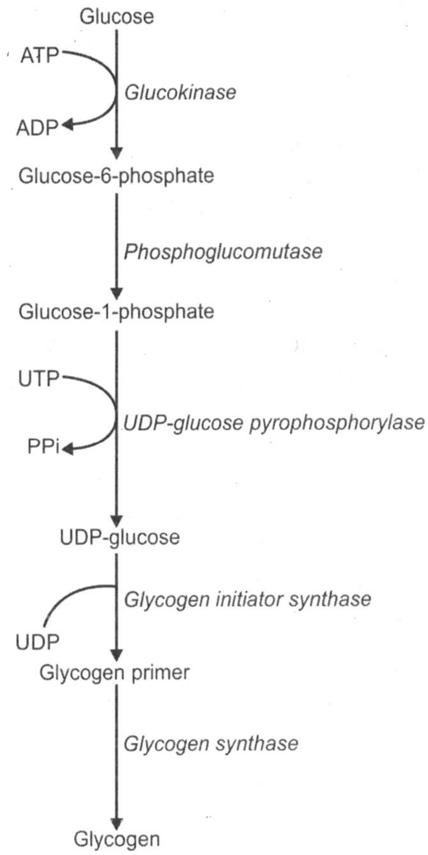

Fig. 3.12: Glycogenesis

Regulation of Gluconeogenesis

Influence of glucagon: This is a hormone, secreted by beta-cells of the pancreatic islets. Glucagon stimulates gluconeogenesis by two mechanisms:

1. Glucagon converts active pyruvate kinase into inactive form. This reduces conversion of PEP to pyruvate and it is diverted for synthesis of glucose.
2. Glucagon reduces concentration of fructose-2,6-bisphosphatase. This allosterically inhibit phosphofructokinase and activates fructose-1,6-bisphosphatase and gluconeogenesis increases.

Availability of Substates

1. Glucogenic aminoacids shows stimulating effect on gluconeogenesis. It is important in diabetes mellitus.
2. Acetyl-CoA promotes gluconeogenesis during starvation.

GLYCOGEN METABOLISM

Glycogen is the storage form of glucose. It is stored mostly in liver and muscle. The prime function of liver glycogen is to maintain the blood glucose levels, particularly between meals. Liver glycogen stores increase in a well-fed state, which is depleted during fasting. Muscle glycogen serves as a fuel reserve for the supply of ATP during muscle contraction.

Glycogenesis

The synthesis of glycogen from glucose is glycogenesis (Fig. 3.12). Glycogenesis takes place in the cytosol and requires ATP and uridine triphosphate (UTP), besides glucose.

Activation of Glucose

The UDP-glucose is formed from glucose-1-phosphate and UTP by the enzyme UDP glucose pyrophosphorylase.

Glycogen Synthase Action

The glucose moiety from UDP-glucose is transferred to a glycogen primer (glycogenin) molecule. Glycogen synthase is responsible for the formation of 1,4-glycosidic linkages. This enzyme transfers the glucose from UDP-glucose to the non-reducing end of glycogen to form alpha-1,4 linkages.

Formation of Branches in Glycogen

The formation of branches is brought about by the action of a branching enzyme, namely glucosyl-4,6-transferase. This enzyme transfers a small fragment of five to eight glucose residues from the non-reducing end of glycogen chain (by breaking alpha-1,4 linkages) to another glucose residue where, it is linked by α-1,6 bold. This leads to the formation of a new non-reducing end, besides the existing one. Glycogen is further elongated and branched, respectively, by the enzymes glycogen synthase and glucosyl-4,6 transferase.

Glycogenolysis

The degradation of stored glycogen in liver and muscle constitutes glycogenolysis. A set of enzymes present in the cytosol carry out glycogenolysis. Glycogen is degraded by breaking alpha-1,4- and alpha-1,6-glycosidic bonds.

Action of Glycogen Phosphorylase

The alpha-1,4-glycosidic bonds are cleaved sequentially by the enzyme glycogen phosphorylase to yield glucose -1-phosphate. It is called phosphorolysis. This is continuous until the formation of limit dextrin.

Action of Debranching Enzyme

Three glucose residues are transferred from the branching point to another chain. The remaining molecule is available for the action of phosphorylase and debranching enzyme.

Formation of Glucose-6-phosphate and Glucose

By the action of glycogen phosphorylase and debranching enzyme, glucose-1-phosphate and free glucose are produced. The former is converted to glucose-6-phosphate by phosphoglucomutase. Hepatic glucose-6-phosphatase hydrolyses glucose-6-phosphate to glucose. The free glucose is released to the bloodstream.

Muscle lacks glucose-6-phosphatase so muscle will not release glucose to the bloodstream.

Regulation of Glycogen Metabolism

Glycogenesis and glycogenolysis are respectively, controlled by the enzymes glycogen synthase and glycogen phosphorylase. Regulation occurs by three mechanisms:

1. Allosteric regulation.
2. Hormonal regulation.
3. Influence of calcium (Ca^{2+}).

Allosteric Regulation of Glycogen Metabolism

There are certain metabolites that allosterically regulate the activities of glycogen synthase and glycogen phosphorylase. Glycogen synthesis is increased when substrate availability and energy levels are high. In a well-fed state, the availability of glucose-6-phosphate is high, which allosterically activates glycogen synthase for glycogen synthesis.

Hormonal Regulation of Glycogen Metabolism

The hormones, through a complex series of reactions, bring about phosphorylation and dephosphorylation of enzyme proteins, which ultimately control glycogen synthesis or its degradation (Fig. 3.13).

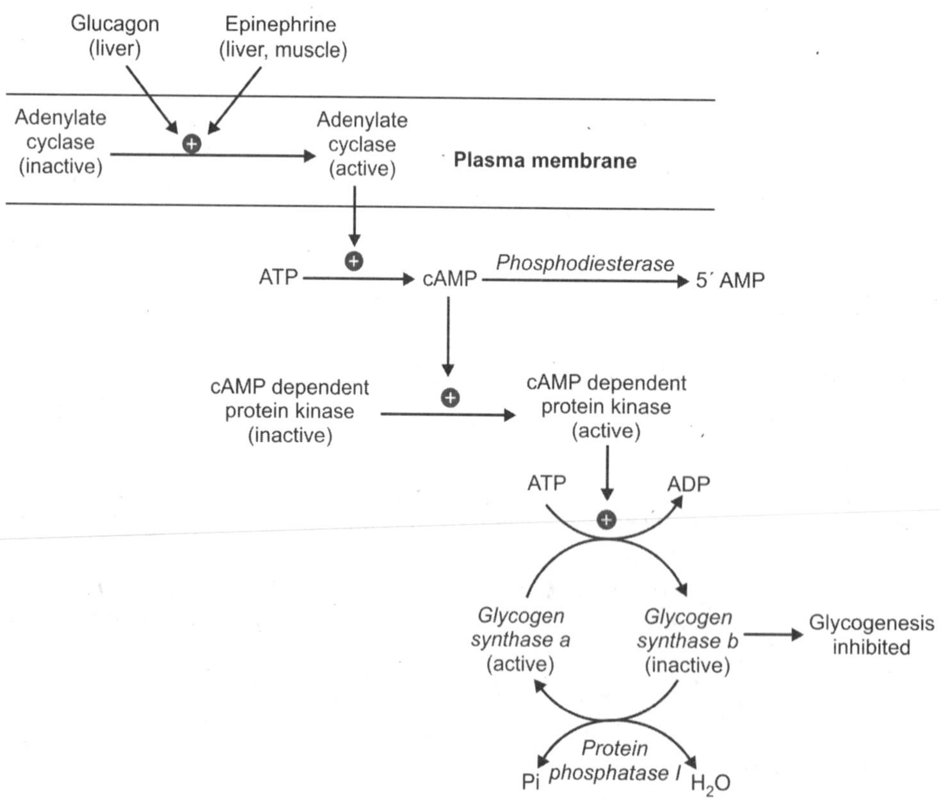

Fig. 3.13: Hormonal regulation of glycogen metabolism

Influence of Calcium

Regulation of glycogen metabolism.

Regulation of Glycogen Synthesis by cAMP

Liver and muscle phosphorylases are activated by cAMP mediated process. Hormones like epinephrine, norepinephrine and glucagon in liver activate adenylate cyclase to increase the production of cAMP.

When the hormone binds to a receptor on the plasma membrane, the enzyme adenylyl cyclase is activated, which converts ATP to cAMP. Increased cAMP activates protein kinase. This enzyme phosphorylates and inactivates glycogen synthase.

Effect of Ca^{2+} Ions on glycogenolysis

When the muscle contracts, Ca^{2+} are released from the sarcoplasmic reticulum. Ca^{2+} binds to calmodulin-calcium modulating protein and directly activates phosphorylase without the involvement of cAMP dependent protein kinase.

Glycogen Storage Diseases

Glycogen storage diseases are inborn-errors of metabolism.
von Gierke disease or glycogen storage disease type-I.

1. Most common type of glycogen storage disease is type-I.
2. Glucose-6-phosphatase is deficient.
3. Fasting hypoglycemia that does not respond to stimulation by adrenaline. The glucose cannot be released from liver during overnight fasting.
4. Hyperlipidemia is due to blockade of gluconeogenesis; more fat is mobilized and results in increased level of free fatty acids and ketone bodies.
5. Glucose-6-phosphate is accumulated, so it is channeled to HMP shunt pathway producing more ribose and more nucleotides. Purines are then catabolized to uric acid leading to hyperuricemia.
6. Glycogen gets deposited in liver. Massive liver enlargement may lead to cirrhosis.
7. Children usually die in early childhood.
8. Treatment is to give small quantity of food at frequent intervals.

Other important disorders are given in Table 3.5.

BLOOD GLUCOSE REGULATION

The plasma glucose level at an instant depends on the balance between glucose entering and leaving the extracellular fluid. Regulation of glucose by pancreatic alpha- and beta-cells are shown in Figure 3.14:

1. Blood glucose regulation during fasting (high glucagon). In fasting state, blood glucose is maintained by glycogenolysis and glucogenesis; further, adipose tissue releases free fatty acids as alternate source of energy.
2. Blood glucose regulation during postprandial state (high insulin). In postprandial state, glucose level is high; then blood glucose level is lowered by tissue oxidation, glycogen synthesis and lipogenesis.

Effect of hyperglycemic and hypoglycemic factors on blood glucose level is depicted in Figure 3.15.

Insulin

Insulin is a polypeptide hormone produced by the beta-cells of islets of Langerhans of pancreas.

Factors stimulating insulin secretion are:

1. Glucose: Most important stimulus for insulin release. A rise in blood glucose level is a signal for insulin secretion.
2. Amino acids: Among the amino acids, arginine and leucine are potent stimulators of insulin release.
3. Gastrointestinal hormones.

Factors inhibiting insulin secretion are:

1. Epinephrine.
2. Alpha-adrenergic stimulation.

Table 3.5: Glycogen storage diseases

Name	Enzyme defect	Features
von Gierke disease (type I)	Glucose-6-phosphatase	Fasting hypoglycemia, hepatomegaly, ketosis hyperlipidemia
Pomper's disease (type II)	Lysosomal maltase	Glycogen accumulates in lysosomes, hepatomegaly
Cori disease/limit dextrinosis (type III)	Debranching enzyme	Branched chain glycogen accumulates, fasting hypoglycemia, hepatomegaly
Andersen's disease (amylopectinoses-type IV)	Branching enzyme	Glycogen with few branches accumulate, liver cirrhosis, hepatosplenomegaly
McArdle's disease (type V)	Muscle phosphorylase	Exercise intolerance, glycogen accumulation in muscles
Hers disease (type VI)	Liver phosphorylase	Hypoglycemia, ketosis, hepatomegaly
Tarui disease (type VII)	Phosphofructokinase	Muscle cramps, hemolysis, glycogen accumulation in muscles

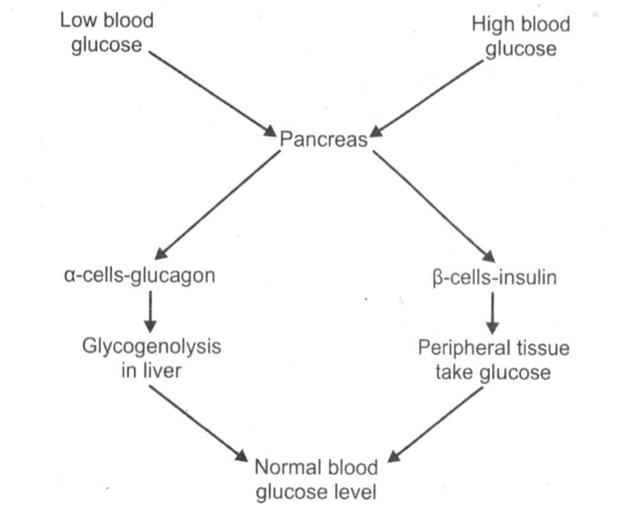

Fig. 3.14: Blood glucose regulation

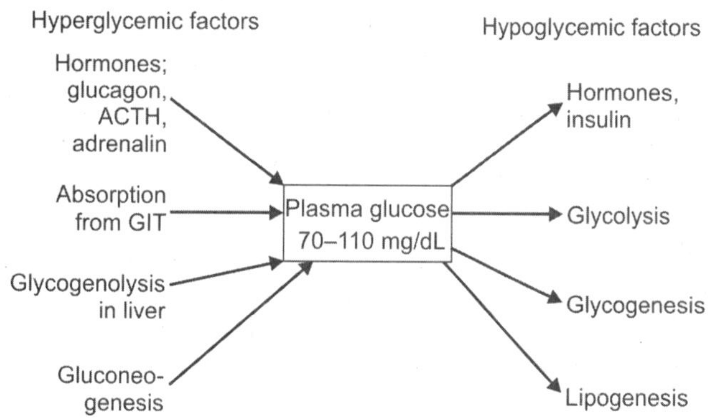

Fig. 3.15: Effect of hyperglycemic and hypoglycemic factors on blood glucose level (ACTH, adrenocorticotropic hormone; GIT, gastrointestinal tract).

Metabolic Effects of Insulin

Insulin lowers blood glucose level (hypoglycemia) by promoting its use and inhibiting its production:

1. Insulin is required for the uptake of glucose by muscle and adipose tissue. Tissues into which glucose can freely enter include brain, kidneys, erythrocytes, retina, nerves, blood vessels and intestinal mucosa.
2. Glucose utilization: Insulin increases glycolysis in muscle and liver.
3. Glucose production: Insulin decreases gluconeogenesis by suppressing the enzymes pyruvate carboxylase, phosphoenolpyruvate carboxykinase and glucose-6-phosphatase. Insulin also inhibits glycogenolysis by inactivating the enzyme glycogen phosphorylase.
4. Insulin acts on lipid and protein metabolism . The net effect of insulin on lipid metabolism is to reduce the release of fatty acids from the stored fat and decrease the production of ketone bodies. It stimulates the entry of amino acids into the cells, enhances protein synthesis and reduces protein degradation.

Mechanism of Action of Insulin

1. Insulin receptor-mediated signal transduction: Insulin receptor is a tetramer consisting of four subunits of two types—alpha and-beta.

   As the hormone insulin binds to the receptor, a conformational change is induced in the alpha subunits of insulin receptor. This results in the generation of signals, which are transduced to beta-subunits. This activates tyrosine kinase activity results in autophosphorylation.
2. Insulin-mediated glucose transport: The glucose transporters are responsible for the insulin-mediated uptake of glucose by the cells.
3. Insulin-mediated enzyme synthesis: Insulin promotes the synthesis of enzymes such as glucokinase, phosphofructokinase and pyruvate kinase.

GLUCAGON

Glucagon, secreted by alpha cells of the pancreas, opposes the actions of insulin. The secretion of glucagon is stimulated by low-blood glucose concentration, amino acids derived from dietary protein and low levels of epinephrine. Increased blood glucose level markedly inhibits glucagon secretion.

Metabolic Effects of Glucagon

Glucagon influences carbohydrate, lipid and protein metabolisms:

1. Glucagon is the most potent hormone that enhances the blood glucose level (hyperglycemic).
2. Primarily, glucagon acts on liver to cause increased synthesis of glucose (gluconeogenesis) and enhanced degradation of glycogen (glycogenolysis).
3. The actions of glucagon are mediated through cyclic AMP.
4. Glucagon binds to the specific receptors on the plasma membrane and acts through the mediation of cyclic AMP, the second messenger.

GLUCOSE TOLERANCE TEST

The ability of a person to metabolize a given load of glucose is referred to as glucose tolerance test (GTT). The diagnosis of diabetes can be made on the basis of individual's response to the oral glucose load, commonly referred to as oral glucose tolerance test (OGTT). Graphical representation of GTT is shown in Figure 3.16.

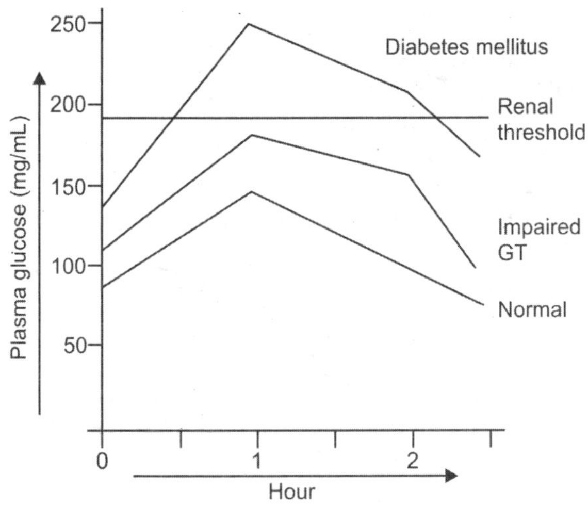

Fig. 3.16: Oral glucosctolerance test

Diagnostic Criteria for OGTT

1. In a normal person, fasting plasma glucose is 70–110 mg/dL.
2. Following the glucose load, the level rises and reaches a peak within 1 hour and then comes down to normal fasting levels by 2–2½ hours (Table 3.6).
3. This is due to the secretion of insulin in response to the elevation in blood glucose.

Indications for OGTT

1. Patient has symptoms suggestive of diabetes mellitus, but fasting blood sugar value is inconclusive (between 100 and 126 mg/dL).

Table 3.6: Diagnostic criteria for OGTT

Condition	Normal (glucose)	Impaired GT	Diabetes
Fasting	< 110 mg/dL	110–126 mg/dL	> 126 mg/dL
1 hour after glucose	< 160 mg/dL	-	-
2 hour after glucose	< 140 mg/dL	140–200 mg/dL	> 200 mg/dL

2. During pregnancy, excessive weight gaining is noticed, with a past history of big baby (> 4 kg) or a past history of miscarriage.
3. To rule out benign renal glucosuria.

Contraindications for OGTT

- Person with confirmed diabetes mellitus
- Acutely ill patients.

Abnormal GTT Curve

1. Impaired glucose tolerance (IGT): Plasma glucose level is above the normal value, but below the diabetic level (110–126 mg/dL, fasting).
2. Alimentary glucosuria: Blood glucose level rises rapidly after meals resulting in its spill over into urine. Seen in patients with hepatic disease, hyperthyroidism and peptic ulcer.
3. Renal glycosuria: Benign condition due to a reduced renal threshold for glucose. Normal threshold is 175–180 mg/dL. When renal threshold is lowered, glucose is excreted in urine. Seen in pregnancy, renal disease, etc.
4. Gestational diabetes mellitus: Carbohydrate intolerance is noticed for the first time during pregnancy. A known diabetic patient who became pregnant is not included in this. It is associated with increased risk of neonatal mortality.

DIABETES MELLITUS

Diabetes mellitus is a metabolic disease, due to absolute or relative insulin deficiency. It is mainly characterized by hyperglycemia.

Diabetes mellitus is broadly divided into two groups, namely insulin-dependent diabetes mellitus (IDDM) and non-insulin dependent diabetes mellitus (NIDDM). This classification is mainly based on the requirement of insulin for treatment.

Insulin-dependent Diabetes Mellitus (Type 1)

The IDDM is also known as juvenile onset diabetes. This disease is characterized by almost total deficiency of insulin due to destruction of beta-cells of pancreas. The beta-cell destruction may be caused by drugs, viruses or autoimmunity. Due to certain genetic variation, the beta-cells are recognized as non-self and they are destroyed by immune mediated injury. The pancreas ultimately fails to secrete insulin in response to glucose ingestion. The patients of IDDM require insulin therapy.

Non-insulin-dependent Diabetes Mellitus (Type 2)

The NIDDM also called adult-onset diabetes. Most common, accounting for 80%–90% of the diabetic population. The causative factors of NIDDM include genetic and environmental. The NIDDM more commonly occurs in obese individuals. Obesity acts as a diabetogenic factor in genetically predisposed individuals by increasing the resistance to the action of insulin. This is due to a decrease in insulin receptors on the insulin responsive (target) cells. The patients of NIDDM may have either normal or even increased insulin levels (Table 3.7).

Table 3.7: Differences between type 1 and type 2 diabetes

Features	IDDM (type 1)	NIDDM (type 2)
Prevalence	10%–20%	80%–90%
Age of onset	Childhood	Adult
Genetic predisposition	Mild or moderate	Very strong
Biochemical defect	Insulin deficiency	Resistance to insulin
Plasma insulin	Decreased	Normal
Auto antibodies	Frequently found	Rare
Ketosis	Common	Rare
Acute complications	Ketoacidosis	Hyperosmolar coma
Oral hypoglycemic drugs	Not useful for treatment	Suitable
Insulin administration	Always required	Not necessary

Clinical Correlation

1. When the blood glucose level exceeds the renal threshold, glucose is excreted in urine (glucosuria).
2. Due to osmotic effect, more water accompanies the glucose (polyuria). To compensate for this loss of water, thirst center is activated, and more water is taken (polydipsia).
3. To compensate the loss of glucose and protein, patient will take more food (polyphagia).
4. The loss and ineffective utilization of glucose leads to breakdown of fat and protein. This would lead to loss of weight.
5. Often the presenting complaint of the patient may be chronic recurrent infections such as boils, abscesses, etc. Any person with recurrent infections should be investigated for diabetes. Tuberculosis is commonly associated with diabetes.

Acute Metabolic Complications

Diabetic Keto Acidosis

Normally the blood level of ketone bodies is less than 1 mg/dL and only traces are excreted in urine. But when the rate of synthesis exceeds the ability of extrahepatic tissues to utilize them, there will be accumulation of ketone bodies in blood. This leads to ketonemia, excretion in urine (ketonuria) and smell of acetone in breath. All these three together constitute the condition known as ketosis.

Chronic Complications

- Vascular diseases—atherosclerosis
- Diabetic retinopathy
- Peripheral neuropathy with paresthesia
- Kimmelstiel-Wilson's syndrome (proteinuria and renal failure)
- Pregnancy—big babies, abortion and premature birth.

Laboratory Investigations in Diabetes

- Plasma glucose level
- Periodic checks of fasting and postprandial plasma glucose are to be done at least once in 3 months
- Complete lipid profile to be done once in 6 months
- Kidney function tests to be done twice an year
- Glycated hemoglobin.

The best index of long-term control of blood glucose level is measurement of glycated hemoglobin or glyco-hemoglobin. Enzymatic addition of any sugar to a protein is called 'glycosylation,' while non-enzymatic process is termed 'glycation.' When there is hyperglycemia, proteins in the body may undergo glycation. It is a non-enzymatic process. Glucose forms a Schiff base with the N-terminal amino group of proteins. This is reversible. Later, Amadori rearrangement takes place to form ketoamines, when the attachment becomes irreversible. The overall reaction is called Maillard reaction. When once attached, glucose is not removed from hemoglobin.

Management of Diabetes Mellitus

- Diet and exercise
- This is the first line of treatment. A diabetic patient is advised to take a balanced diet with high-protein content, low calories, devoid of refined sugars and low-saturated fat, adequate PUFA, and fiber rich diet.
- Oral hypoglycemic agents
- Sulfonylurea and biguanides. They are mainly used in type 2 diabetes.
- Insulin injections
- In type 1 disease. Short acting and long acting preparations are available.

Hypoglycemia

A fall in plasma glucose less than 50 mg/dL. Hypoglycemia is fatal.

Causes

Causes of hypoglycemia:
- Overdose of insulin
- Postprandial hypoglycemia
- Insulinoma: Insulin secreting tumors
- von Gierke disease.

PENTOSE PHOSPHATE PATHWAY

Pentose phosphate pathway (HMP shunt) provides NADPH (serves as e^- donor) and forms ribose 5-phosphate (nucleotide synthesis).

Pathway active in tissues that synthesize fatty acids or sterols because large amounts of NADPH needed.

In muscle and brain, little pentose phosphate pathway (PPP) activity. All reactions are cytosolic. Divided into two stages:

1. Oxidative:
   - Glucose-6-phosphate + 2 $NADP^+$ + H_2O ⟶ Ribulose-5-phosphate + 2 NADPH + CO_2 + $2H^+$
2. Non-oxidative:
   - Uses transketolases (transfers 2-C units) and transaldolases (transfers 3-C units)
   - Links PPP with glycolysis
   - Used to catalyze these types of reactions:
     - C5 + C5 ⟷ C7 + C3
     - C7 + C3 ⟷ C4 + C6
     - C5 + C4 ⟷ C3 + C6

All reactions are reversible ⟶ very flexible pathway.

For example:

1. If ribose-5-phosphate needed, fructose-6-phosphate + glyceraldehyde-3-phosphate taken from glycolysis and channeled through PPP to make product.
2. If NADPH is needed, then ribulose-5-phosphate is converted to glyceraldehyde-3-phosphate and fructose-6-phosphate ⟶ converted to glucose-6-phosphate more NADPH made.
3. If use PPP, 1 glucose can be completely oxidized to 12 NADPH and $6CO_2$.
4. If NADPH and ATP are needed, ribulose-5-phosphate converted into ⟶ glyceraldehyde-3-phosphate and fructose-6-phosphate ⟶ glycolysis ⟶ pyruvate.

Regulation of Pentose Phosphate Pathway

- Controlled by levels of $NADP^+$
- Controlled step is dehydrogenation of glucose-6-phosphate to 6-phosphogluconolactone
- Enzyme stimulated by high [$NADP^+$]
- Non-oxidative branch controlled primarily by substrate availability.

Significance

Generation of Reducing Equivalents

The major metabolic role of the pathway is to provide cytoplasmic NADPH for reductive biosynthesis of fatty acids, cholesterol and steroids.

Free Radical Scavenging

Free radicals are inactivated by superoxide dismutase (SOD), peroxidase, glutathione reductase (GR). Reduced GR is regenerated with the help of NADPH.

Erythrocyte Membrane Integrity

The NADPH, glutathione and glutathione reductase together will preserve the integrity of RBC membrane.

Detoxification of Drugs

Most of the drugs and other foreign substances are detoxified by the liver microsomal P450 enzymes, with the help of NADPH.

Prevention of Methemoglobinemia

The NADPH is required to keep the iron of hemoglobin in the reduced (ferrous) state and to prevent the accumulation of met-hemoglobin.

Lens of Eye

The NADPH is required for preserving the transparency of lens.

Macrophage Bactericidal Activity

The NADPH is required for production of reactive oxygen species (ROS) by macrophages to kill bacteria.

Availability of Ribose

Ribose and deoxyribose are required for DNA and RNA synthesis. Reversal of non-oxidative phase is present in all tissues by which ribose could be made available.

Adenosine Triphosphate

The ATP is neither utilized nor produced by the HMP shunt pathway.

Clinical Correlation

1. GPD deficiency: The defect is transmitted as an X-linked recessive trait. It will lead to drug-induced hemolytic anemia. The deficiency is manifested only when exposed to certain drugs or toxins, e.g. intake of antimalarial drugs like primaquine. Sulfa drugs and furadantin precipitate the hemolysis and lead to jaundice and severe anemia. The enzyme deficiency offers resistance to Plasmodium infection.
2. Methemoglobinemia: The GPD deficient persons will show increased met-hemoglobin in circulation.

3. Thiamine deficiency: The occurrence and manifestation of Wernicke's Korsakoff's syndrome (encephalopathy), which is seen in alcoholics and those with thiamine deficiency is due to a genetic defect in the enzyme transketolase.

GLUCURONIC ACID PATHWAY OF GLUCOSE METABOLISM

Glucuronic acid pathway provides, UDP-glucuronic acid, which is the active form of glucuronic acid.

Uses

Uses are:
- Conjugation of bilirubin
- Conjugation of steroids
- Conjugation of various drugs
- Synthesis of glycosaminoglycans (GAG).

Essential Pentosuria

- It is one of the members of the Garrod's tetrad
- It is an inborn error of metabolism
- L-xylulose is converted to D-xylulose by two enzymes, xylitol dehydrogenase and xylulose reductase, absence of any of these enzymes leads to the pentosuria
- Barbiturates, aminopyrine, etc. will induce uronic acid pathway and will increase xylulosuria in such patients
- Positive Benedict's test.

POLYOL PATHWAY OF GLUCOSE

Polyol pathway involves the reduction of glucose by aldose reductase to sorbitol, which can then be oxidized to fructose (Fig. 3.17).

Glucose when converted to sorbitol cannot diffuse out of the cell easily and gets trapped there. Sorbitol is normally present in lens of eyes. But in diabetes mellitus, when glucose level is high, the sorbitol concentration also increases in the lens. This leads to osmotic damage of the tissue and development of cataract.

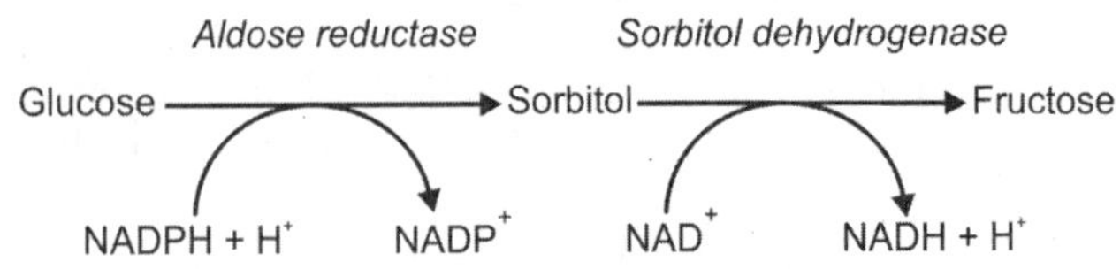

Fig. 3.17: Polyol pathway

FRUCTOSE METABOLISM

Fructose is a ketohexose present in fruits, honey and sucrose.

Fructose is phosphorylated by fructokinase, an enzyme present in liver with a high affinity for fructose. Fructokinase phosphorylates the substrate at first position, whereas hexokinase action is on the sixth position. Fructokinase is not dependent on insulin. So fructose is more rapidly utilized in normal persons. The fructose-1-phosphate is cleaved by the enzyme aldolase-B (Fig. 3.18).

Fructose is mainly metabolized by liver, but free fructose is seen in large quantities in seminal plasma.

Hereditary Fructose Intolerance

- Hereditary fructose intolerance (HFI) is an autosomal recessive inborn error of metabolism
- The defect is in aldolase-B; hence fructose-1-phosphate cannot be metabolized
- Accumulation of fructose-1-phosphate will inhibit glycogen phosphorylase; this leads to accumulation of glycogen in liver and associated hypoglycemia
- Positive Benedict's test
- Associated with vomiting, loss of appetite, hepatomegaly, jaundice and liver damage
- Common in infants.

Fructosuria

Fructosuria is a benign metabolic defect due to deficiency of fructokinase. There is excretion of fructose in urine. Urine gives positive Benedict's tests and Seliwanoffs tests.

GALACTOSE METABOLISM

Galactose is a constituent of lactose of milk sugar. Galactose is metabolized almost exclusively by the liver. The UDP galactose is the active donor of galactose during synthetic reactions. Galactose is necessary for synthesis of lactose, glycosaminoglycans, cerebrosides, glycoproteins (Fig. 3.19):

1. Galactokinase reaction: Galactose is first phosphorylated by galactokinase to galactose-1-phosphate.
2. Galactose-1-phosphate uridyl transferase: This is the rate limiting enzyme in the galactose metabolism.
3. Epimerase reaction: By this reaction, galactose is channelled to the metabolism of glucose. The reaction is freely reversible.
4. Alternate pathway: The galactose-1-phosphate pyrophosphorylase in liver becomes active only after 4 or 5

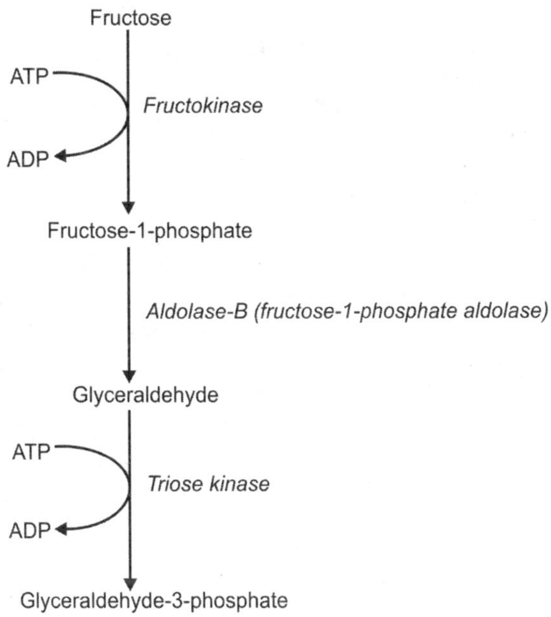

Fig. 3.18: Fructose metabolism

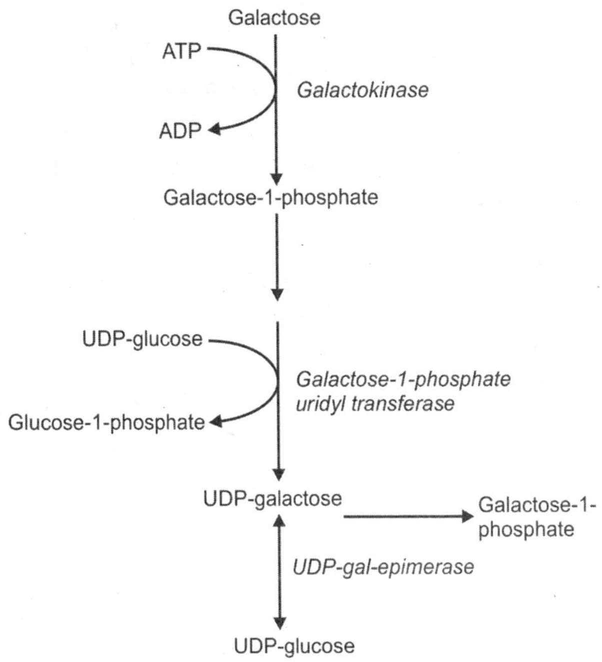

Fig. 3.19: Galactose metabolism

years of life. The enzyme will produce UDP-galactose directly, which can be epimerized to UDP-glucose.

Galactosemia

1. There is deficiency of enzyme galactose-1-phosphate uridyl transferase. It is an inborn error of metabolism.
2. Due to the block in this enzyme, galactose-1-phosphate will accumulate in liver. This will inhibit galactokinase as well as glycogen phosphorylase—hypoglycemia occurs.
3. Unconjugated bilirubin level is increased in blood.
4. Enlargement of liver, jaundice and severe mental retardation occurs.
5. Free galactose accumulates, leading to galactosemia. It is partly excreted in urine (galactosuria).
6. Galactose is reduced to dulcitol. The accumulation of dulcitol in the lens results in congenital cataract due to its osmotic effect.
7. Galactose-1-phosphate may get deposited in renal tubules, producing tubular damage leading to generalized amino aciduria.

Diagnosis

Clinical manifestation including congenital cataract and presence of galactose in urine as well as elevated blood galactose levels will help in the diagnosis. Amniocentesis may be useful in prenatal diagnosis.

Treatment

If lactose is withdrawn from the diet, most of the symptoms recede. But mental retardation, when established, will not improve. Hence, early detection is most important. For affected infant lactose-free diet is given.

METABOLISM OF ALCOHOL

Alcohol absorption starts from the stomach itself, but most of it is absorbed by intestine. Major fraction of the alcohol is oxidized in the liver (Fig. 3.20).

Alcohol Dehydrogenase

Alcohol dehydrogenase (ADH) is an NAD^+ dependent cytoplasmic enzyme that oxidizes ethanol to acetaldehyde.

Aldehyde Dehydrogenase

Acetaldehyde is further oxidized to acetate by a mitochondrial NAD^+ dependent enzyme.

Metabolic Changes

1. In the cytoplasm, the high NADH level favors conversion of pyruvate to lactate, leading to lactic acidosis. Deficiency of pyruvate leads to inadequate formation of oxaloacetate. This results in depression of gluconeogenesis, leading to hypoglycemia.

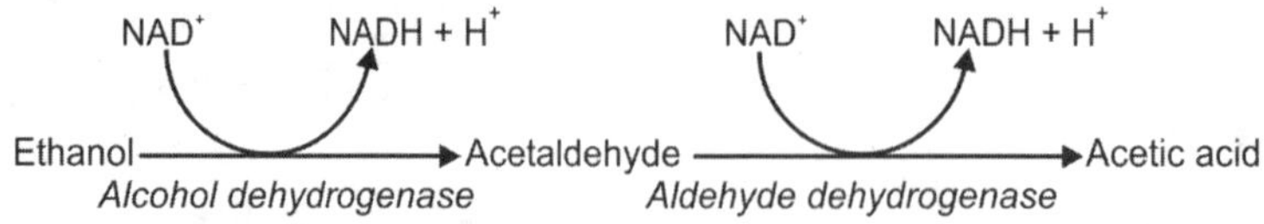

Fig. 3.20: Metabolism of alcohol

2. Acetyl-CoA is accumulated, which favors ketogenesis. Increased level of acetyl-CoA causes increased fatty acid synthesis, resulting in fatty liver and steatosis.
3. Alcohol also increases the release of ROS, leading to mitochondrial damage and apoptosis.
4. Lactic acidosis causes decreased excretion of uric acid, resulting in acute attack of gout.
5. Alcohol causes CNS depression by inhibiting excitatory receptors and by potentiating inhibitory neurotransmitter (GABA) receptors.

Chronic Alcoholism

Accumulation of fat in liver cells leading to fatty liver. This is followed by replacement by fibrous tissue. Fibrosis of liver is called cirrhosis. In chronic alcoholics, the brain ventricles are enlarged, neurons are lost, neurodegenerative changes set in the memory is affected. In alcoholics, combined thiamine deficiency leads to Wernicke's disease. Aldehyde inhibits pyridoxal phosphate; hence neuritis is very common in alcoholics.

Chapter

4

Proteins and Amino Acids

AMINO ACIDS

All proteins are polymers of amino acids. Proteins are composed of a number of amino acids linked by peptide bonds.

Classification

Based on Structure

1. Aliphatic amino acids:
   a. Monoamino monocarboxylic acids:
      - Simple amino acids: Glycine, alanine
      - Branched-chain amino acids: Valine, leucine, isoleucine
      - Hydroxy amino acids: Serine, threonine
      - Sulfur-containing amino acids BCA: Cysteine, methionine
      - Amino acids with amide group: Asparagine, glutamine.

   b. Monoamino dicarboxylic acids: Aspartic acid, glutamic acid.
   c. Dibasic monocarboxylic acids: Lysine, arginine.
2. Aromatic amino acids: Phenylalanine, tyrosine.
3. Heterocyclic amino acids: Tryptophan, histidine.
4. Imino acid: Proline.
5. Derived amino acids:
   a. Derived amino acids found in proteins: After the synthesis of proteins, some of the amino acids are modified, e.g. hydroxyproline, hydroxylysine, γ-carboxyglutamic acid.
   b. Derived amino acids not seen in proteins (non-protein amino acids), e.g. ornithine, citrulline, homocysteine.
   c. Non-α amino acids: Gamma-aminobutyric acid (GABA) is derived from glutamic acid. β-alanine, is a constituent of pantothenic acid (vitamin) and coenzyme A.

Based on Side Chain

1. Amino acids having non-polar side chains: These include alanine, valine, leucine, isoleucine, methionine, proline, phenylalanine and tryptophan. The groups are hydrophobic and lipophilic.
2. Amino acids having uncharged or non-ionic polar side chains: Glycine, serine, threonine, cysteine, tyrosine, glutamine and asparagine.
3. Amino acids having charged or ionic polar side chains:
   a. Acidic amino acids: Aspartic acid, glutamic acid.
   b. Basic amino acids: Lysine, arginine, histidine.

Based on Metabolism

1. Purely ketogenic: Leucine.
2. Ketogenic and glucogenic: Lysine, isoleucine, phenylalanine, tyrosine, tryptophan.
3. Purely glucogenic: Remaining 14 amino acids.

Based on Nutrition

1. Essential amino acids: Isoleucine, leucine, threonine, lysine, methionine, phenylalanine, tryptophan, valine.
2. Semi-essential: Histidine, arginine.
3. Nonessential: Remaining 10 amino acids.

Structure

There are 20 common amino acids called α-amino acids because they all have an amino (NH_3^+) group and a carboxyl group (COOH) attached to C-2 carbon (α-carbon).

At pH of 7, amino group is protonated ($-NH_3^+$) and carboxyl group is ionized (COO–). The amino acid is called zwitterion.

- pKa of a carboxyl group = 1.8–2.5
- pKa of a amino group = 8.7–10.7.

The α-carbon is chiral or asymmetric (four different groups are attached to the carbon; exception is glycine).

Amino acids exist as stereoisomers (same molecular formula, but differ in arrangement of groups). Designated as D (right) or L (left). Amino acids used in nature are of L configuration.

Ionization of Amino Acids

All amino acids are having a neutral net charge at physiological pH (7.4). The carboxyl and amino groups or any other ionizable groups determine charge. Each amino acid has 2 or 3 pKa values (seven amino acids have side chains that are ionizable). This complicates the basic titration curve, so that there are three inflection points rather than two. At a given pH, amino acids have different net charges. Titration curves can be used for amino acids to show ionizable groups.

The isoelectric point (pI) is the pH at which the amino acid has no net charge = zwitterion:

- If pH > pI, amino acid would be negatively charged
- If pH < pI, amino acid would be positively charged
- If pH is = pI, amino acid would have no charge.

If pH is more than pKa, there is a greater ionization and a greater amount of amino acid can use Henderson-Hasselbalch equation to calculate the fraction of group ionized at a given pH:

- A carboxyl group pKa 1.8–2.5
- A amino group pKa 8.7–10.7.

If pH is less than pKa, a greater amount of the group is protonated (NH_3^+ or COOH). Unprotonated or anion form (NH_2 or COO^-).

If pH = pKa, then [conjugate base] = [weak acid].

Reactions of Amino Acids

Decarboxylation

The amino acids will undergo α-decarboxylation to form the corresponding amine. For example:

Histidine ⟶ Histamine + CO_2
Tyrosine ⟶ Tyramine + CO_2
Tryptophan ⟶ Tryptamine + CO_2
Lysine ⟶ Cadaverine + CO_2
Glutamic acid ⟶ Gamma-aminobutyric acid + CO_2

Amide Formation

The -COOH group of dicarboxylic amino acids (other than α-carboxyl) can combine with ammonia to form the corresponding amide. For example:

Aspartic acid + NH_3 ⟶ Asparagine
Glutamic acid + NH_3 ⟶ Glutamine

Transamination

The α-amino group of amino acid can be transferred to α-keto acid to form the corresponding new amino acid and α-keto acid. This is an important reaction in the body for the interconversion of amino acids and for synthesis of non-essential amino acids.

Oxidative Deamination

The α-amino group is removed from the amino acid to form the corresponding keto acid and ammonia. Glutamic acid undergoes oxidative deamination.

Formation of Carbamino Compound

Carbon dioxide adds to the α-amino group of amino acids to form carbamino compounds.

Transmethylation

The methyl group of methionine, after activation, may be transferred to an acceptor, which becomes methylated.

Methionine + Acceptor ⟶ Methylated acceptor + Homocysteine.

Ester Formation by the -OH Group

The hydroxyl amino acids can form esters with phosphoric acid. In this manner, the serine and threonine residues of proteins are involved in the formation of phosphoproteins.

Reaction of the Amide Group

The amide groups of glutamine and asparagine can form N-glycosidic bonds with carbohydrate residues to form glycoproteins.

Reactions of -SH Group

Cysteine has a sulfhydryl (SH) group and it can form a disulfide (S-S) bond with another cysteine residue. The two cysteine residues can connect two polypeptide chains by the formation of interchain disulfide bonds. The dimer formed by two cysteine residues is sometimes called cystine.

Amino Acid Derivatives

1. Gamma-aminobutyric acid (derivative of glutamic acid) and dopamine (derived from tyrosine) are neurotransmitters.

2. Histamine (synthesized from histidine) is the mediator of allergic reactions.
3. Thyroxine (from tyrosine) is an important thyroid hormone.
4. Cycloserine, a derivative of serine is an antituberculosis drug. Azaserine inhibits reactions where amide groups are added and so acts as an anticancer drug.
5. Histidine residues are important in the buffering activity of proteins.
6. Ornithine and citrulline are derivatives of arginine, and are essential for urea synthesis.

PROTEINS

Proteins are polypeptides of amino acids linked by peptide bond.

Structure of Proteins

Primary Structure

Primary structure of protein denotes the number and sequence of amino acids in the protein and location of disulfide bonds if any. Primary structure determines biological activity. It is maintained by the covalent peptide bonds. The peptide bond is a partial double bond. The C—N bond is 'trans' in nature and there is no freedom of rotation because of the partial double bond character. The side chains are free to rotate on either side of the peptide bond. The angles of rotation are known as Ramachandran angles. At one end, a free α-amino group is present, this end is called amino terminal (N-terminal). Other end with free carboxyl group is called carboxy-terminal end (C-terminal).

Primary structure of insulin: It has two polypeptide chains. The chain (glycine chain) has 21 amino acids and B (phenylalanine) chain has 30 amino acids. They are held together by two interchain disulfide bonds. There is another intrachain disulfide bond between 6th and 11th cysteine residues of A chain. Proinsulin has an additional C peptide (connecting peptide) which is removed during maturation (Figs 4.1A and B).

Secondary Structure

Secondary structure is the steric relationship of amino acids, close to each other. They are preserved by non-covalent forces or bonds like hydrogen bonds, electrostatic bonds, hydrophobic interactions and van der Waals forces. Three types are there (Fig. 4.2).

Alpha helix: It is the most common and stable conformation for a polypeptide chain. In proteins like hemoglobin and myoglobin, the α-helix is abundant. The α-helix is a spiral structure. The α-helix is generally right handed. Left handed α-helix is rare, because amino acids found in proteins are of L-variety.

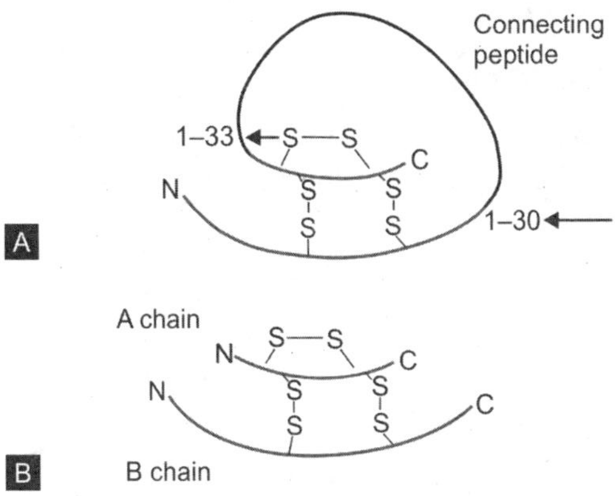

Figs 4.1A and B: Primary structure of insulin. **A.** Proinsulin; **B.** Active insulin.

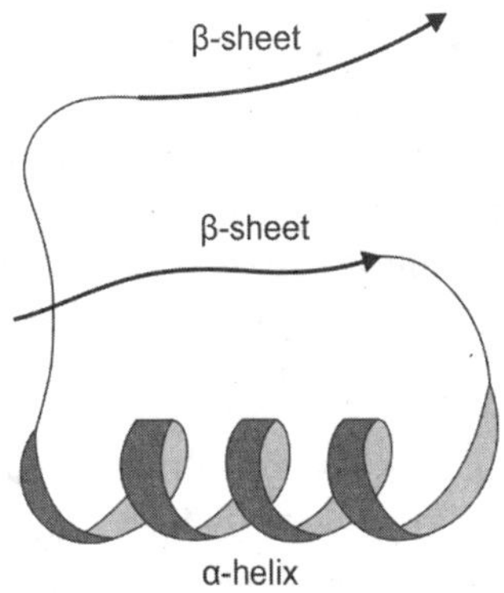

Fig. 4.2: Secondary structure of protein

Beta-pleated sheet: The polypeptide chains in β-pleated sheet is almost fully extended. β-pleated sheet is the major structural motif in proteins like silk fibroin (antiparallel), flavodoxin (parallel) and carbonic anhydrase (both).

Collagen helix: It is a triple helical structure found in collagen.

Tertiary Structure

Tertiary structure denotes the overall arrangement and inter-relationship of the various regions or domains of a single polypeptide chain. The tertiary structure is maintained by non-covalent interactions such as hydrophobic bonds, electrostatic bonds and van der Waals forces. Domain is the term used to denote a compact globular functional unit of a protein.

Quaternary Structure

Quaternary structure results when the proteins consist of two or more polypeptide chains held together by non-covalent forces. They are functional proteins. Examples are hemoglobin, immunoglobulin, etc.

Classification of Proteins

Based on Functions

1. Contractile proteins, e.g. myosin, actin.
2. Transport proteins, e.g. hemoglobin, myoglobin, albumin, transferrin.
3. Regulatory proteins or hormones, e.g. adrenocorticotropic hormone (ACTH), insulin growth hormone.
4. Genetic proteins, e.g. histones.
5. Protective proteins, e.g. immunoglobulins, interferons, clotting factors.
6. Catalytic proteins, e.g. enzymes.
7. Structural proteins, e.g. collagen, elastin.

Based on Composition and Solubility

1. Simple proteins: They contain only amino acids:
   a. Albumins: They are soluble in water and coagulated by heat, e.g. human serum albumin, lactalbumin of milk and egg albumin.
   b. Globulins: These are insoluble in pure water, but soluble in dilute salt solutions. They are also coagulated by heat, e.g. egg globulin, serum globulins, legumin of peas.
   c. Protamines: These are soluble in water, dilute acids and alkalis. They contain large number of arginine and lysine residues, and so are strongly basic, e.g. protamine zinc insulinate.
   d. Prolamins: They are soluble in alcohol. They are rich in prolines, but lack, in lysine, e.g. zein from corn, gliadin of wheat, hordein of barley.
   e. Lectins: These are precipitated by ammonium sulfate. They have high affinity to sugar groups.
   f. Scleroproteins: They are insoluble in water, salt solutions and organic solvents; soluble only in hot strong acids. They form supporting tissues. For example, collagen of bone, cartilage and tendon, keratin of hair, horn, nail and hoof.
2. Conjugated proteins: They are combinations of protein with a non-protein part called prosthetic group:
   a. Glycoproteins: These are proteins combined with carbohydrates. Blood group antigens and many serum proteins are glycoproteins.
   b. Lipoproteins: These are proteins loosely combined with lipid components.
   c. Nucleoproteins: These are proteins attached to nucleic acids, e.g. histones.
   d. Chromoproteins: These are proteins with colored prosthetic groups, e.g. hemoglobin (heme, red).
   e. Phosphoproteins: These contain phosphorus casein of milk and vitellin of egg yolk, e.g.
   f. Metalloproteins: They contain metal ions. For example, hemoglobin (iron), cytochrome (iron), tyrosinase (copper) and carbonic anhydrase (zinc).
3. Derived proteins: They are degradation products of native proteins.

Based on the Shape

1. Globular proteins: Spherical or oval in shape and easily soluble, e.g. albumins, globulins and protamines.
2. Fibrous proteins: Elongated or needle-shaped, and solubility is minimum; they resist digestion, e.g. collagen, elastin and keratins.

Based on Nutritional Value

1. Nutritionally rich proteins (complete proteins or first class proteins): They contain all the essential amino acids in the required proportion, e.g. casein.
2. Incomplete proteins: They lack one essential amino acid. Proteins from pulses are deficient in methionine, while proteins of cereals lack lysine.
3. Poor proteins: They lack in many essential amino acids. Zein from corn lacks tryptophan and lysine.

Biologically Important Peptides

1. Thyrotropin-releasing hormone (TRH) is a tripeptide with the sequence of Glu-His-Pro.
2. Glutathione is a tripeptide. It is γ-glutamyl-cysteinyl-glycine. It is involved in erythrocyte membrane integrity and is important in keeping enzymes in active state.
3. Oxytocin and vasopressin antidiuretic hormone (ADH) are nanopeptides with nine amino acids.
4. Angiotensin.

METABOLISM OF AMINO ACIDS

Amino acids are either derived from diet or are synthesized by the body. The body amino acid pool is always in a steady state, the rate of synthesis of proteins balances the rate of degradation.

Digestion of Proteins

The major proteolytic enzymes are:
1. Endopeptidases: Pepsin, trypsin, chymotrypsin.
2. Exopeptidases: Carboxypeptidases, aminopeptidases.

1. Gastric Digestion of Proteins

In the stomach, hydrochloric acid is secreted. It makes the pH optimum for the action of pepsin and also activates pepsin.

The acid also denatures the proteins. Rennin, otherwise called chymosin, is active in infants and is involved in the curdling of milk. It is absent in adults. Milk protein, casein is converted to paracasein by the action of rennin. Pepsin is secreted by the chief cells of stomach as inactive pepsinogen. The optimum pH for activity of pepsin is around 2.

2. Pancreatic Digestion of Proteins

The optimum pH for the activity of pancreatic enzymes (pH 8) is provided by the alkaline bile and pancreatic juice. The secretion of pancreatic juice is stimulated by the peptide hormones, cholecystokinin and pancreozymin. Pancreatic juice contains the important endopeptidases namely trypsin, chymotrypsin, elastase and carboxypeptidase. Trypsinogen is activated by enterokinase, which activates trypsin.

3. Intestinal Digestion of Proteins

Complete digestion of the small peptides to amino acids is by enzymes present in intestinal juice (succus entericus). Leucine aminopeptidase, proline aminopeptidase, dipeptidases and tripeptidases are involved.

Absorption of Amino Acids

Five different carriers are involved for the transport of amino acids:

- Neutral amino acids (alanine, valine, leucine, methionine, phenylalanine, tyrosine, isoleucine)
- Basic amino acids (Lys, Arg and cysteine)
- Imino acids and glycine
- Acidic amino acids (Asp, Glu)
- Beta-amino acids (β-alanine).

Amino Acid Pool

Amino acid pool of the body depends on the input and output of amino acids (Fig. 4.3).

Metabolism of Ammonia

Ammonia is a toxic product released during amino acid metabolism. Sources and fate of ammonia are shown in Figure 4.4. Detoxification of ammonia is by conversion to urea and excretion through urine.

1. Transamination

Transamination is the exchange of the α-amino group between one α-amino acid and another α-keto acid, forming a new α-amino acid (Fig. 4.5).

Significance of transamination: These are the following:

1. In this first step, ammonia is removed and the carbon skeleton of the amino acid enters into catabolic pathway.
2. By means of transamination, all non-essential amino acids can be synthesized. For example, pyruvate can be transaminated to synthesize alanine.
3. Interconversion of amino acids.
4. Transamination is reversible and requires pyridoxal phosphate.
5. Exception: Lysine, threonine and proline are not transaminated. They follow direct degradative pathways.
6. Aspartate aminotransferase (AST) and alanine aminotransferase (ALT) are induced by glucocorticoids, which favor gluconeogenesis. AST and ALT are markers of liver injury.

2. Transdeamination

a. The amino group of most of the amino acids is released by a coupled reaction, transdeamination, i.e. transamination followed by oxidative deamination. Transamination takes place in the cytoplasm. The amino group is transported to liver as glutamic acid, which is finally oxidatively deaminated in the mitochondria of hepatocytes.
b. Only liver mitochondria contain glutamate dehydrogenase (GDH), which deaminates glutamate to α-ketoglutarate plus ammonia. So, all amino acids are first transaminated to glutamate, which is then finally deaminated (transdeamination).

Urea Cycle

Urea is the end product of protein metabolism. The nitrogen in amino acid is converted into toxic ammonia, which

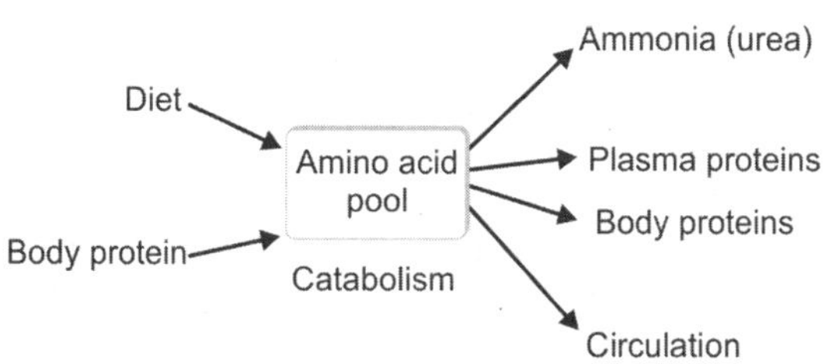

Fig. 4.3: Amino acid pool

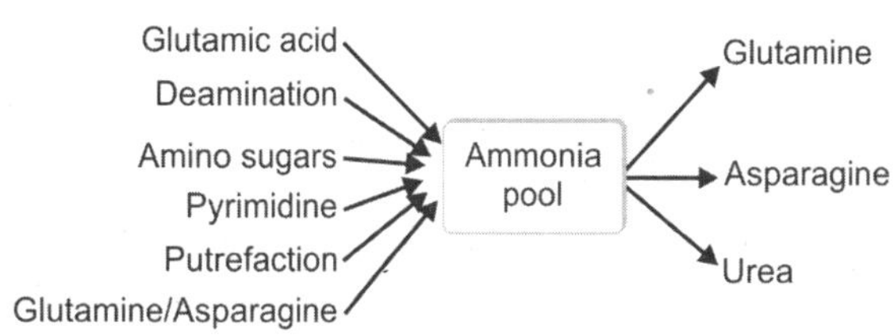

Fig. 4.4: Fate of ammonia

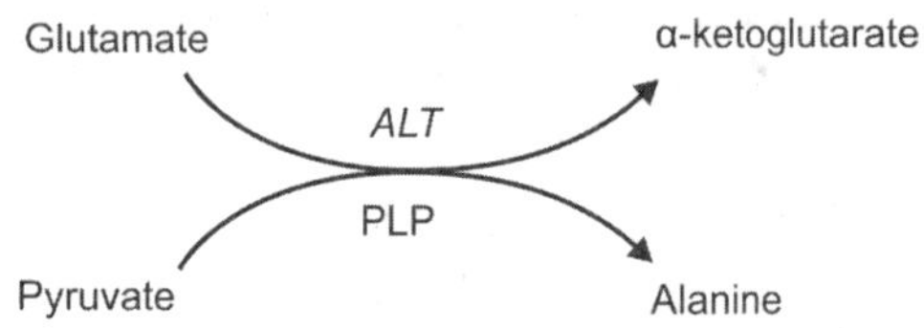

Fig. 4.5: Transamination (ALT, alanine aminotransferase; PLP, pyridoxal phosphate).

then detoxifies to urea by urea cycle. The urea cycle is the first metabolic pathway to be elucidated. The cycle is known as Krebs-Henseleit urea cycle. As ornithine is the first member of the reaction, it is also called ornithine cycle (Fig. 4.6).

Steps

Urea synthesis is a five-step cyclic process, with five distinct enzymes. The first two enzymes are present in mitochondria, while the rest are localized in cytosol.

Step 1: Formation of carbamoyl phosphate

One molecule of ammonia condenses with CO_2 in the presence of two molecules of adenosine triphosphate (ATP) to form carbamoyl phosphate. The reaction is catalyzed by the mitochondrial enzyme carbamoyl phosphate synthetase I (CPS I). An entirely different cytoplasmic enzyme, carbamoyl phosphate synthetase II, (CPS II) is involved in pyrimidine nucleotide synthesis. CPS I reaction is the rate-limiting step in urea formation. It is irreversible and allosterically regulated.

Step 2: Formation of citrulline

Citrulline is synthesized from carbamoyl phosphate and ornithine by ornithine transcarbomylase. Ornithine is regenerated and used in urea cycle. The citrulline leaves the mitochondria and further reactions are taking place in cytoplasm.

Step 3: Synthesis of argininosuccinate

Argininosuccinate synthase condenses citrulline with aspartate to produce argininosuccinate. The second amino group of urea is incorporated in this reaction. This step requires ATP, which is cleaved to adenosine monophosphate (AMP) and inorganic pyrophosphate (PPi). The PPi is an inhibitor of this step.

Step 4: Formation of arginine

Argininosuccinate is cleaved by argininosuccinate lyase (argininosuccinate) to arginine and fumarate. The enzyme is inhibited by fumarate. The fumarate formed may be funneled into TCA cycle to be converted to malate and then to oxaloacetate to be transaminated to aspartate. Thus the urea cycle is linked to tricarboxylic acid (TCA) cycle through fumarate.

$$\text{Citrulline} + \text{Aspartate} \longrightarrow \text{Arginine} + \text{Fumarate}$$

Step 5: Formation of urea

The final reaction of the cycle is the hydrolysis of arginine to urea and ornithine by arginase. The ornithine returns to the mitochondria to react with another molecule of carbamoyl phosphate, so that the cycle will proceed. Thus, ornithine may be considered as a catalyst, which enters the reaction and is regenerated.

Overall Reaction and Energetics of Urea Cycle

The urea cycle is irreversible and consumes four ATP. Two ATP are utilized for the synthesis of carbamoyl phosphate. One ATP is converted to AMP and PPi to produce argininosuccinate, which equals to two ATP. Four ATP are actually consumed.

$$NH_4^+ + CO_2 + \text{Aspartate} + 3ATP \longrightarrow \text{urea} + \text{Fumarate} + 2ADP + 2Pi + AMP + PPi$$

Regulation of the Urea Cycle

Coarse regulation: The enzyme levels change with the protein content of diet. During starvation, the activity of urea cycle enzymes is elevated to meet the increased rate of protein catabolism.

Fine regulation: The major regulatory step is catalyzed by CPS I, where the positive effector is N-acetylglutamate (NAG). It is formed from glutamate and acetyl-CoA. Arginine is an activator of NAG synthase.

Compartmentalization: The urea cycle enzymes are located in such a way that the first two enzymes are in the mitochondrial matrix. The inhibitory effect of fumarase on its own formation is minimized because argininosuccinate lyase is in the cytoplasm, while fumarase is in mitochondria.

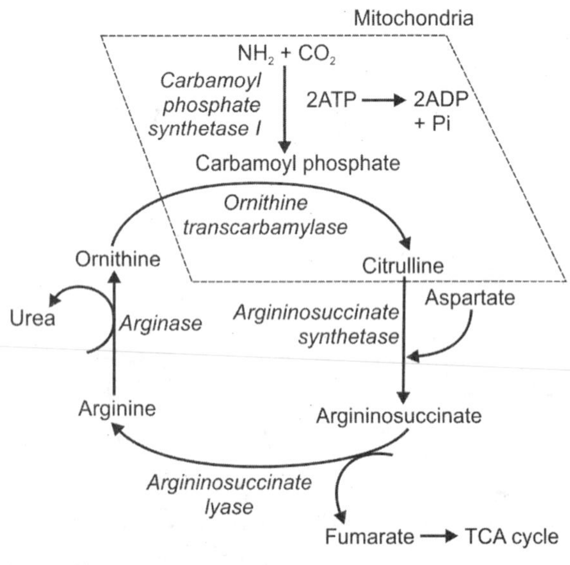

Fig. 4.6: Urea cycle (ADP, adenosine diphosphate; ATP, adenosine triphosphate; TCA, tricarboxylic cycle; Pi, inorganic phosphate).

Disorders of Urea Cycle

Disorders of urea cycle are summarized in Table 4.1.

Urea Level in Blood

In clinical practice, blood urea level is taken as an indicator of renal function. The normal urea level in plasma is from 20 to 40 mg/dL. Urinary excretion of urea is 15–30 g/day (6–15 g nitrogen/day).

Elevation of blood urea may be broadly classified as:

1. **Pre-renal:** This is associated with increased protein breakdown leading to a negative nitrogen balance, as seen after major surgeries, prolonged fever, diabetic coma, etc.
2. **Renal:** In renal disorders like acute glomerulonephritis, chronic nephritis, nephrosclerosis, polycystic kidney, blood urea is increased.
3. **Postrenal:** When there is obstruction in urinary tract, blood urea is elevated. This is due to increased reabsorption of urea from renal tubules.
4. **Uremia:** Increased blood urea levels mostly due to renal failure.
5. **Azotemia:** A condition with elevation in blood urea or other nitrogen metabolites, which may or may not be associated with renal disease.

ONE-CARBON METABOLISM

The different one-carbon groups of the 'one-carbon pool' of the body are:

- Formyl group
- Formimino group
- Methenyl group
- Hydroxymethyl group
- Methylene group
- Methyl group.

The one-carbon groups, except methyl group, are carried by tetrahydrofolic acid (THFA). The THFA is produced from folic acid. Generation of one-carbon group is shown in Figure 4.7.

Generation of One-carbon Groups

The one-carbon groups are contributed to the one-carbon pool by amino acids:

1. Serine to glycine (serine hydroxymethyltransferase reaction) is the primary contributor for methylene THFA.
2. Glycine cleavage system also produces methylene groups.
3. Histidine contributes to N^5-formimino THFA through formiminoglutamic acid (FIGLU).
4. Tryptophan donates formyl-THFA.
5. Choline and betaine are donors of hydroxymethyl groups.

As serine is converted to choline, three one-carbon units are used up. During the conversion of choline to glycine, these methyl groups are recovered. Hence, this pathway is called 'salvage pathway' for one-carbon units.

Role of Methionine and Vitamin B_{12} in One-carbon Metabolism

Methyl ($-CH_3$) group is an important one-carbon unit. After the release of methyl group, methionine is converted to homocysteine. For the regeneration of methionine, free homocysteine and N-methyltetrahydrofolate (THF) are required and this reaction is dependent on methylcobalamin (vitamin B_{12}). The one-carbon pool, under the control of THF, is linked with methionine metabolism (transmethylation) through vitamin B_{12}. Hence vitamin B_{12} is also involved in one-carbon metabolism (refer Fig. 4.7).

Utilization of One-carbon Groups

The carbon units are used for synthesis of the following compounds:

Table 4.1: Disorders of urea cycle

Diseases	Enzyme deficit	Features
Hyperammonemia type I	Carbamoyl phosphate synthetase I	High NH_3 level in blood, autosomal recessive, mental retardation
Hyperammonemia type II	Ornithine transcarbamylase	High NH_3 level in blood, orotic aciduria
Hyperornithinemia	Defective ornithine transporter protein	Hyperornithinemia, hyperammonemia Homocitrullinuria Autosomal recessive
Citrullinemia	Argininosuccinate synthetase	Autosomal recessive, citrullinuria, high blood levels of NH_3 and citrulline
Argininosuccinic aciduria	Argininosuccinate lyase	Argininosuccinate in blood and urine
Hyperargininemia	Arginase	Arginine increased in blood and cerebrospinal fluid (CSF); cysteine and lysine in urine

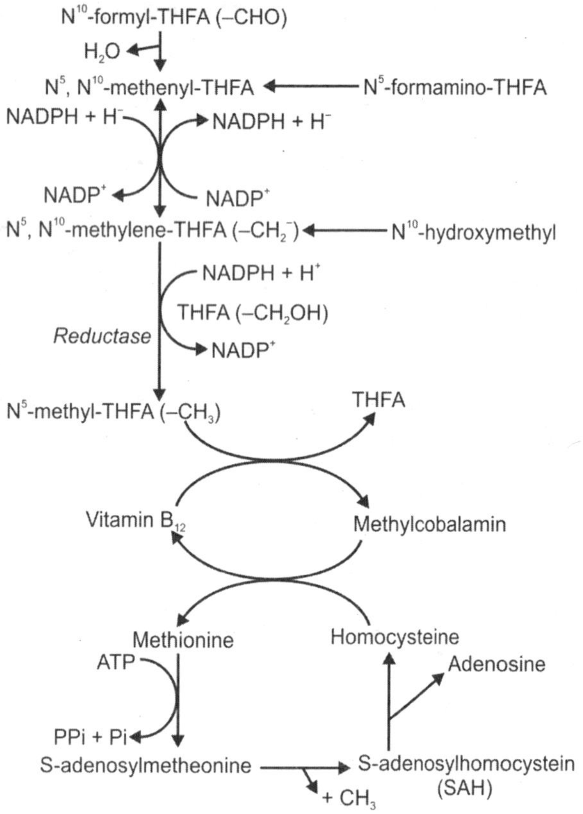

Fig. 4.7: One-carbon metabolism (ATP, adenosine triphosphate; NADPH, nicotinamide adenine dinucleotide phosphate; THFA, tetrahydrofolic acid).

- C2 of purine
- Formylation of methionyl-tRNA
- C8 of purine
- Glycine
- Serine
- Choline
- Deoxythymidine monophosphate (TMP)
- Transmethylation reactions including creatine, choline and epinephrine synthesis
- Excreted as carbon dioxide.

AMINO ACID METABOLISM

Glycine (G)

Glycine (G) is the simplest amino acid. It is non-essential and glucogenic.

Synthesis of Glycine

1. From serine: The β-carbon of serine is channeled into the one-carbon pool, carried by THFA. The α-carbon of serine becomes the α-carbon of glycine.

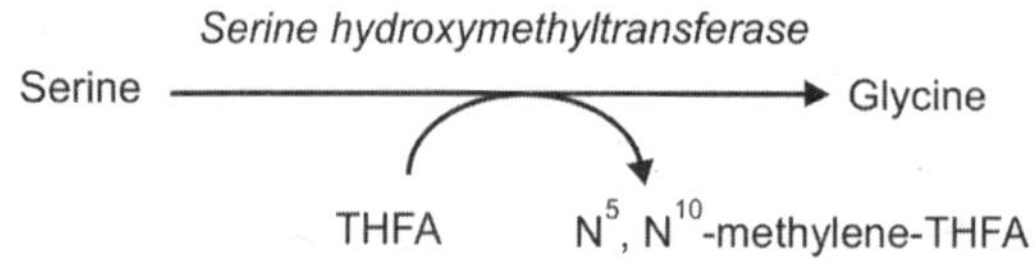

2. From threonine by the activity of threonine aldolase.

$$\text{Threonine} \xrightarrow{\textit{Threonine aldolase}} \text{Glycine} + \text{Acetaldehyde}$$

3. From glycine synthase: Glycine can be synthesized by the glycine synthase reaction from CO_2, NH_3 and one carbon unit. This is the reversal of the glycine cleavage system.

Metabolism of Glycine

1. From glycine cleavage system: Glycine undergoes oxidative deamination (reversal of glycine synthase) to form NH_3, CO_2 and one-carbon unit methylene-THFA. This pathway is the major catabolic route for glycine (Fig. 4.8). It consist of:
   a. Glycine decarboxylase with pyridoxal phosphate (PLP).
   b. Lipoamide-containing amino methyltransferase.
   c. Methylene THFA-synthesizing enzyme.
   d. NAD+-dependent lipoamide dehydrogenase.
2. Glucogenic pathway: Glycine is mainly channeled into the glucogenic pathway by getting first converted to serine. This is the reversal of serine hydroxymethyltransferase reaction. The serine is then converted to pyruvate by serine dehydratase.
3. Creatine and creatine phosphate: Creatine constitutes about 0.5% of total muscle weight. It is synthesized from three amino acids, glycine, arginine and methionine (Fig. 4.9).
4. Synthesis of heme: The enzyme aminolevulinic acid (ALA) synthase condenses glycine with succinyl-CoA to form delta ALA. It is the key enzyme of heme synthesis.
5. Synthesis of purines: The whole molecule of glycine is incorporated into the purine ring (C_4, C_5 and N_7).

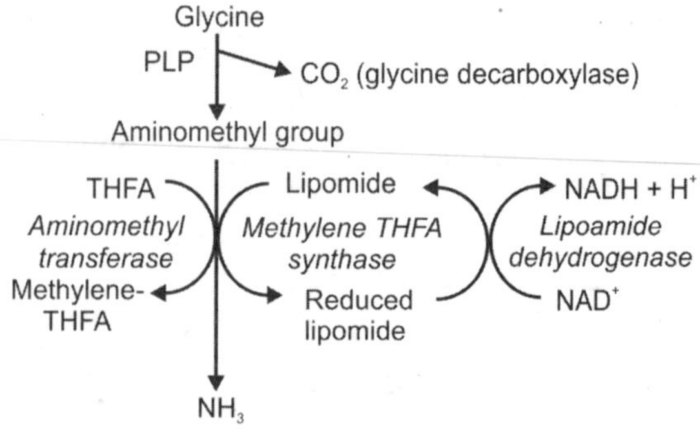

Fig. 4.8: Glycine cleavage (NADH, nicotinamide adenine dinucleotide; PLP, pyridoxal phosphate; THFA, tetrahydrofolic acid)

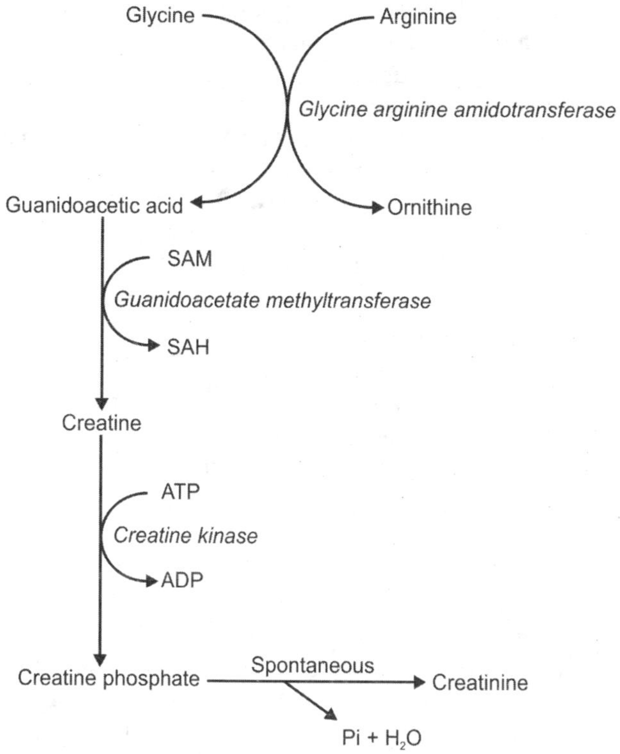

Fig. 4.9: Creatine metabolism (ADP, adenosine diphosphate; ATP, adenosine triphosphate; SAH, S-adenosylhomocysteine; SAM, S-adenosylmethionine).

6. Synthesis of glutathione: Glutathione is a tripeptide formed from glutamic acid, cysteine and glycine.
7. Glycine as a conjugating agent:
   a. Bile acids: Glycine is used to conjugate bile acids, to produce bile salts.
   b. Benzoic acid: It is used in small amounts as preservative in foods. Glycine is used for detoxification of benzoic acid to form hippuric acid.
8. Glycine as a neurotransmitter: Glycine is seen in the brainstem and spinal cord. Glycine opens chloride-specific channels. In moderate levels, glycine inhibits neuronal traffic; but at high levels, it causes overexcitation.
9. Glycine as a constituent of protein: Glycine is seen where the polypeptide chain bends or turns (β-bends or loops). In collagen, every third amino acid is glycine.

Clinical Correlation

1. Normal serum creatinine level is 0.7–1.4 mg/dL and serum creatine level is 0.2–0.4 mg/dL.
2. Creatinine level in blood is a sensitive indicator of renal function.
3. Urine contains negligible amounts of creatine in normal males.
4. But in muscular dystrophies, the blood creatine and urinary creatinine are increased.

The enzyme creatine kinase (CK) is elevated in myocardial infarction.

Sulfur-containing Amino Acids

The sulfur-containing amino acids are methionine, cysteine and cystine. Among these, only methionine is essential. It serves as a precursor for the synthesis of cysteine and cystine, which are therefore nonessential.

Methionine

Metabolism of methionine may be divided into three parts:
1. Utilization of methionine for transmethylation reactions.
2. Conversion of methionine to cysteine and cystine.
3. Degradation of cysteine and its conversion to specialized products.

Transmethylation: The transfer of methyl group (-CH3) from active methionine to an acceptor is known as transmethylation. Methionine has to be activated to S-adenosylmethionine (SAM) or active methionine to donate the methyl group.

Significance of transmethylation
1. Transmethylation is of great biological significance since many compounds become functionally active only after methylation.
2. Protein (amino acid residues) methylation helps to control protein turnover. In general, methylation protects the proteins from immediate degradation.
3. In plants, S-adenosylmethionine is the precursor for the synthesis of a plant hormone, ethylene, which regulates plant growth and development, and is involved in the ripening of fruits.

Cysteine

Formation of cysteine: This is by using the carbon skeleton contributed by serine and sulfur-originating from methionine (Fig. 4.10).

Methionine ⟶ SAM ⟶ SAH ⟶ Homocysteine ⟶ Cystathionine ⟶ Cysteine

Degradation of cysteine: This includes the following:
1. Transamination: Cysteine is transaminated to form β-mercaptopyruvic acid and finally pyruvate. The β-mercaptopyruvate can transfer the S to CN to form thiocyanate (SCN).
2. Cysteine on decarboxylation gives β-mercaptoethanolamine. This is used for synthesis of CoA.

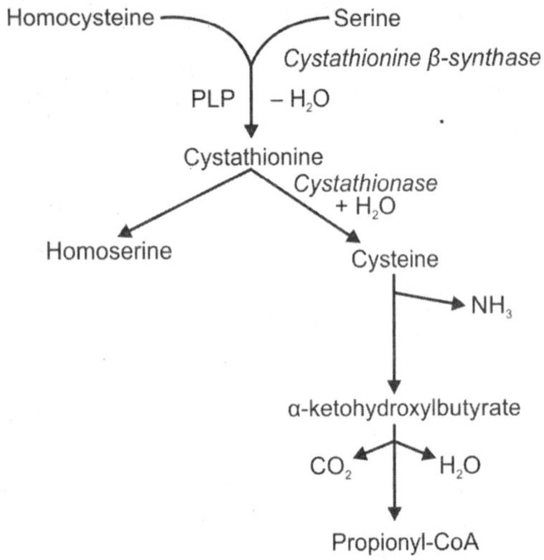

Fig. 4.10: Cysteine formation (PLP, pyridoxal phosphate)

Metabolic functions of cysteine: Are as follows:

1. **Formation of glutathione**
   Glutathione is gamma-glutamylcysteinylglycine. Glutathione is generally abbreviated as GSH, to indicate the reactive SH group.
   Glutamate + Cysteine ⟶ Gamma-glutamylcysteine
   Glutamylcysteine + Glycine ⟶ Glutathione
2. **Coenzyme role**
   Metabolic role of GSH is mainly in reduction reactions:
   2GSH ⟶ GS-SG + H_2
   (Reduced) (Oxidized)
   The hydrogen released is used for reducing other substrates. A few examples are shown below:
   Maleylacetoacetate ⟶ Fumarylacetoacetate
   Cysteic acid ⟶ Taurine
3. **Red blood cell (rbc) membrane integrity**
   Glutathione is present in the red blood cells (RBCs). This is for inactivation of free radicals formed inside RBC. The enzyme is glutathione peroxidase, selenium-containing enzyme. The glutathione is regenerated by an NADPH-dependent glutathione reductase. The NADPH is derived from the glucose-6-phosphate (GPD) shunt pathway. The occurrence of hemolysis in GPD deficiency is attributed to decreased regeneration of reduced glutathione.
4. **Methemoglobin**
   The methemoglobin is unavailable for oxygen transport. The GSH is necessary for the reduction of methemoglobin (ferric state) to normal hemoglobin (ferrous state).
5. **Conjugation for detoxification**
   Glutathione helps to detoxify several compounds by transferring cysteinyl group, such as:
   - Organophosphorus compounds
   - Halogenated compounds
   - Nitrogenous substances
   - Heavy metals.

   The reaction is catalyzed by glutathione S-transferase (GST). The GST is seen in all tissues, especially in liver. GST is a dimer and each chain may be any one out of four polypeptides, so there are six isoenzymes. These are named as A, B, C, D, E and AA. Moreover, many polymorphic forms of GST are also described.
6. **Activation of enzymes**
   Many enzymes having -SH groups in the active site are kept in the active form by the glutathione. Such enzymes are active in the reduced form. Glutathione keeps the enzymes in reduced and active state.
7. **Taurine**
   Cysteine is oxidized to cysteic acid and then decarboxylated to form taurine. Alternatively cysteine is oxidized to cysteine sulfinic acid. It is then decarboxylated by a decarboxylase to hypotaurine, which in turn is oxidized to taurine. Taurine is used for conjugation of bile acids.
   Taurine + Cholyl-CoA ⟶ Taurocholate + CoASH
   Taurine is a modulator of calcium fluxes, calcium binding and movement. In the central nervous system (CNS) it is an inhibitory neurotransmitter.
8. **Formation of active sulfate**
   Active sulfate or phosphoadenosine phospho-5′-sulfate (PAPS) is formed by the reaction between ATP and SO_4, and the sulfate is attached to the ribose-5′-phosphate. The PAPS is used for various sulfuration reactions, e.g. synthesis of sulfatides, glycosaminoglycans, etc.

Cystinuria

Cystinuria is one of the inborn errors of metabolism included in the Garrod's tetrad. It is an autosomal recessive condition. The disorder is attributed to the deficiency in transport of amino acids. Signs and symptoms include:

1. Abnormal excretion of cystine and to a lesser extent lysine, ornithine and arginine. Hence, the condition is also called cystine-lysinuria.
2. Crystalluria: In acidic pH, cystine crystals are formed in urine.
3. Obstructive uropathy, which may lead to renal insufficiency.

Treatment is to increase urinary volume by increasing fluid intake. Solubility of cystine is increased by alkalinization of urine by giving sodium bicarbonate.

Cystinosis

Cystinosis is a familial disorder characterized by the widespread deposition of cystine crystals in the lysosomes. Cystine accumulates in liver, spleen, bone marrow, white blood cells (WBCs) kidneys, cornea and lymph nodes.

Homocystinuria

Normal homocysteine level in blood is 5–15 μmol/L. In diseases, it may be increased to 50–100 times. Moderate increase is seen in aged persons, vitamin B_{12} or B_6 deficiency, tobacco smokers, alcoholics and hypothyroid patients.

Large amounts of homocysteine are excreted in urine. In plasma, homocysteine with -SH group disulfide –SS group exists. Both if present in urine, it will be in homocysteine form. If homocysteine level in blood is increased, there is increased risk for coronary artery diseases (Fig. 4.11).

Causes of congenital homocystinuria

1. Cystathionine β-synthase deficiency: It causes elevated plasma levels of methionine and homocysteine, and increased excretion of both in urine.
2. General symptoms are mental retardation and Charlie Chaplin gait.
3. In eyes, ectopia lentis (subluxation of lens), myopia and glaucoma may be observed.
4. Homocysteine may lead to increased platelet adhesiveness and life-threatening intravascular thrombosis.
5. Cyanide-nitroprusside test will be positive in urine.
6. Treatment is a diet low in methionine and rich in cysteine.

Glutamic Acid

Glutamic acid is one of the non-essential amino acids, which is acidic in nature. By the reversible reaction catalyzed by glutamate dehydrogenase, glutamic acid is formed in the liver from α-ketoglutaric acid and ammonia.

Metabolic Fate of Glutamic Acid

1. Glutamic acid is a precursor of a number of biologically active compounds.
2. By a transamination reaction, α-amino group of glutamate becomes available for the synthesis of several non-essential amino acids.

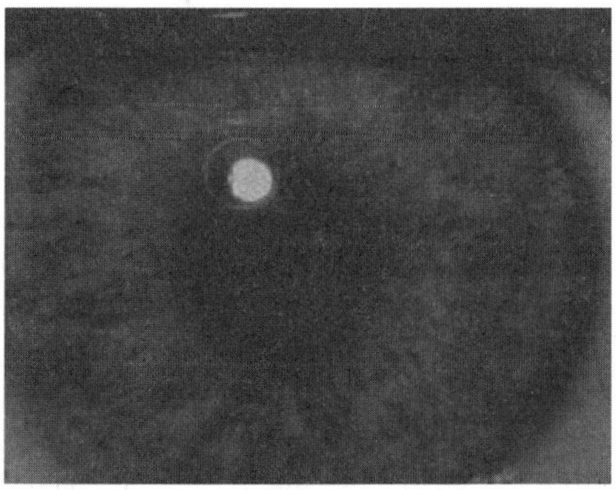

Fig. 4.11: Homocystinuria

3. Glutamic acid, in the presence of glutamine synthetase and ATP, reacts with ammonia and forms glutamine.
4. Oxidative deamination: Deamination occurs with the help of NAD^+.

$$\text{Glutamic acid} \xrightarrow{\text{Glutamate dehydrogenase}} \text{Alpha-ketoglutarate} + NH_3$$

5. Glutathione: Glutamate is a constituent of the tripeptide glutathione.

Gamma-aminobutyric Acid

1. Metabolism: Glutamic acid on decarboxylation gives rise to GABA. Part of the glutamate in the brain can be shunted through the GABA pathway and catabolized to succinate.
2. The GABA is an inhibitory neurotransmitter and it opens the chloride channels in postsynaptic membranes in CNS.
3. Pyridoxal phosphate: Both the formation and catabolism of GABA requires PLP as coenzyme. Therefore in pyridoxine deficiency, the metabolism of glutamate by the GABA shunt pathway is affected.
4. The GABA is an inhibitory transmitter, a low level of GABA or deficiency of PLP would lead to convulsions.

Glutamine

Glutamic acid reacts with ammonia and forms its amide glutamine. The reaction is catalyzed by the enzyme glutamine synthetase, which is a mitochondrial enzyme. This is the major pathway for the metabolic disposal of ammonia, chiefly in the brain.

Metabolic Fates of Glutamine

1. Glutamine is transported to the liver for the conversion of its ammonia to urea, and to the kidney. The latter reaction is catalyzed excretion of its amide nitrogen as ammonia (NH_4^+) in the urine by enzyme glutaminase. It thus protects the brain by fixing ammonia (with glutamate), which is very toxic.
2. It is a principle source of free ammonia in the urine and thus plays an important role in the maintenance of acid-base balance.
3. In the CNS, glutamine also helps in the transport of K^+
4. Glutamine is also important for the synthesis of purines in the cytoplasm and contributes to N_3 and N_9 of a purine ring.
5. In humans and other primates, glutamine conjugates with phenylacetate and forms phenylacetylglutamine.

Aromatic Amino Acids

Phenylalanine and Tyrosine

Phenylalanine and tyrosine are structurally related aromatic amino acids. Phenylalanine is essential amino acid, while tyrosine is nonessential. The need for phenylalanine becomes minimal, if adequate tyrosine is supplied in the food. This is called sparing action of tyrosine on phenylalanine. Catabolism of phenylalanine and tyrosine is given in Figure 4.12.

Important products from tyrosine

- Melanin
- Catecholamines (epinephrine)
- Thyroxine.

Synthesis of melanin: In the melanocytes, tyrosine is used for synthesis of melanin. By the enzyme tyrosinase (copper containing protein), tyrosine is first converted to dihydroxyphenylalanine (DOPA) and then to DOPA quinone. Subsequently, DOPA quinone forms melanin, a brown-black pigment found in skin, hair and retina (Fig. 4.13).

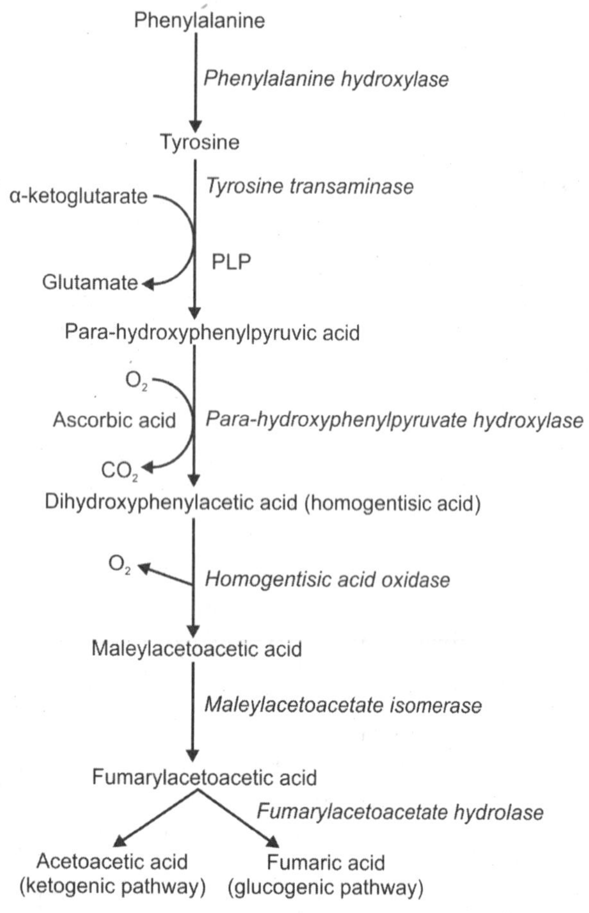

Fig. 4.12: Catabolism of phenylalanine (PLP, pyridoxal phosphate)

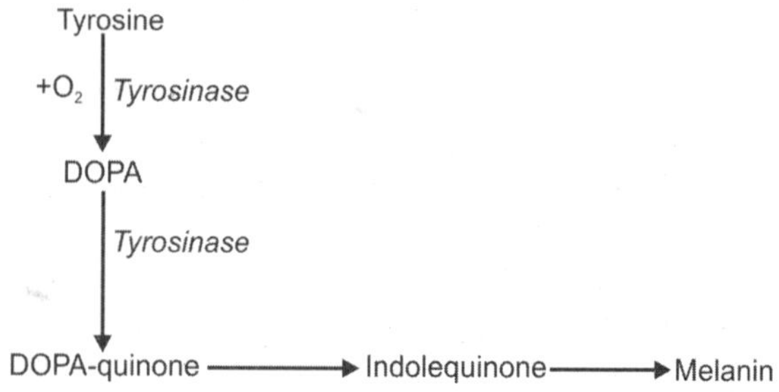

Fig. 4.13: Melanin synthesis (DOPA, dihydroxyphenylalanine)

Clinical correlation of melanin: These include the following:

1. Copper deficiency: Since tyrosinase is a copper-containing enzyme, there may be disturbances in pigmentation during copper deficiency. Hair synthesized at the time of deficiency may be depigmented.
2. Malignant melanoma: Melanoblasts, especially in junctional nevi, may multiply to give rise to malignant melanoma.
3. Leukoderma: When tyrosinase or melanin-forming cells or both are absent from epidermis, leukoderma (white patches) results.
4. Albinism: Albinism and leukoderma are different. In albinism, tyrosinase is absent in melanocytes all over the body.

Synthesis of catecholamines: The catecholamines are derived from tyrosine. They include epinephrine, norepinephrine and dopamine.

Vanillylmandelic Acid Estimation

Vanillylmandelic acid (VMA) is the major end product of adrenaline degradation (Fig. 4.14).

Normal level of excretion of VMA is 2–6 mg/24 h. It is increased in pheochromocytoma (epinephrine excess) and in neuroblastoma (norepinephrine excess).

Phenylketonuria

Deficiency of phenylalanine hydroxylase is the cause for this disease. The genetic mutation may be such that either the enzyme is not synthesized or a non-functional enzyme is synthesized. It is a recessive condition. Frequency of phenylketonuria (PKU) was considered to be 1 in 10,000 births (Fig. 4.15).

Types: There are five types of PKU described. It is due to phenylalanine hydroxylase deficiency. Types II and III are due to deficiency of dihydrobiopterin reductase. Type IV and V are due to the deficiency of the enzyme synthesizing biopterin.

Biochemical abnormalities: Phenylalanine could not be converted to tyrosine. So phenylalanine accumulates. Phenylalanine level in blood is elevated.

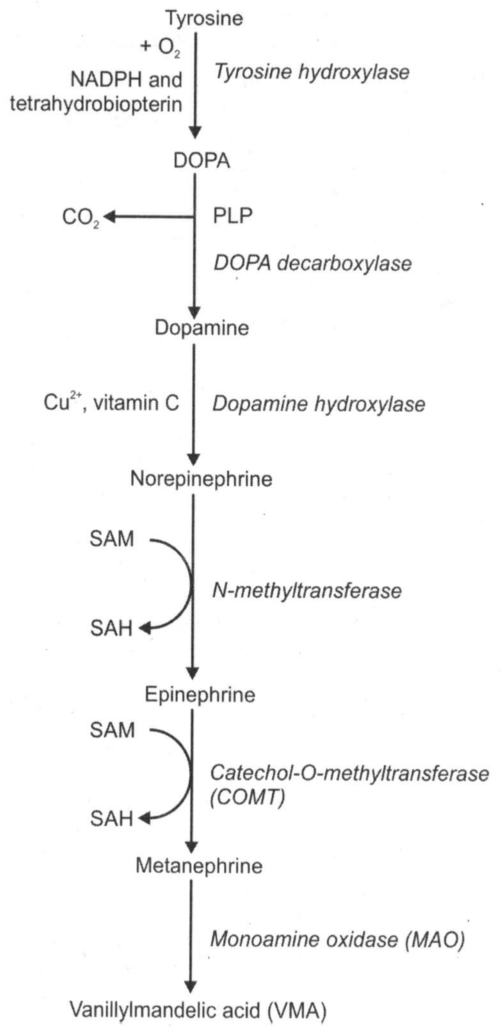

Fig. 4.14: Synthesis of catecholamines (DOPA, dihydroxyphenylalanine; SAH, S-adenosylhomocysteine; SAM, S-adenosylmethionine)

Clinical manifestations: The classical PKU child is mentally retarded with an IQ of 50.

- Agitation, hyperactivity, tremors and convulsions are often manifested
- The child often has hypopigmentation
- ousy body odor.

Laboratory diagnosis: These include the following:

1. Blood phenylalanine: Normal level is 1 mg/dL, but in PKU, the level is greater than 20 mg/dL.
2. Tandem mass spectroscopy is the most reliable test; but is costly.
3. *Guthrie test* is a rapid screening test.
4. *Ferric chloride test*: Urine of the patient contains phenyl ketones about 500–3,000 mg/day. This could be detected by adding a drop of ferric chloride to the urine. A transient blue-green color is a positive test. But this is a less reliable test.

Treatment: Early detection is very important. About 5 units of IQ are lost for each 10-week delay in starting the treatment.

The treatment is to provide a diet containing low phenylalanine (10–20 mg/kg body weight per day). Food based on tapioca (cassava) will have low-phenylalanine content.

Alkaptonuria

The term alkaptonuria arises from the Arabic word alkapton for 'alkali' and Greek word `to suck up-oxygen greedily in alkali. Alkaptonuria and albinism are two inborn errors included under Garrod's tetrad; the other two being pentosuria and cystinuria. Garrod introduced the term 'inborn errors of metabolism'.

Biochemical defect: Alkaptonuria is an autosomal recessive condition with an incidence of 1 in 250,000 births.

The metabolic defects are the deficiency of homogentisate oxidase. This results in excretion of homogentisic acid in urine.

Clinical manifestations: Blackening of urine due to formation of black-colored alkapton bodies formed by oxidation of homogentisic acid to benzoquinone acetate by polyphenol oxidase.

Ochronosis (deposition of alkapton bodies in intervertebral disks, cartilages of nose, pinna of ear) arthritis.

Diagnosis: Urine becomes black on standing when it becomes alkaline. Blackening is accelerated on exposure to sunlight and oxygen. The urine when kept in a test tube will start to blacken from the top layer.

Ferric chloride test will be positive for urine. Benedict's test is strongly positive.

Albinism

Albinism is an autosomal recessive disease with an incidence of 1 in 20,000 population.

Cause: Tyrosinase is completely absent, leading to defective synthesis of melanin.

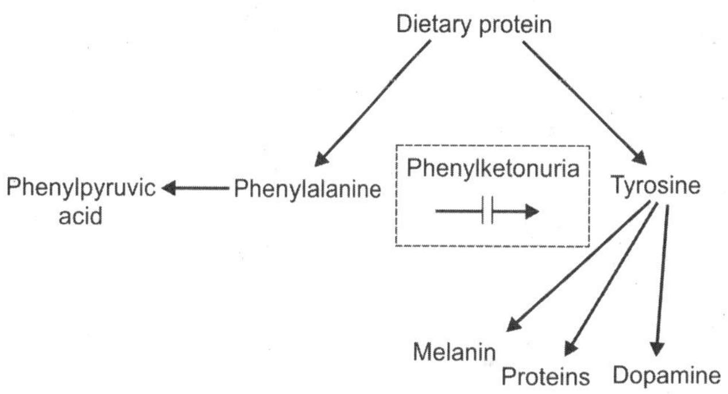

Fig. 4.15: Phenylketonuria

Clinical manifestations: The ocular fundus is hypopigmented and iris may be gray or red with photophobia, nystagmus and decreased visual acuity. Skin may show presence of nevi and melanomas; hair will be white.

Albinism may be produced by the following causes:

- Melanocyte deficiency secondary to a failure of melanoblasts to colonize the skin
- Failure of melanocytes to form melanosomes
- Due to tyrosinase deficiency, melanin is not produced in the melanosomes
- Failure of melanosomes to form melanin owing to substrate deficiency
- Failure of melanosomes to store melanin or to transport melanin to keratinocytes
- Excessive destruction of functional melanosomes.

Tryptophan

Tryptophan (Trp) was the first to be identified as an essential amino acid. It contain an indole ring and chemically it is α-amino-β-indolepropionic acid. Tryptophan is both glucogenic and ketogenic in nature.

The metabolism of tryptophan is divided into:

- Kynurenine (kynurenine-anthranilate) pathway
- Serotonin pathway.

Kynurenine Pathway

Kynurenine (kynurenine-anthranilate) pathway is shown in Figure 4.16.

Clinical correlation

Xanthurenic aciduria: Several enzymes of the tryptophan-kynurenine pathway, such as kynureninase are dependent on PLP.

In B_6 deficiency, kynurenine and 3-hydroxykynurenine are alternatively catabolized to kynurenic acid and xanthurenic acid respectively. Increased excretion of xanthurenic acid imparts a greenish yellow color to the urine and the condition is known as xanthurenic aciduria.

Serotonin Pathway

Pathway of serotonin metabolism is given in Figure 4.17.

Functions of serotonin

1. Serotonin is an important neurotransmitter in brain. 5-hydroxytryptamine (5-HT) is an antidepressant.
2. When carbohydrate-rich diet is taken, insulin secretion is increased, this will lower the amino acid concentration in blood. So, tryptophan easily enters the brain cells. When tryptophan is available in brain in excess quantity, serotonin may be generated to induce sleep.
3. Carbohydrate will induce sleep, while protein-rich food will cause alertness.
4. Serotonin level is found to be low in patients with depressive psychosis. Serotonin is involved in mood, sleep, appetite and temperature regulation. It increases gastrointestinal motility.

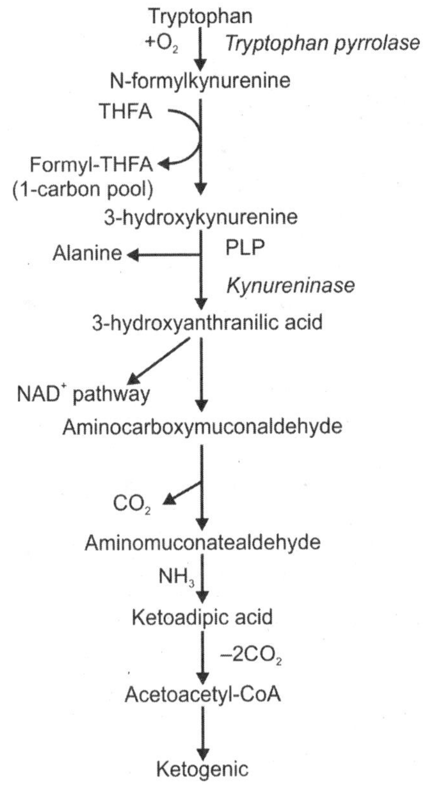

Fig. 4.16: Kynurenine pathway (PLP, pyridoxal phosphate; THFA, tetrahydrofolic acid)

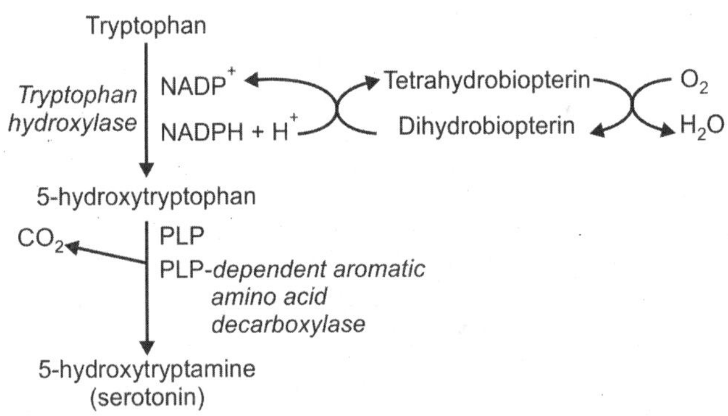

Fig. 4.17: Serotonin pathway (NADH, nicotinamide adenine dinucleotide; PLP, pyridoxal phosphate)

Clinical correlation

Hartnup disease

1. Hartnup disease is an inherited autosomal recessive disease.
2. Absorption of aromatic amino acids from intestine as well as reabsorption from renal tubules are defective. So, amino acids are excreted in urine.
3. Excretion of indican is increased in urine. Indican is the potassium salt of indoxyl sulfate. The foul smell of feces and the natural color of urine is due to this compound.
4. The pellagra-like symptoms and the common manifestations are dermatitis and ataxia.
5. A diagnosis is based on aminoaciduria and increased excretion of indole compounds are detected by Obermeyer test.
6. A patient may improve with supplementation of niacin and minimum exposure to sunlight.

Branched-chain Amino Acids

Valine (Val) or (V) is glucogenic; leucine (Leu) or (L) is ketogenic, while isoleucine (Ile) or (I) is both ketogenic and glucogenic. All the three are essential amino acids. Leucine is the major ketogenic amino acid.

Clinical Correlation

Maple syrup urine disease (MSUD): It is also called branched-chain ketonuria. The name originates from the characteristic smell of urine (similar to burnt sugar or maple sugar due to excretion of branched-chain keto acids.

The basic biochemical defect is deficient decarboxylation of branched-chain keto acids (BKA). Disease starts in the 1st week of life. It is characterized by convulsion, severe mental retardation, vomiting.

Laboratory Findings

Urine contains BKA, valine, leucine and isoleucine; Rothera's test is positive. Diagnosis depends on enzyme analysis in cells.

Treatment

Giving a diet low in branched-chain amino acids; mild variant called intermittent branched-chain ketonuria, will respond to high doses of thiamine. This is because the decarboxylation of the BKA enzyme requires thiamine.

These amino acids serve as an alternate source of fuel for the brain especially under conditions of starvation.

Chapter

5

Lipids

CHEMISTRY OF LIPIDS

Lipids may be regarded as organic substances relatively insoluble in water, soluble in organic solvents (alcohol, ether, etc.), actually or potentially related to fatty acids and utilized by the living cells.

FUNCTIONS OF LIPIDS

Lipids perform several important functions:

1. They are the concentrated fuel reserve of the body (triacylglycerols).
2. Lipids are the constituents of membrane structure and regulate the membrane permeability (phospholipids and cholesterol).
3. They serve as a source of fat-soluble vitamins (A, D, E and K).
4. Lipids are important as cellular metabolic regulators (steroid hormones and prostaglandins).
5. Lipids protect the internal organs, serve as insulating materials, and give shape and smooth appearance to the body.

CLASSIFICATION OF LIPIDS

Simple Lipids

- Triacylglycerol
- Waxes.

Compound Lipids

1. Phospholipids-containing phosphoric acid:
   a. Nitrogen-containing glycerophosphatides:
      - Lecithin [phosphatidylcholine (PI)]
      - Cephalin (phosphatidylethanolamine)
      - Phosphatidylserine.
   b. Non-nitrogen glycerophosphatides:
      - Phosphatidylinositol
      - Phosphatidylglycerol
      - Diphosphatidylglycerol (cardiolipin).
   c. Plasmalogens, having long chain alcohol:
      - Choline plasmalogen
      - Ethanolamine plasmalogen.
   d. Phosphosphingosides with sphingosine:
      - Sphingomyelin.
2. Non-phosphorylated lipids:
   a. Glycosphingolipids (carbohydrate):
      - Cerebrosides (ceramide monohexosides)
      - Globosides (ceramide oligosaccharides)
      - Gangliosides.
   b. Sulfolipids or sulfatides:
      - Sulfated cerebrosides
      - Sulfated globosides
      - Sulfated gangliosides.

Derived Lipids

Fatty acids, steroids, prostaglandins, leukotrienes, terpenes and dolichols.

Lipids Complexed to Other Compounds

Proteolipids and lipoproteins.

FATTY ACIDS

Fatty acids are included in the group of derived lipids. It is the most common component of lipids in the body. They are generally found in ester linkage in different classes of lipids. In the human body, free fatty acids (FFAs) are formed only during metabolism. Fatty acids are aliphatic carboxylic acids and have the general formula R-COOH, where COOH (carboxylic group) represents the functional group. Depending on the R group (the hydrocarbon chain), the physical properties of fatty acids may vary.

Clinical Correlations

1. Excessive fat deposits causes obesity. Truncal obesity is a risk factor for heart attack.
2. Abnormality in cholesterol and lipoprotein metabolism leads to atherosclerosis and cardiovascular diseases.
3. In diabetes mellitus, the metabolisms of fatty acids and lipoproteins are deranged, leading to ketosis.

Classification of Fatty Acids

1. Depending on total number of carbon atoms:
   a. Even chain: They have carbon atoms 2, 4, 6 and similar series. Most of the naturally occurring lipids contain even chain fatty acids.
   b. Odd chain: They have carbon atoms 3, 5, 7, etc. Odd numbered fatty acids are seen in microbial cell walls. They are also present in milk.
2. Depending on length of hydrocarbon chain:
   a. Short chain with 2–6 carbon atoms.
   b. Medium chain with 8–14 carbon atoms.
   c. Long chain with 16–22 carbon atoms.
   d. Very long-chain fatty acids (more than 24 carbon).
3. Depending on nature of hydrocarbon chain:
   a. Saturated fatty acids.
   b. Unsaturated fatty acids—which may be subclassified into monounsaturated (monoenoic) having single double bond or polyunsaturated (polyenoic) with two or more double bonds.
   c. Branched-chain fatty acids.
   d. Hydroxy fatty acids.

Saturated and Unsaturated Fatty Acids

Saturated fatty acids do not contain double bonds, while unsaturated fatty acids contain one or more double bonds. Both saturated and unsaturated fatty acids almost equally occur in the natural lipids. Fatty acids with one double bond are monounsaturated and those with two or more double bonds are collectively known as polyunsaturated fatty acids (PUFA).

Physical and Chemical Properties of Fatty Acids

1. Generally, short-chain fatty acids (between C4 and C8) are liquid, while long-chain fatty acids (more than C15) are solid at room temperature.
2. Fatty acids present in various oils react with alkali and form salts. Salts of various acids are used as soaps and emulsifying agents.
3. Unsaturated fatty acids undergo reduction and are converted to saturated fats such as hydrogenation of a vegetable oil results in the formation of ghee.
4. Unsaturated fatty acids exhibit cis-trans isomerism, due to the presence of double bond.
5. Various fatty acids can be separated from a mixture by gas-liquid chromatography.

Essential Fatty Acids

The fatty acids that cannot be synthesized by the body and therefore should be supplied in the diet are known as essential fatty acids (EFA). Chemically, they are polyunsaturated fatty acids, namely linoleic acid and linolenic acid. Arachidonic acid becomes essential, if its precursor linoleic acid is not provided in the diet in sufficient amounts.

Biochemical basis for essentiality: Linoleic acid and linolenic acid are essential, since humans lack the enzymes that can introduce double bonds beyond carbons 9 and 10.

Functions of EFA: Essential fatty acids are required for the membrane structure and function, transport of cholesterol, formation of lipoproteins, prevention of fatty liver, etc. They are also needed for the synthesis of another important group of compounds namely eicosanoids.

Deficiency of EFA: The deficiency of EFA results in phrynoderma or toad skin, characterized by the presence of horny eruptions on the posterior and lateral parts of limbs, on the back and buttocks, loss of hair and poor wound healing.

Clinical Correlation

1. Linoleic and linolenic acids are polyunsaturated fatty acids.
2. They are called essential fatty acids because they cannot be synthesized by the body and have to be supplied in the diet.
3. Unsaturated fatty acids are also designated omega-3 (ω3) family—linolenic acids, ω6 family—linoleic and arachidonic acids, ω9 family—oleic acid.
4. Arachidonic acid is the precursor of prostaglandins and can be synthesized in the body, if the essential fatty acids are supplied in the diet.
5. The pentaenoic acid present in fish oils is of great nutritional importance (ω3 unsaturated fatty acid).
6. Eicosanoids (eicosa = twenty) are derived from C20 arachidonic acid. They are polyenoic fatty acids.

Phospholipids

Phospholipids are complex or compound lipids containing phosphoric acid, in addition to fatty acids, nitrogenous base and alcohol. There are two classes of phospholipids:

1. Glycerophospholipids (phosphoglycerides) that contain glycerol as the alcohol.
2. Sphingophospholipids (sphingomyelins) that contain sphingosine as the alcohol.

Glycerophospholipids

Glycerophospholipids are the major lipids that occur in biological membranes. They consist of glycerol 3-phosphate esterified at its C1 and C2 with fatty acids. Usually, C1 contains a saturated fatty acid, while C2 contains an unsaturated fatty acid:

1. Phosphatidic acid: This is the simplest phospholipid. It does not occur in good concentration in the tissues. Basically, phosphatidic acid is an intermediate in the synthesis of triacylglycerols and phospholipids.
2. Lecithins (phosphatidylcholine): These are the most abundant group of phospholipids in the cell membranes. Chemically, lecithin is a phosphatidic acid with choline as the base. Phosphatidylcholines represent the storage form of body's choline:
   a. Dipalmitoyl lecithin is an important phosphatidylcholine found in lungs. It is a surface active agent and prevents the adherence of inner surface of the lungs due to surface tension.
   b. Lysolecithin is formed by removal of the fatty acid either at C1 or C2 of lecithin.
3. Cephalins: Ethanolamine is the nitrogenous base present in cephalins. Thus, lecithin and cephalin differ with regard to the base.
4. Phosphatidyl inositol: The stereoisomer myoinositol is attached to phosphatidic acid to give PI. This is an important component of cell membranes. The action of certain hormones (e.g. oxytocin, vasopressin) is mediated through PI.
5. Phosphatidyl serine: The amino acid serine is present in this group of glycerophospholipids.
6. Plasmalogens: When a fatty acid is attached by an ether linkage at C1 of glycerol in the glycerophospholipids, the resultant compound is plasmalogen. Choline, inositol and serine may substitute ethanolamine to give other plasmalogens.
7. Cardiolipin: It is so named as it was first isolated in heart muscle. It is an important component of inner mitochondrial membrane. Cardiolipin is the only phosphoglyceride that possesses antigenic properties.

Sphingomyelin (Sphingophospholipids)

Sphingosine is an amino alcohol present in sphingomyelins (sphingophospholipids). They do not contain glycerol at all. Sphingosine is attached by an amide linkage to a fatty acid to produce ceramide. Sphingomyelins are important constituents of myelin and are found in good quantity in brain and nervous tissues.

Functions of Phospholipids

1. Structural component of cell membrane and regulate membrane permeability.
2. Lecithin, cephalin and cardiolipin in mitochondria are responsible for maintaining the conformation of electron transport chain (ETC) and cellular respiration.
3. Helps in absorption of fat from intestine and participate in lipid transport.
4. Fatty liver can be prevented by phospholipids, hence known as lipotropic factors.
5. Phospholipids act as surfactants (agents lowering surface tension). Dipalmitoylphosphatidylcholine is an important surfactant.
6. Cephalins are important in blood clotting.
   a. Liposome: These are microscopic spherical vesicles. When mixed with water under special conditions, the phospholipids arrange themselves to form a bilayer membrane, which encloses some of the water in a phospholipid sphere.

Glycolipids

Glycolipids are seen widely in nervous tissues. This group of lipids does not contain phosphoric acid; instead they contain carbohydrates and ceramide:

1. Globosides (Ceramide Oligosaccharides): They contain two or more hexoses or hexosamines, attached to a ceramide molecule. Lactosylceramide is a component of erythrocyte membrane.
2. Gangliosides: They are formed when ceramide oligosaccharides have at least one molecule of NANA (N-acetylneuraminic acid) (sialic acid) attached to them. Gangliosides contribute to stability of paranodal junctions and ion channel clusters in myelinated nerve fibers.

Metabolism of Fatty Acids

Digestion of Lipids

The major dietary lipids are triacylglycerol, cholesterol and phospholipids. The average normal Indian diet contains

Table 5.1: Enzymes involved in lipid digestion

Enzyme	Site of action	Action
Lingual lipase	Mouth	Triglyceride → Fatty acids, monoglycerides, glycerol
Lipase/Colipase	Pancreas	Triglyceride → Fatty acids, monoglycerides, glycerol
Phospholipase A/B	Pancreas	Lecithin → Fatty acid, lysolecithin
Cholesterol esterase	Pancreas	Cholesterol ester → Cholesterol, fatty acid
Retinyl ester hydrolase	Pancreas	Retinyl ester → Retinol, fatty acid
Monoglyceride lipase	Small intestine	Monoglyceride → glycerol + fatty acid
Lecithinase	Small intestine	Lecithin → Fatty acids, glycerol, phosphoric acid, choline

about 20–30 g of lipids per day. Western diet generally contains two or three times more than this quantity. Several enzymes are involved in lipid digestion (Table 5.1).

Clinical Correlation

Lipuria: Ingestion of large amounts of lipids may lead to a condition called alimentary lipuria (adiposuria). The urine of such individuals becomes opalescent, turbid or sometimes even milky. In rare instances, when its lipid content is very high, a peculiar creamy layer is also seen. Lipuria may also be observed in lipemia of diabetes mellitus, lipoid nephrosis, fractures of the long bones with injury to the bone marrow and in phosphorous poisoning.

Steps in Lipid Absorption

There are six steps in lipid absorption, which are as follows:

1. Minor digestion of triacylglycerols in mouth and stomach by lingual (acid stable) lipase.
2. Major digestion of all lipids in the lumen of the duodenum/jejunum by pancreatic lipolytic enzymes.
3. Bile acid facilitated formation of mixed micelles (when phospholipids are distributed in water, their hydrophobic parts keep away from water forming molecular aggregates called micelle).
4. Passive absorption of the products of lipolysis from the mixed micelle into the intestinal epithelial cell.
5. Re-esterification of 2-monoacylglycerol with free fatty acids inside the intestinal enterocyte.
6. Assembly of chylomicrons containing very low-density lipoprotein (VLDL) (apo) B-48, triacylglycerol, cholesterol esters and phospholipids and export from intestinal cells. Overview of fat metabolism is shown in Figure 5.1.

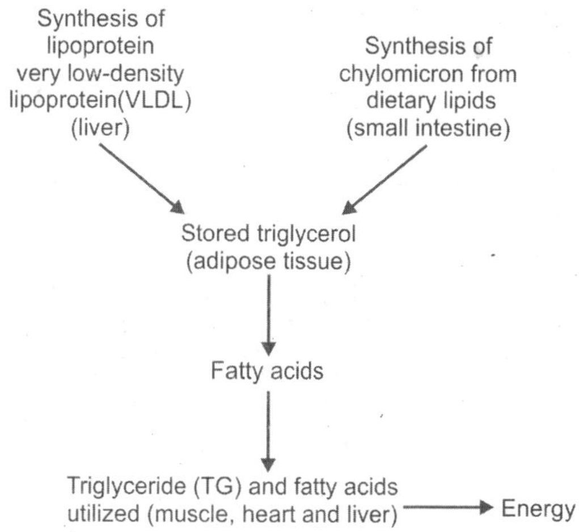

Fig. 5.1: Overview of fat and metabolism

Beta-oxidation

The fatty acids in the body are mostly oxidized by β-oxidation. β-oxidation (Fig. 5.2) may be defined as the oxidation of fatty adds on the β-carbon atom. This results in the sequential removal of two carbon fragment acetyl-CoA.

Fatty Acid Activation

Fatty acids are activated to acyl-CoA by thiokinases or acyl-CoA synthetases. The reaction occurs in two steps and requires ATP, coenzyme A (CoA) and Mg^{2+}. In the activation, two high energy phosphates are utilized, since ATP is converted to pyrophosphate (PPi). The enzyme inorganic pyrophosphatase hydrolyzes PPi to phosphate (P1). The immediate elimination of PPi makes this reaction totally irreversible.

Transport of Acyl-CoA

The inner mitochondrial membrane is impermeable to fatty acids. A specialized carnitine carrier system (carnitine shuttle) operates to transport activated fatty acids from cytosol to mitochondria. This occurs in four steps:

1. Acyl group of acyl-CoA is transferred to carnitine (β-hydroxy-gamma-trimethyl aminobutyrate), catalysed by carnitine acyltransferase present on the outer surface of inner mitochondrial membrane.
2. The acylcarnitine is transported across the membrane to mitochondrial matrix by a specific carrier protein.
3. Carnitine acyltransferase II found on the inner surface of mitochondrial membrane, converts acyl-carnitine to acyl-CoA.
4. The carnitine released returns to cytosol for reuse.

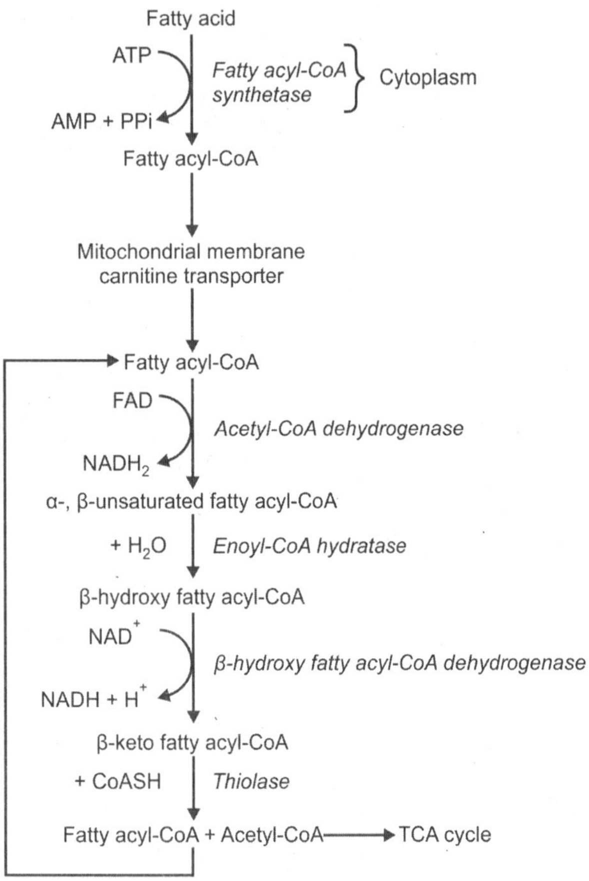

Fig. 5.2: Beta-oxidation

Beta-oxidation Proper

Each cycle of β-oxidation liberating a two carbon unit-acetyl-CoA, occurs in a sequence of four reactions:

1. Oxidation: Acyl-CoA undergoes dehydrogenation by a flavin adenine dinucleotide (FAD)-dependent flavoenzyme acyl-CoA dehydrogenase. A double bond is formed between α- and β-carbons.
2. Hydration: Enoyl-CoA hydratase brings about the hydration of the double bond to form β-hydroxyacyl-CoA.
3. Oxidation: β-hydroxyacyl-CoA dehydrogenase catalize the second oxidation and generates NADH. The product formed is β-ketoacyl-CoA.
4. Cleavage: The final reaction in β-oxidation is the liberation of a two carbon fragment, acetyl-CoA from acyl-CoA. This occurs by a thiolytic cleavage catalyzed by β-ketoacyl-CoA thiolase.

Clinical Correlation

Heart muscles utilize free fatty acids as their primary fuel via β-oxidation. Patients suffering from angina pectoris, parts of the heart muscles become ischemic. Under these conditions, one of the aims of treatment is to shift the metabolic fuel of heart muscles from fatty acids to glucose, which also helps to reduce the accompanying acidosis.

Oxidation of Palmitoyl-CoA

Palmitoyl-CoA + 7 CoASH + 7 FAD + 7 NAD^+ + $7H_20$ → 8 Acetyl-CoA + 7 $FADH_2$ + 7 NADH + $7H^+$.

Palmitoyl-CoA undergoes seven cycles of β-oxidation to yield eight acetyl-CoA. Acetyl-CoA can enter citric acid cycle and get completely oxidized to CO_2 and H_2O.

Energetics of Beta-oxidation

The ultimate aim of fatty acid oxidation is to generate energy. The energy obtained from the complete oxidation of palmitic acid (16 carbon) is given in Table 5.2.

Table 5.2: Oxidation of palmitic acid

Mechanism	ATP yield
β-oxidation 7 cycles 7 $FADH_2$ (oxidized by electron transport chain) 7 NADH (oxidized by ETC[*], each NADH[†] liberates 3 ATP)	7 × 1.5 ATP = 10.5 7 × 2.5 ATP = 17.5
From 8 acetyl-CoA oxidized by citric acid cycle, each acetyl-CoA provides 12 ATP	8 × 10 ATP = 80

[*]ETC, electron transport chain; [†]NADH, nicotinamide adenine dinucleotide.

Clinical Correlation

Sudden infant death syndrome (SIDS): It is an unexpected death of healthy infants, usually overnight. It is now estimated that at least 10% of SIDS is due to deficiency of medium-chain acyl-CoA dehydrogenase. The sudden death in infants is due to a blockade in β-oxidation caused by a deficiency in medium chain acyl-CoA dehydrogenase (MCAD):

- Total energy from one mole of palmitoyl-CoA = 108
- Energy utilized for activation (formation of palmitoyl-CoA) = –2
- Net yield of oxidation of one molecule of palmitate = 106.

OXIDATION OF ODD-CHAIN FATTY ACIDS

The odd-chain fatty acids are oxidized exactly in the same manner as even chain fatty acids. However, after successive removal of 2-carbon units at the end, one 3-carbon unit, propionyl-CoA is produced.

Alpha-oxidation

Alpha-oxidation is a process by which fatty acids are oxidized by removing carbon atoms, one at a time, from the carboxyl end. The process is important in brain.

Refsum's Disease

Refsum's disease is a rare, but severe neurological disorder with cerebral ataxia and peripheral neuropathy. There will be accumulation of an unusual fatty acid and phytanic acid.

Phytanic acid undergoes initial α-oxidation and this is followed by β-oxidation. Refsum's disease is caused by a defect in α-oxidation, due to deficiency of phytanic acid α oxidase. The patient should not consume diet containing chlorophyll.

Omega-oxidation

Omega (ω)-oxidation is a minor pathway taking place in microsomes with the help of hydroxylase enzymes involving NADPH and cytochrome P450. ω-oxidation becomes important when β-oxidation is defective and dicarboxylic acids (6C and 8C acids) are excreted in urine causing dicarboxylic aciduria.

Fatty Acid Synthase Complex

Fatty acid synthase is a multienzyme complex form a dimer with identical subunits (Fig. 5.3).

Advantages of Multienzyme Complex

1. Intermediates of the reaction can easily interact with the active sites of the enzymes.
2. One gene codes all the enzymes, so all the enzymes are in equimolecular concentrations.
3. The efficiency of the process is enhanced.

First Domain or Condensing Unit

Condensing unit is the initial substrate binding site. The enzymes involved are beta-ketoacyl synthase or condensing enzyme (CE), acetyl transferase (AT) and malonyl transacylase (MT).

Second Domain or Reduction Unit

Reduction unit contains the dehydratase (DH), enoyl reductase (ER), β-ketoacyl reductase (KR) and acyl carrier protein (ACP). The acyl carrier protein is a polypeptide chain having a phosphopantotheine group to which the acyl groups are attached in thioester linkage. So, ACP acts like the CoA carrying fatty acyl groups.

Third Domain or Releasing Unit

Releasing unit is involved in the release of the palmitate synthesized. It contains thioesterase (TE).

De novo Synthesis of Fatty Acids (Lynen Cycle)

De novo synthesis of fatty acids occurs in liver, kidney, adipose tissue, etc. The enzyme machinery for fatty acids production is located in cytosomal fraction (Fig. 5.4).

The steps in fatty acid synthesis are:

- Production of acetyl-CoA and NADPH
- Conversion of acetyl-CoA to malonyl-CoA
- Reactions of fatty acid synthase complex.

Production of Acetyl-CoA and NADPH

Acetyl-CoA and NADPH are the prerequisites for fatty acid synthesis. Acetyl-CoA is produced in the mitochondria by the oxidation of pyruvate and fatty acids. Degradation of carbon skeleton of certain amino acids and ketone bodies.

Acetyl-CoA condenses with oxaloacetate in mitochondria to form citrate. Citrate is freely transported to cytosol where it is cleaved by citrate lyase to liberate acetyl-CoA and oxaloacetate. Oxaloacetate in the cytosol is converted to malate.

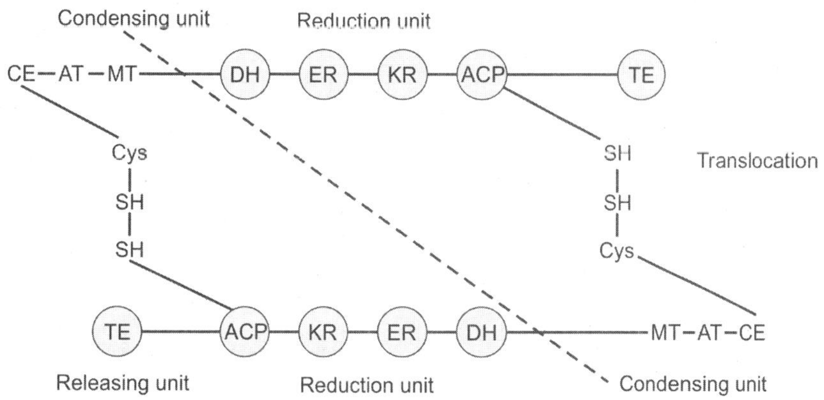

Fig. 5.3: Fatty acid synthase complex (ACP, acyl carrier protein; AT, Acetyltrans acylase; CE, condensing enzyme; DH, dehydratase; ER, enoyl reductase; KR, ketoacylreductase; MT, malonyl transacylase; TE, thioesterase)

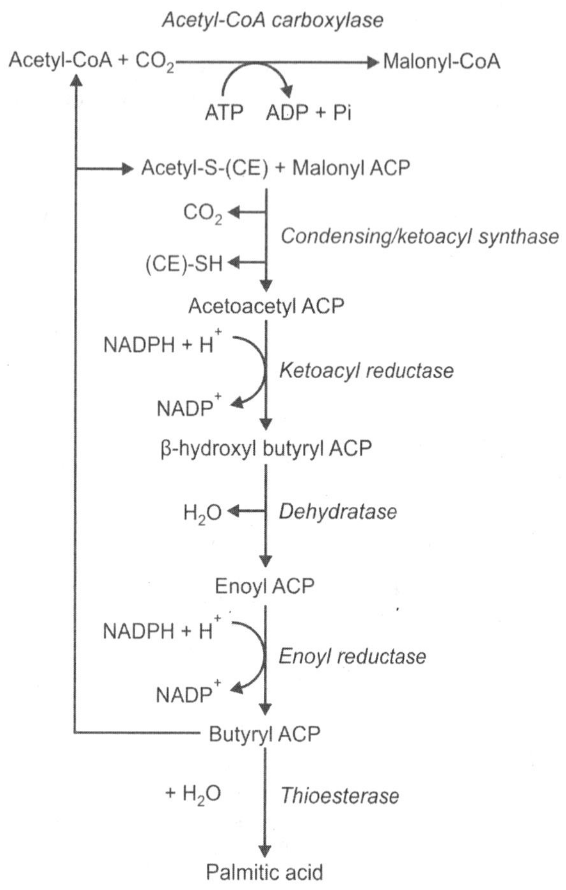

Fig. 5.4: De novo synthesis of fatty acids

Formation of Malonyl-CoA

Acetyl-CoA is carboxylated to malonyl-CoA by the enzyme acetyl-CoA carboxylase. This is an ATP-dependent reaction and requires biotin for CO_2 fixation. The mechanism of action of acetyl-CoA carboxylase is similar to that of pyruvate carboxylase. Acetyl-CoA carboxylase is a regulatory enzyme in fatty acid synthesis.

Reaction of Fatty Acid Synthase Complex

The remaining reactions are catalyzed by a multifunctional enzyme, fatty acid synthase complex:

1. The two carbon fragment of acetyl-CoA is transferred to ACP of fatty acid synthase, catalyzed by the enzyme acetyl-CoA-ACP transacylase. The acetyl unit is then transferred from ACP to cysteine residue of the enzyme. Thus, ACP site falls vacant.
2. The enzyme malonyl-CoA-ACP transacylase transfers malonate from malonyl-CoA to bind to ACP.
3. The acetyl unit attached to cysteine is transferred to malonyl group (bound to ACP). The malonyl moiety loses CO_2, which was added by acetyl-CoA carboxylase. Thus, CO_2 is never incorporated into fatty acid carbon chain. The decarboxylation is accompanied by loss of free energy, which allows the reaction to proceed forwards. This reaction is catalyzed by β-ketoacyl ACP synthase.
4. The β-ketoacyl ACP reductase reduces ketoacyl group to hydroxyacyl group. The reducing equivalents are supplied by NADPH.
5. The β-hydroxyacyl ACP undergoes dehydration. A molecule of water is eliminated and a double bond is introduced between α- and β-carbons.
6. A second NADPH-dependent reduction catalyzed by enoyl-ACP reductase occurs to produce acyl-ACP. The 4-carbon unit attached to ACP is butyryl group.
7. The enzyme palmitoyl thioesterase separates palmitate from fatty acid synthase. This completes the synthesis of palmitate.

Regulation

1. Acetyl-CoA carboxylase: This enzyme controls a committed step in fatty acid synthesis.
2. Hormonal influence: Hormones regulate acetyl-CoA carboxylase by phosphorylation and dephosphprylation of the enzyme.
3. Dietary regulation: Consumption of high carbohydrate or fat-free diet increases synthesis of acetyl-CoA carboxylase and fatty acid synthase, which promote fatty acid formation.
4. Availability of NADPH: The reducing equivalents for fatty acid synthesis are provided by NADPH, which come either from citrate transport on hexose-monophosphate (HMP) shunt. NADPH obtained from HMP shunt influences fatty acid synthesis.

TRIACYLGLYCEROLS

Triacylglycerols (formerly triglycerides) are the esters of glycerol with fatty acids. They are insoluble in water and nonpolar in character and commonly known as neutral fats.

Fats as Stored Fuel

Triacylglycerols are the most abundant group of lipids that primarily function as fuel reserves of animals.

Fats Primarily Occur in Adipose Tissue

Adipocytes of adipose tissue are predominantly found in the subcutaneous layer and in the abdominal cavity, and are specialized for storage of triacylglycerols.

Structures of Acylglycerols

Monoacylglycerols, diacylglycerols and triacylglycerols, respectively consisting of one, two and three molecules of fatty acids esterified to a molecule of glycerol:

1. Simple triacylglycerols contain the same type of fatty acid residue at all the three carbons, e.g. tristearoyl glycerol or tristearin.
2. Mixed triacylglycerols are more common. They contain two or three different types of fatty acid residues. In general, fatty acid attached to C1 is saturated that attached to C2 is unsaturated, while that on C3 can be either. Triacylglycerols are named according to placement of acyl radical on glycerol, e.g. 1,3-palmitoyl-2-linoleoyl glycerol.

Properties of Triacylglycerols

1. Hydrolysis: Triacylglycerols undergo stepwise enzymatic hydrolysis to finally liberate free fatty acids and glycerol. The process of hydrolysis catalyzed by lipases is important for digestion of fat in the gastrointestinal tract and fat mobilization from the adipose tissues.
2. Saponification: The hydrolysis of triacylglycerols by alkali to produce glycerol and soaps is known as saponification.
   Triacylglycerol + 3 NaOH → Glycerol + 3R-COONa (soaps)
3. Rancidity: It is the term used to represent the deterioration of fats and oils resulting in an unpleasant taste. Fats containing unsaturated fatty acids that are more susceptible to rancidity. Rancidity occurs when fats and oils are exposed to air, moisture, light, bacteria, etc.:
   a. Hydrolytic rancidity occurs due to partial hydrolysis of triacylglycerols by bacterial enzymes.
   b. Oxidative rancidity is due to oxidation of unsaturated fatty acids.
   Antioxidants: The substances, which can prevent the occurrence of oxidative rancidity are known as antioxidants. Trace amounts of antioxidants such as tocopherols, hydroquinone are added to the commercial preparation of fats and oils to prevent rancidity.
4. Lipid peroxidation in vivo: In the living cells, lipids undergo oxidation to produce peroxides and free radicals, which can damage the tissue. It can cause inflammatory diseases, aging, cancer, atherosclerosis, etc.
5. Iodine number: Number of iodine absorbed by 100 g of fat or oil. It is useful to know the relative unsaturation of fat and is directly proportional to content of unsaturated fatty acids.

Synthesis of Triglycerides

Liver and adipose tissue are the major sites of triglycerides (TAG) synthesis. The TAG synthesized by esterification of fatty acyl-CoA with glycerol-3-phosphate or dihydroxyacetone phosphate (DHAP). In adipose tissue, glycerol kinase is deficient and the major source is DHAP derived from glycolysis (Fig. 5.5).

Metabolism of Adipose Tissue

1. Adipose tissue in well-fed condition:
   a. Esterification of fatty acyl-CoA with glycerol phosphate to form TAG occurs at rapid rate.
   b. Glycerol phosphate is derived from metabolism of glucose by channeling DHAP, an intermediate of glycolysis.
2. Adipose tissue in fasting condition:
   a. Synthesis of TAG occurs side by side with lipolysis, FFA level is increased in plasma.
   b. Glycerol phosphate is derived from DHAP formed during gluconeogenesis.
3. Adipose tissue and diabetes mellitus:
   a. Lipolysis is enhanced and high FFA level in plasma in diabetes mellitus.
   b. The insulin acts through receptors on the cell surface of adipocytes.
   c. Receptors are decreased, leading to insulin insensitivity in diabetes.
4. Adipose tissue and obesity:
   a. Fat content can increase depending on the amount of excess calories taken in.
   b. This leads to obesity.

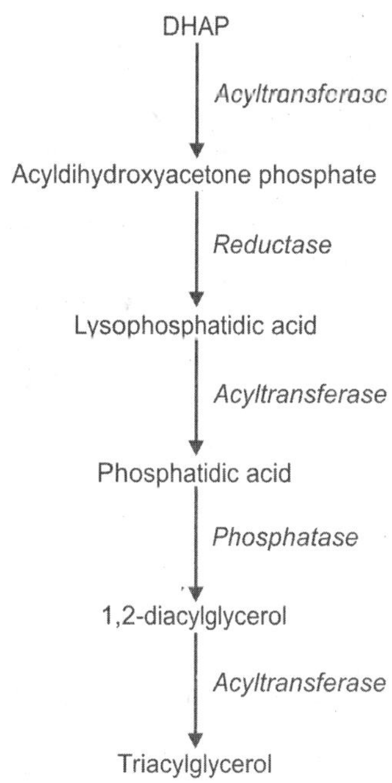

Fig. 5.5: Synthesis of triglycerides

Fatty Liver and Lipotropic Factors

Fatty liver refers to the deposition of excess triglycerides in the liver cells. The balance between the factors causing fat deposition in liver versus factors causing removal of fat from liver determines the outcome.

Causes of fatty liver

1. Excessive mobilization of fat: The capacity of liver to take up the fatty acids from blood far exceeds its capacity for excretion as VLDL. So, fatty liver can occur in diabetes mellitus and starvation due to increased lipolysis in adipose tissue.
2. Excess calorie intake: Excess calories either in the form of carbohydrates or fats are deposited as fat. Hence, obesity may be accompanied by fatty liver.
3. Toxic injury to liver: It is due to poisoning by compounds like carbon tetrachloride, arsenic, lead, etc. The capacity to synthesize VLDL affected leading to fatty infiltration of liver. In protein calorie malnutrition, amino acid required to synthesize apoproteins may be lacking. Occurrence of fatty liver in protein energy malnutrition (PEM) may be due to defective apoprotein synthesis. Hepatitis B virus infection reduces the function of hepatic cells, leads to fatty liver.
4. Alcoholism: It is the most common cause of fatty liver and cirrhosis in India. Alcohol is oxidized to acetaldehyde. This reaction produces increased quantities of NADH, which converts oxaloacetate to malate. As the availability of oxaloacetate reduced, the oxidation of acetyl-CoA through citric acid cycle is reduced. So, fatty acid accumulates leading to TAG deposits in liver.
5. Non-alcoholic fatty liver disease (NAFLD) and non-alcoholic steatohepatitis (NASH): NAFLD is the most common liver disease where fat is accumulated in hepatocytes. High-fat diet and uncontrolled diabetes mellitus are the most common causes. As the disease progresses inflammatory reaction occurs, which is then termed as NASH.
6. Fatty liver progresses to cirrhosis: Fat molecules infiltrate the cytoplasm of the cell (fatty infiltration). These are seen as fat droplets, which are merged together so that most of the cytoplasm becomes laden with fat.

The nucleus is pushed to a side of the cell. Nucleus disintegrates (karyorrhexis) and ultimately the hepatic cell is lysed. As a healing process, fibrous tissue is laid down, causing fibrosis of liver, otherwise known as cirrhosis. Liver function tests show abnormal values.

Lipotropic factors

They are required for the normal mobilization of fat from liver. Deficiency of these factors results in fatty liver. They can afford protection against the development of fatty liver:

1. Choline: Feeding of choline has been able to reverse fatty changes in animals.
2. Lecithin and methionine: They help in synthesis of apoprotein and choline formation. The deficiency of methyl groups for carnitine synthesis may also hinder fatty acid oxidation.
3. Vitamin E and selenium give protection due to their antioxidant effect.
4. Omega 3 fatty acids present in marine oils have protective effect against fatty liver.

KETONE BODIES

The compounds acetone, acetoacetate and β-hydroxyl butyrate are known as ketone bodies. They are water soluble and energy yielding.

Ketogenesis

Synthesis of ketone bodies in liver is known as ketogenesis. Acetoacetate is the primary ketone body, while β-hydroxy butyrate and acetone are secondary ketone bodies. Ketogenesis occurs through the following reactions (Fig. 5.6).

Step 1 condensation: Two molecules of acetyl-CoA are condensed to form acetoacetyl-CoA.

Step 2 production of HMG-CoA: One more acetyl-CoA is added to acetoacetyl-CoA to form HMG-CoA. The enzyme is HMG-CoA synthase.

Step 3 lysis: The HMG-CoA is lysed to form acetoacetate. HMG-CoA lyase is present only in liver.

Step 4 reduction: The β-hydroxy butyrate is formed by reduction of acetoacetate. Ratio between acetoacetate and

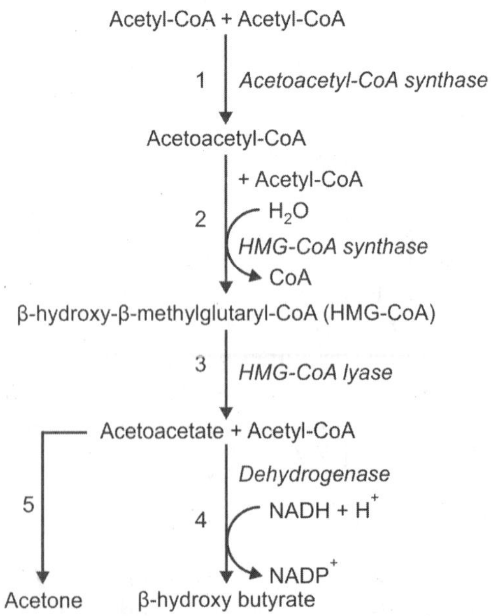

Fig. 5.6: Ketogenesis

*β-hydroxy butyrate is decided by the cellular NAD:*NADH ratio.

Step 5 Spontaneous decarboxylation: Acetone is formed.

Regulation of Ketogenesis

Ketone body formation occurs due to nonavailability of carbohydrates to tissues. This is an outcome of excessive utilization of fatty acids to meet the energy requirements of the cell. The hormone glucagon stimulates ketogenesis, but insulin inhibits. The increased ratio of glucagon/insulin in diabetes promotes ketogenesis. This is due to disturbances caused in carbohydrate and lipid metabolism in diabetes.

Ketolysis

The ketone bodies are formed in the liver, but they are utilized by extrahepatic tissues. The heart muscle and renal cortex prefer the ketone bodies to glucose as fuel. Tissues like skeletal muscle and brain can also utilize the ketone bodies as alternate sources of energy, if glucose is not available. Acetoacetate is activated to acetoacetyl CoA by thiophorase enzyme.

$$\text{Acetoacetate + succinyl-CoA} \xrightarrow{\textit{Thiophorase}} \text{Acetyl-CoA + succinate}$$

Ketosis

1. Normally the rate of synthesis of ketone bodies by the liver is such that they can be easily metabolized by the extrahepatic tissues. Hence, the blood level of ketone bodies is less than 1 mg/dL and only traces are excreted in urine.
2. But when the rate of synthesis exceeds, the ability of extrahepatic tissues to utilize them, there will be accumulation of ketone bodies in blood.
3. This leads to **ketonemia,** excretion in urine **(ketonuria)** and **smell of acetone** in breath. All these three together constitute the condition known as ketosis.

Causes for Ketosis

1. Diabetes mellitus: Uncontrolled diabetes mellitus is the most common cause for ketosis. Even though glucose is in plenty, the deficiency of insulin causes accelerated lipolysis and more fatty acids are released into circulation. Oxidation of these fatty acids increases the acetyl-CoA pool. Enhanced gluconeogenesis restricts the oxidation of acetyl-CoA by tricarboxylic acid (TCA) cycle, since availability of oxaloacetate is less.
2. Starvation: In starvation, the dietary supply of glucose is decreased. Available oxaloacetate is channeled to gluconeogenesis. The increased rate of lipolysis is to provide alternate source of fuel. The excess acetyl-CoA is converted to ketone bodies. The high glucagon level favors ketogenesis. The brain derives 60%–75% of energy from ketone bodies under conditions of prolonged starvation. Hyperemesis (vomiting) in early pregnancy may also lead to starvation-like condition and may lead to ketosis.

Salient Features of Ketosis

1. Metabolic acidosis—acetoacetate and β-hydroxyl butyrate, which are acids accumulates and results in metabolic acidosis.
2. Reduced buffers—the plasma bicarbonate is used for buffering these acids.
3. Kussmaul's respiration—hyperventilation present.
4. Smell of acetone—in patients breath.
5. Osmotic diuresis—induced by ketonuria may lead to dehydration.
6. Sodium loss—ketone bodies are excreted in urine as their sodium salts leading to lose of cations.
7. Dehydration and comma.

CHOLESTEROL AND LIPOPROTEINS

Cholesterol is found exclusively in animals, hence it is often called animal sterol. Cholesterol is amphipathic in nature, since it possesses both hydrophilic and hydrophobic regions in the structure. It has a cyclopentano perhydro phenanthrene ring system (Fig. 5.7).

Functions of Cholesterol

1. Cholesterol is essential to life, as it performs a number of important functions.
2. It is a structural component of cell membrane.
3. Cholesterol is the precursor for the synthesis of all other steroids in the body. These include steroid hormones, vitamin D and bile acids.

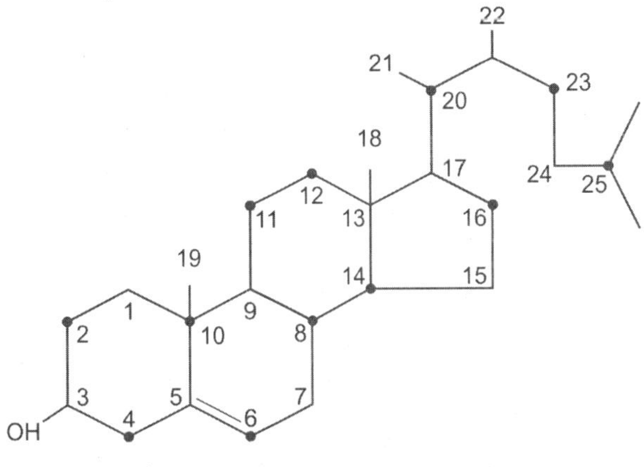

Fig. 5.7: Structure of cholesterol

4. It is an essential ingredient in the structure of lipoproteins in which form the lipids in the body are transported.
5. Fatty acids are transported to liver as cholesteryl esters for oxidation.

Cholesterol Biosynthesis

The largest contribution is made by liver (50%), the enzymes involved in cholesterol synthesis are found in the cytosol and microsomal fractions of the cell. Acetate of acetyl-CoA provides all the carbon atoms in cholesterol. The reducing equivalents are supplied by NADPH, while ATP provides energy. For the production of one mole of cholesterol, 18 moles of acetyl-CoA, 36 moles of ATP and 16 moles of NADPH are required.

The synthesis of cholesterol may be learnt in five stages (Fig. 5.8):

1. Synthesis of HMG-CoA.
2. Formation of mevalonate (6C).
3. Production of isoprenoid units (5C).
4. Synthesis of squalene (30C).
5. Conversion of squalene to cholesterol (27C).

Synthesis of β-hydroxy-beta-methylglutaryl-CoA (HMG-CoA): Two moles of acetyl-CoA condense to form acetoacetyl-CoA. Another molecule of acetyl-CoA is then added to produce HMG-CoA. There exist two pools of HMG-CoA in the cell.

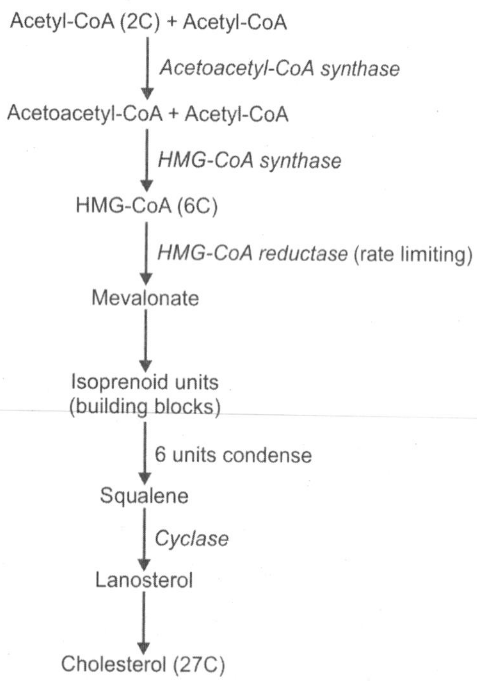

Fig. 5.8: Cholesterol synthesis

Formation of mevalonate: HMG-CoA reductase is the rate limiting enzyme in cholesterol biosynthesis. It catalyzes the reduction of HMG-CoA to mevalonate. The reducing equivalents are supplied by NADPH.

Production of isoprenoid units: In a three-step reaction catalyzed by kinases, mevalonate is converted to 3-phospho -5-pyrophosphomevalonate, which on decarboxylation forms isopentenyl pyrophosphate (IPP). The latter isomerizes to dimethylallyl pyrophosphate (DPP). Both IPP and DPP are 5-carbon isoprenoid units.

Synthesis of squalene: IPP and DPP condense to produce a 10-carbon geranyl pyrophosphate (GPP). Another molecule of IPP condenses with GPP to form a 15-carbon farnesyl pyrophosphate (FPP). Two units of farnesyl pyrophosphate unite and get reduced to produce a 30-carbon squalene.

Conversion of squalene to cholesterol: Squalene undergoes hydroxylation and cyclization utilizing O_2 and NADPH, and gets converted to lanosterol. The following are the most important reactions:

1. Reducing the carbon atoms from 30 to 27.
2. Removal of two methyl groups from C4 and one methyl group from C14.
3. Shift of double bond from C8 to C5.
4. Reduction in the double bond present between C24 and C25.

The penultimate product is 7-dehydrocholesterol, which on reduction finally yields cholesterol.

Regulation of Cholesterol Synthesis

Feedback control: End product cholesterol controls its own synthesis by a feedback mechanism. Increase in the cellular concentration of cholesterol, reduces the synthesis of the enzyme HMG-CoA reductase. This is achieved by decreasing the transcription of the gene responsible for the production of HMG-CoA reductase (Fig. 5.9).

Hormonal regulation: The enzyme HMG-CoA reductase exists in two interconvertible forms. The dephosphorylated form of HMG-CoA reductase is more active, while the phosphorylated form is less active. The hormones exert their influence through cAMP by a series of reactions. The net effect is that glucagon and glucocorticoids favor the formation of inactive HMG-CoA reductase (phosphorylated form) and thus, decrease cholesterol synthesis. On the other hand, insulin and thyroxine increase cholesterol production by enhancing the formation of active HMG-CoA reductase (dephosphorylated form).

Inhibition by drugs: The drugs compactin and lovastatin (mevinolin) are fungal products. They are used to decrease the serum cholesterol level in patients with hypercholesterolemia. Compactin and lovastatin are competitive inhibitors

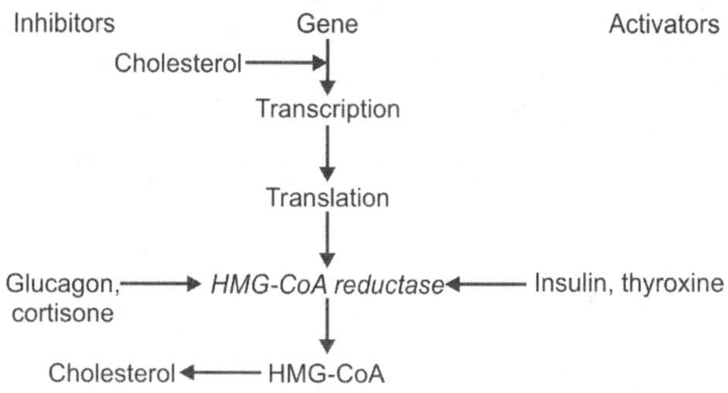

Fig. 5.9: Regulation of cholesterol synthesis

of the enzyme HMG-CoA reductase. HMG-CoA reductase activity is inhibited by bile acids. Fasting also reduces the activity of this enzyme.

Degradation of Cholesterol

Cholesterol (50%) is converted to bile acids, excreted in feces, serves as a precursor for the synthesis of steroid hormones, vitamin D, coprostanol and cholestanol.

Synthesis of bile acids: The bile acids are amphipathic in nature since they possess both polar and non-polar groups. They serve as emulsifying agents in the intestine and actively participate in the digestion and absorption of lipids.

The synthesis of primary bile acids takes place in the liver and involves a series of reactions. The step catalyzed by 7 α-hydroxylase is inhibited by bile acids and this is the rate limiting reaction. Cholic acid and chenodeoxycholic acid are the primary bile acids. On conjugation with glycine or taurine, conjugated bile acids (glycocholic acid, taurocholic acid, etc.) are formed, which are more efficient in their function as surfactant. Conjugated bile acids exist as sodium and potassium salts known as bile salts.

Synthesis of steroid hormones: Cholesterol is the precursor for the synthesis of all the five classes of steroid hormones:

- Glucocorticoids (e.g. cortisol)
- Mineralocorticoids (e.g. aldosterone)
- Progestins (e.g. progesterone)
- Androgens (e.g. testosterone)
- Estrogens (e.g. estradiol).

Synthesis of cholesterol: 7-dehydrocholesterol, an intermediate in the synthesis of cholesterol is converted to cholecalciferol (vitamin D_3) by ultraviolet rays in the skin.

Plasma Lipid Profile

Normal values of lipid fractions are given in Table 5.3.

LIPOPROTEINS

Lipoproteins are molecular complexes that consist of lipids and proteins. They function as transport vehicle for lipids in blood plasma. Lipoproteins deliver lipid components (cholesterol, triglycerides) to various tissues for utilization.

Table 5.3: Plasma lipid profile (normal values)

Analyte	Normal value
Total plasma lipids	400–600 mg/dL
Total cholesterol	140–200 mg/dL
HDL cholesterol, male	30–60 mg/dL
HDL cholesterol, female	35–75 mg/dL
LDL cholesterol, 30–39 years	80–130 mg/dL
Triglycerides, male	50–150 mg/dL
Triglycerides, female	40–150 mg/dL
Phospholipids	150–200 mg/dL
Free fatty acids (FFA) (NEFA)	10–20 mg/dL

Classification of Lipoproteins

Depending on the density, the lipoproteins in plasma are classified into five major types:

1. Chylomicrons contain apoprotein B-48.
2. Very low-density lipoproteins or pre-beta lipoproteins. Main apoprotein is B-100.
3. Intermediate-density lipoproteins (IDL) or broad β-lipoproteins.
4. Low-density lipoproteins (LDL) or β-lipoproteins. Major apoprotein in LDL is B-100.
5. High-density lipoproteins (HDL) or α-lipoproteins. Major apoprotein in HDL is apoA.

Apolipoproteins

The protein part of lipoprotein is called apolipoprotein (apoLp) or apoprotein:

1. Apo-A-I: It activates lecithin-cholesterol acyltransferase (LCAT). It is the ligand for HD receptor. It is antiatherogenic.
2. Apo-B-100: It is a component of LDL; it binds to LDL receptor on tissues. Apo-B-10 is one of the biggest proteins.
3. Apo-B-48: It is synthesized in intestinal cells. It is the structural component of chylomicrons.
4. Apo-C-II: It activates lipoprotein lipase.
5. Apo-E: It is an arginine-rich protein. It is present in chylomicrons, LDL and VLDL.

Overview of lipoprotein metabolism is shown in Figure 5.10.

Chylomicrons

Chylomicrons are formed in the intestinal mucosal cells and secreted into the lacteals of lymphatic system. They are rich in triglyceride.

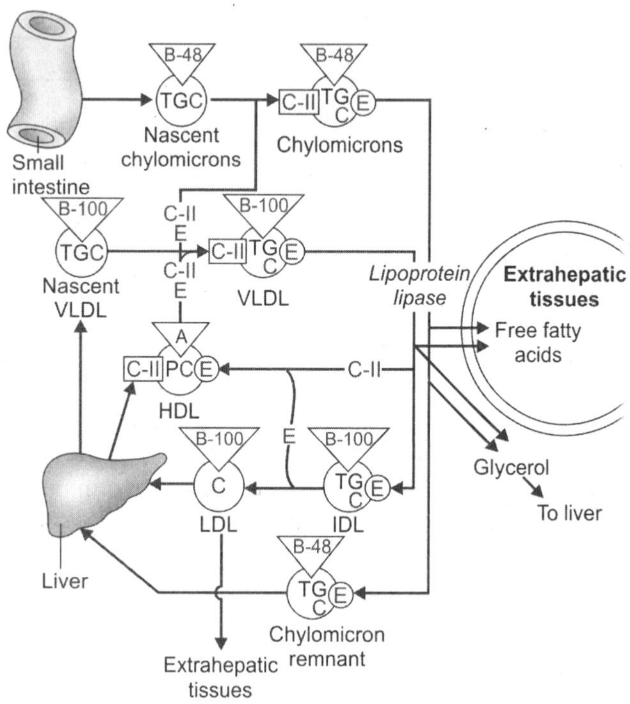

Fig. 5.10: Metabolism of lipoproteins (HDL, high-density lipoprotein; LDL, low-density lipoprotein; VLDL, very low-density lipoprotein)

Metabolism of chylomicrons

1. Main sites of metabolism of chylomicrons are adipose tissue and skeletal muscle.
2. The enzyme lipoprotein lipase (LPL) is located at the endothelial layer of capillaries of adipose tissue, muscles and heart, but not in liver. Apo-C-II present in the chylomicrons activates the LPL. The LPL hydrolyzes triglycerides present in chylomicrons into fatty acids and glycerol. Muscle or adipose tissue cells take up the liberated fatty acids.
3. Following injection of heparin, the LPL is released from the tissues and lipemia is thus cleared. This is called post-heparin lipolytic activity. Insulin increases LPL activity.
4. Liver takes up chylomicron remnants.

Function of chylomicrons

Chylomicrons are the transport form of dietary triglycerides from intestines to the adipose tissue for storage and to muscle or heart for their energy needs.

Very Low-density Lipoproteins

Very low-density lipoproteins are synthesized in the liver from glycerol and fatty acids and incorporated into VLDL along with hepatic cholesterol, apo-B-100, C-II and E. Apo-B-100 is the major lipoprotein present in VLDL when it is secreted. Apo-E and C-II are obtained from HDL in plasma.

Metabolism of VLDL

When they reach the peripheral tissues, apo-C-II activates LPL, which liberates fatty acids that are taken up by adipose tissue and muscle.

The remnant is now designated as IDL. The major fraction of IDL further loses triglyceride, so as to be converted to LDL. This conversion of VLDL to IDL and then to LDL is referred to as lipoprotein cascade pathway. A fraction of IDL is taken up by the hepatic receptors.

Function of VLDL

It carries triglycerides (endogenous triglycerides) from liver to peripheral tissues for energy needs.

Low-density Lipoproteins

Low-density lipoproteins transports cholesterol from liver to peripheral tissues. The only apoprotein present in LDL is apo-B-100. Most of the LDL particles are derived from VLDL, but a small part is directly released from liver.

Metabolism of LDL and LDL receptors

The LDL receptors are located in specialized regions called clathrin-coated pits. Binding of LDL to the receptor is by apo-B-100 and uptake of cholesterol from LDL is a highly regulated process. When apo-B-100 binds to its receptor, the receptor-LDL complex is internalized by endocytosis.

Function of LDL

1. About 75% of the plasma cholesterol is incorporated into the LDL particles. LDL transports cholesterol from liver to the peripheral tissues. The cholesterol thus liberated in the cell has three major fates:
   a. It is used for the synthesis of other steroids like steroid hormones.
   b. Cholesterol may be incorporated into the membranes.
   c. Cholesterol may be esterified to a monounsaturated fatty acid (MUFA) by acyl cholesterol acyltransferase (ACAT) for storage.

Clinical correlation

The LDL concentration in blood has positive correlation with incidence of cardiovascular diseases. It result in atherosclerosis leading to myocardial infarction. Since, LDL cholesterol is deposited in tissues, the LDL variety is called 'bad cholesterol' and LDL as 'lethally dangerous lipoprotein'.

High-density Lipoprotein

High-density lipoprotein are synthesized in liver, also known as good cholesterol.

Metabolism of HDL

1. The intestinal cells synthesize components of HDL and release into blood.
2. The free cholesterol derived from peripheral tissue cells are taken up by the HDL. The apo-A-I of HDL activates lecithin cholesterol acyltransferase (LCAT) present in the plasma. The LCAT then binds to the HDL disk. The cholesterol from the cell is transferred to HDL by a cholesterol efflux regulator protein, which is an ABC proteins.
3. Lecithin is a component of phospholipid bilayer of the HDL disk. The second carbon of lecithin contains one molecule of polyunsaturated fatty acid (PUFA). The esterified cholesterol, which is more hydrophobic, moves into the interior of the HDL disk.
4. This reaction continues, till HDL becomes spherical with a lot of cholesterol esters are formed. This HDL particle designated as HDL-3.
5. Mature HDL spheres are taken up by liver cells by apo-A-I mediated receptor mechanism HDL is taken up by hepatic scavenger receptor B1. Hepatic lipase hydrolyzes HDL phospholipid and TAG, and cholesterol esters are released into liver. It is used for synthesis of bile acids.
6. When the HDL-3 remains in circulation, the cholesterol ester from HDL is transferred to VLDL, IDL and LDL by a cholesterol ester transfer protein (CETP).
7. The efflux of cholesterol from peripheral cells to HDL is mediated by the ABC transporters.

Functions of HDL

The HDL is the main transport form of cholesterol from peripheral tissue to liver, which is later excreted through bile. This is called reverse cholesterol transport by HDL. The only excretory route of cholesterol from the body is the bile.

Clinical correlation

The HDL level in serum is inversely related to myocardial infarction. Due to its antiatherogenic or protective nature, HDL is known as good cholesterol.

Disorders of Plasma Lipoproteins

1. Hyperlipoproteinemias: Elevation in one or more of the lipoprotein fractions constitutes hyperlipoproteinemias. Frederickson's classification based on electrophoretic pattern of lipoproteins, divides hyperlipoproteinemias into six categories:
   a. Type I: Familial lipoprotein lipase deficiency. Increase in chylomicron and TAG levels.
   b. Type IIa (hyperbetalipoproteinemia): Defect in LDL receptors.
   c. Type IIb: LDL and VLDL increase along with plasma cholesterol and TAG, and overproduction of Apo-B.
   d. Type III (broad-β disease): Increase in intermediate density lipoprotein.
   e. Type IV: Overproduction of endogenous TAG with rise in VLDL.
   f. Type V: Chylomicrons and VLDL are elevated.
2. Hypolipoproteinemias: Low levels of plasma lipids are associated with certain abnormalities, they are:
   a. Familial hypobetalipoproteinemias—due to impaired synthesis of Apo-B. LDL level is affected.
   b. Abetalipoproteinemias—defective synthesis of apoprotein B. There is total absence of LDL in plasma. TAG accumulate in liver and intestine.
   c. Familial α-lipoproteinemia (Tangier disease)—plasma HDL is almost absent. Reverse transport of cholesterol is severely affected leading to accumulation in tissues.

FREE FATTY ACIDS

1. It is also known as non-esterified fatty acids (NEFA). It is complexed with albumin in plasma.
2. The FFA is derived from lipolysis of triglycerides by hormone sensitive lipase. FFA may be long chain saturated or unsaturated fatty acids.
3. The FFA molecules are transported to heart, skeletal muscle, liver and other soft tissues. They are either oxidized for energy or incorporated into tissue lipids by esterification.
4. In tissue cells, FFA-albumin complex is dissociated, FFA binds with a fatty acid transport protein. It is a co-transporter with sodium. After entry to cells, FFA bounds to fatty acid binding protein.
5. Half-life of FFA in plasma is very short. During starvation, 50% of energy need of body is met by FFA oxidation.
6. Blood level of FFA is very low in fully fed condition, high in starved state, very high in uncontrolled diabetes mellitus.

POLYUNSATURATED FATTY ACIDS

The important polyunsaturated fatty acids (PUFA) are:

1. Linoleic acid (18C, 2 double bonds).
2. Linolenic acid (18C, 3 double bonds).
3. Arachidonic acid (20C, 4 double bonds):
   a. The PUFAs are seen in vegetable oils.
   b. They are nutritionally essential and are called essential fatty acids.
   c. Prostaglandins, thromboxanes and leukotrienes are produced from arachidonic acid.

d. The PUFAs form integral part of mitochondrial membranes. In deficiency of PUFA, the efficiency of biological oxidation is reduced.
e. They are components of membranes. Arachidonic acid is 10%–15% of the fatty acids of membranes.
f. As double bonds are in cis configuration, the PUFA molecule cannot be closely packed. So, PUFAs will increase the fluidity of the membrane.
g. As PUFAs are easily liable to undergo peroxidation, the membranes containing PUFAs are more prone for damage by free radicals.
h. The production of docosahexaenoic acid (DHA) from α-linolenic acid is limited. DHA is present in high concentrations in fish oils. DHA is present in high concentrations in retina, cerebral cortex and sperms.

EICOSANOIDS

Eicosanoids are 20C compounds derived from arachidonic acid. They are:

1. Prostanoids containing:
   a. Prostaglandins (PGs).
   b. Prostacyclins (PGIs).
   c. Thromboxanes (TXs).
2. Leukotrienes (LTs).

Prostaglandins

Prostaglandins (PGs) were originally isolated from prostate issue and hence the name. But they are present in almost all tissues. They are the most potent biologically active substances, as low as 1 ng/mL of PG will cause smooth muscle contraction. The diverse physiological roles of prostaglandins confer on them are the status of local hormones.

Synthesis of Prostaglandins

Arachidonic acid is the precursor for most of the prostaglandins in humans. The biosynthesis of PGs occurs in the endoplasmic reticulum in the following stages:

1. Release of arachidonic acid from membrane-bound phospholipids by phospholipase A_2. This reaction occurs due to specific stimuli by hormones such as epinephrine or bradykinin.
2. Oxidation and cyclization of arachidonic acid to PGG_2, which is then converted to PGH_2 by a reduced glutathione-dependent peroxidase.
3. The PGH_2 serves as immediate precursor for the synthesis of a number of PGs, including prostacyclins and thromboxanes.

The above pathway is known as cyclic pathway of arachidonic acid.

Cyclooxygenase is a suicide enzyme capable of undergoing self-catalyzed destruction to switch off PG synthesis.

Inhibition of PG synthesis: A number of structurally unrelated compounds can inhibit prostaglandin synthesis:

1. Corticosteroids prevent the formation of arachidonic acid by inhibiting the enzyme phospholipase A_2.
2. Many non-steroidal anti-inflammatory drugs inhibit the synthesis of prostaglandins, prostacyclins and thromboxanes.
3. Aspirin irreversibly inhibits the enzyme cyclooxygenase and inhibits PG synthesis.

Biochemical Actions

Prostaglandins act as local hormones in their function. Prostaglandins are involved in a variety of biological functions:

1. Regulation of blood pressure: The prostaglandins (PGE_2, PGA and PGI_2) are vasodilator in function. This results in increased blood flow and decrease peripheral resistance to lower the blood pressure. PGs serve as agents in the treatment of hypertension.
2. Inflammation: Prostaglandins PGE_1 and PGE_2 induce the symptoms of inflammation (redness, swelling, edema, etc.) due to arteriolar vasodilation.
3. Reproduction: Prostaglandins have widespread applications in the field of reproduction. PGE_2 and PGF_2 are used for the medical termination of pregnancy and induction of labor.
4. Pain and fever: It is believed that pyrogens (fever producing agents) promote prostaglandin biosynthesis leading to the formation of PGE_2 in the hypothalamus, the site of regulation of body temperature. PGE_2 along with histamine and bradykinin cause pain. Migraine is also due PGE_2. Aspirin and other non-steroidal drugs inhibit PG synthesis, and thus control fever and relieve pain.
5. Regulation of gastric secretion: PGs are used for the treatment of gastric ulcers. However, PGs stimulate pancreatic secretion and increase the motility of intestine, which often causes diarrhea.
6. Influence on immune system: Macrophages secrete PGE, which decreases the immunological functions of B and T lymphocytes.
7. Effects on metabolism: PGs influence certain metabolic reactions, probably through the mediation of CAMP.

Leukotrienes

Leukotrienes (LTs) are produced from arachidonic acid. LTB_4 is produced in neutrophils, it is the most potent chemotactic agent (factor attracting cells to the inflammatory site). The 12-lipoxygenase in platelets produces 12-hydroxy-eicosatetraenoic acid (12-HETE) and 15-lipoxygenase in eosinophils produce 15-HETE. The slow reacting substance of anaphylaxis (SRS-A) contains LTC_4, LTD_4 and LTE_4. They cause smooth muscle contraction, constrict the bronchioles, increase capillary permeability, activate leukocytes and produce vasoconstriction. SRS is the mediator of hypersensitivity reactions such as asthma (Fig. 5.11).

SPHINGOLIPIDOSES OR LIPID STORAGE DISEASES

Sphingolipidoses form a group of lysosomal storage diseases. The diseases result from failure of breakdown of a particular sphingolipid due to deficiency of a single enzyme. The children afflicted by these diseases are severely mentally retarded and seldom survive for long. All these diseases can be diagnosed prenatally by amniocentesis and culture of amniotic fluid cells. The common features of lipid storage diseases include:

1. Only one type of sphingolipid accumulates.
2. Rate of synthesis of the lipid is normal, only degradation is affected.
3. Extent of the enzyme deficiency is same in all tissues.

Gaucher's Disease

Gaucher's disease is an inborn error of metabolism due to failure of degradation of glucocerebrosides. The enzyme β-glucosidase is deficient in this condition. The salient features are as follows:

- Three types—adult, infantile and juvenile
- Hepatosplenomegaly
- Erosion of bone
- Moderate anemia
- Pigmentation of skin
- Mental retardation.

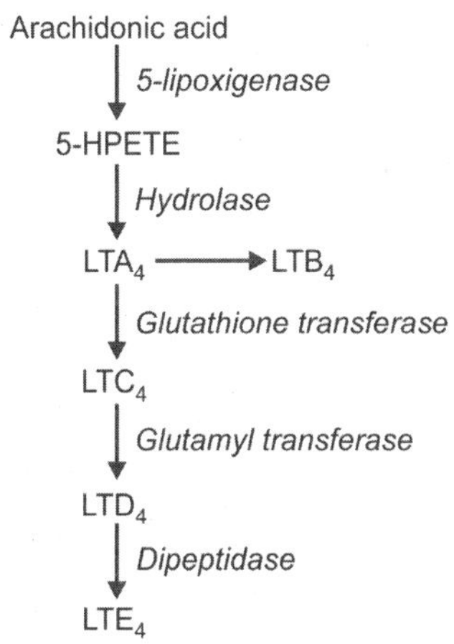

Fig. 5.11: Leukotriene synthesis

Tay-Sachs Disease

Tay-Sachs disease is an inborn error of metabolism due to failure of degradation of gangliosides. The enzyme hexosaminidase A is deficient in this condition. The salient features are as follows:

- Mental retardation
- Cherry-red spot in the macula
- Progressive deterioration
- Death by 3–4 days.

Krabbe's Disease

Defect in β-galactosidase results in accumulation of galactocerebrosides. The salient features are as follows:

- Absence of myelin formation
- Hepatosplenomegaly
- Mental retardation.

Niemann-Pick Disease

Defect in sphingomyelinase enzyme. The salient features are as follows:

- Hepatomegaly
- Mental retardation.

HYPERCHOLESTEROLEMIA

Increase in plasma cholesterol (> 200 mg/dL) concentration is known as hypercholesterolemia and is observed in many disorders:

1. Diabetes mellitus: Due to increased cholesterol synthesis since, the availability of acetyl-CoA is increased.
2. Hypothyroidism (myxedema): This is believed to be due to decrease in the HDL receptors on hepatocytes.
3. Obstructive jaundice: Due to an obstruction in the excretion of cholesterol through bile.
4. Nephrotic syndrome: Increase in plasma globulin concentration is the characteristic feature of nephrotic syndrome.

Control of Hypercholesterolermia

1. Consumption of PUFA: Dietary intake of polyunsaturated fatty acids (PUFA) reduces the plasma cholesterol level.
2. Dietary cholesterol: The cholesterol is found only in animal foods and not in plant foods. Dietary cholesterol influence on plasma cholesterol is minimal.
3. Plant sterols: Certain plant sterols and their esters (e.g. sitostanol esters) reduce plasma cholesterol levels.
4. Dietary fiber: Decreases the cholesterol absorption.

5. Avoiding high carbohydrate diet.
6. Moderate alcohol consumption.
7. Use of drugs: Drugs such as lovastatin, which inhibit HMG-CoA reductase and decrease cholesterol synthesis are used. Clofibrate increases the activity of lipoprotein lipase and reduces the plasma cholesterol, and triacylglycerols.

ATHEROSCLEROSIS

1. Atherosclerosis is a pathological process involving the arterial wall. It starts with repeated subtle injuries to the endothelium followed by migration of blood monocytes into the tunica media and accumulation as modified macrophages, accumulation of cholesterol and its esters in the macrophages (known as lipid-laden foam cells), smooth muscle cell proliferation, plaque formation and luminal narrowing.
2. Major risk factors include hypercholesterolemia, diabetes mellitus, hypertension, tobacco smoking, high plasma lipoprotein (a) and hyperhomocysteinemia, while the accessory risk factors are high calorie diet, sedentary lifestyle, obesity, alcohol, stress, estrogen supplements, etc.
3. The risk of developing atherosclerosis is directly related to the plasma concentration of LDL cholesterol, but inversely related to HDL cholesterol. Therefore, LDL cholesterol is called 'bad cholesterol', while the HDL cholesterol is referred to as the 'good cholesterol', although chemically there is only one cholesterol.
4. The most feared complications of atherosclerosis result from stenosis (narrowing) of arteries or the formation of thrombus on the plaque, or dislodging of the thrombus as an embolus or rupture of the plaque itself, leading to acute myocardial infarction, stroke, peripheral vascular disease and accelerated hypertension with organ damage (Fig. 5.12).

Class 1: Modifiable Risk Factors, Interventions have Been Proved to Lower CAD Risk

- Cigarette smoking
- High total cholesterol
- High LDL cholesterol
- Low HDL cholesterol
- High fat/cholesterol diet
- Left ventricular hypertrophy (LVH)
- Thrombogenic factors.

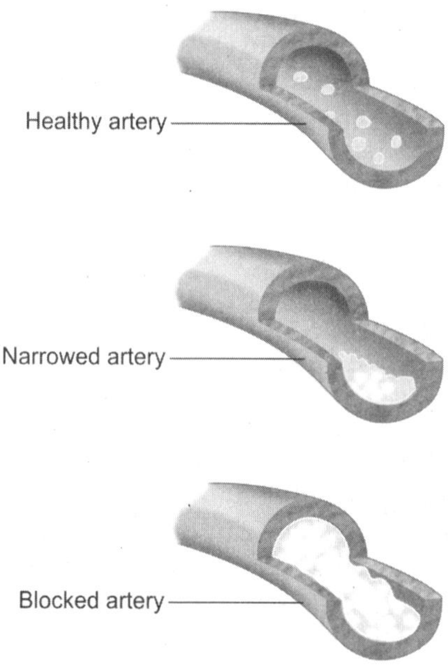

Fig. 5.12: Atherosclerosis

Class 2: Modifiable Risk Factors, Interventions are Likely to Lower CAD Risk

- Lipoprotein (a) or Lp(a)
- Diabetes mellitus
- Hypertension
- Physical inactivity
- Obesity
- High triglycerides
- High homocysteine
- Increased high sensitivity-CRP (hs-CRP)
- Stress.

Class 3: Non-modifiable Risk Factors

- Age
- Male gender
- Family history of cardiovascular disease (CAD).

Prevention

- Reduce dietary cholesterol—less than 200 mg/day
- Vegetable oils and PUFA—reduces cholesterol level
- Moderation in fat intake
- Use green leafy vegetables
- Avoid sucrose and cigarette
- Regular moderate exercise
- Hypolipidemic drugs—HMG-CoA reductase inhibitors (statins), bile acid binding resins, probucol, nicotinic acid, Aspirin and vitamin E.

Chapter 6

Cellular Energetics

Bioenergetics or biochemical thermodynamics is the study of the energy changes accompanying biochemical reactions. Biological systems are essentially isothermic and use chemical energy to power living processes.

CITRIC ACID CYCLE

The tricarboxylic acid cycle (TCA cycle also known as the citric acid cycle or Krebs cycle) is a cyclic metabolic pathway in the mitochondrial matrix. In eight-steps, it oxidizes acetyl residues (CH_3–CO–) to carbon dioxide (CO_2).

Reactions of Tricarboxylic Acid Cycle

The Krebs cycle starts with reaction between the acetyl moiety of acetyl-CoA and the four-carbon dicarboxylic acid oxaloacetate, forming a six-carbon tricarboxylic acid (citrate). In the subsequent reactions, two molecules of CO_2 are released and oxaloacetate is regenerated (Fig. 6.1).

Significance

- Complete oxidation of acetyl-CoA
- Adenosine triphosphate (ATP) generation

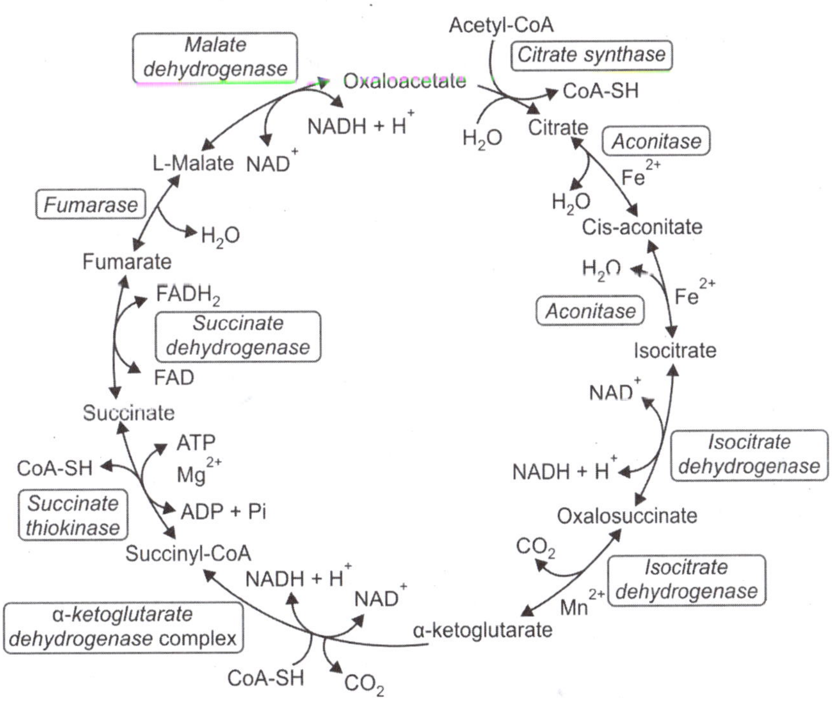

Fig. 6.1: Tricarboxylic acid cycle

- Final common oxidative pathway
- Integration of major metabolic pathways
- Fat is burned on the wick of carbohydrates
- Excess carbohydrates are converted as neutral fat
- No net synthesis of carbohydrates from fat
- Carbon skeletons of amino acids finally enter citric acid cycle
- Amphibolic pathway
- Anaplerotic role.

Complete Oxidation of Acetyl-CoA

Carbon Dioxide Removal Steps

During the citric acid cycle, two carbon dioxide molecules are removed in the following reactions (Table 6.1):

- The two carbon atoms of acetyl-CoA are removed as CO_2 in steps 3 and 4
- Net result is that acetyl-CoA is completely oxidized during one turn of cycle.

ATP Generating Steps in TCA Cycle

Importance

Alpha-ketoglutarate dehydrogenase reaction is the only one *irreversible* step in the cycle. Free energy changes of the reactions are such that the cycle will operate spontaneously in the clockwise direction (Table 6.2).

Final Common Oxidative Pathway

Citric acid cycle may be considered as the final common oxidative pathway of all foodstuffs and all the major ingredient of foodstuffs are finally oxidized through TCA cycle.

Integration of Major Metabolic Pathways

1. Carbohydrates are metabolized through glycolytic pathway to pyruvate and then converted to acetyl-CoA, which enters the citric cycle.
2. Fatty acids through beta-oxidation are broken down to acetyl-CoA and then enter this cycle.
3. Glucogenic amino acids after transamination enter at some points in this cycle. Ketogenic amino acids are converted into acetyl-CoA.
4. The integration of metabolism is achieved at junction points by key metabolites. Ketogenic amino acids are converted into acetyl-CoA. Several pathways can converge at this point with the result that carbon atoms from one source can be used for synthesis of another. Important intermediates are *acetyl-CoA* and *oxaloacetate.*

Carbohydrates are Required for Oxidation of Fats

In the body, oxidation of fat (acetyl-CoA) needs the help of oxaloacetate and oxidizes acetyl-CoA to two CO_2 molecules. Here, oxaloacetate acts as a true catalyst. The major source of oxaloacetate is pyruvate (carbohydrate). Hence, carbohydrates are absolutely required for oxidation of fats.

Excess Carbohydrates are Converted to Neutral Fat

Excess calories are deposited as fat in adipose tissue. The pathway is glucose to pyruvate to acetyl-CoA to fatty acid. However, *fat cannot be converted to glucose* because pyruvate dehydrogenase reaction (pyruvate to acetyl-CoA) is an absolutely irreversible step.

Table 6.1: Carbon dioxide removal steps

Step No	Reaction	Enzyme involved
3	Isocitrate to α-ketoglutarate	Isocitrate dehydrogenase
4	α-ketoglutarate to succinyl-CoA	α-ketoglutarate dehydrogenase

Table 6.2: ATP generating steps

Step No	Reactions	Coenzyme	ATPs
3	Isocitrate to α-ketoglutarate	NADH*	2.5
4	α-ketoglutarate to succinyl-CoA	NADH	2.5
5	Succinyl-CoA to succinate	GTP† (substrate level phosphorylation)	1
6	Succinate to fumarate	$FADH_2$‡	1.5
8	Malate to oxaloacetate	NADH	2.5
			Total 10

*NADH, nicotinamide adenine dinucleotide; †GTP, guanosine triphosphate; ‡$FADH_2$, flavin adenine dinucleotide

Amino Acids Finally Enter the TCA

The acetyl-CoA molecules either enter the TCA cycle and are completely oxidized or are channeled to ketone body formation. Hence, they are called *ketogenic amino acids*. Glucogenic amino acids also get converted to intermediates of TCA cycle.

Amphibolic Pathway

The tricarboxylic acid cycle has both catabolic and anabolic functions—it is amphibolic.

As a *Catabolic pathway*, it initiates the '*terminal oxidation*' of energy substrates. Many catabolic pathways lead to intermediates of the tricarboxylic acid cycle or supply metabolites such as pyruvate and acetyl-CoA that can enter the cycle where their C atoms are oxidized to CO_2.

The tricarboxylic acid cycle also supplies important precursors for anabolic pathways (Fig. 6.2).

Intermediates in the cycle are converted into:

- Glucose (gluconeogenesis, precursors oxaloacetate and malate)
- Porphyrins
- Amino acids
- Fatty acids and isoprenoids.

After the oxidation of acetyl-CoA to CO_2, they are constantly regenerated and their concentrations therefore remain constant, averaged over time.

Anabolic pathways, which remove intermediates of the cycle (e.g. gluconeogenesis) would quickly use up the

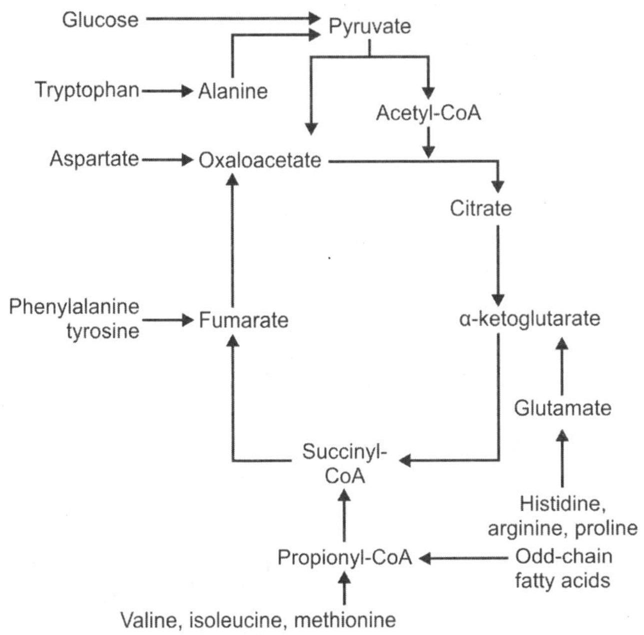

Fig. 6.2: Anabolic pathway

small quantities present in the mitochondria, if metabolites did not re-enter the cycle at other sites to replace the compounds consumed.

Processes that replenish the cycle in this way are called *anaplerotic reactions*. The degradation of most amino acids is anaplerotic because it produces either intermediates of the cycle or pyruvate (*glucogenic amino acids*). A particularly important anaplerotic step in animal metabolism leads from pyruvate to oxaloacetic acid. This ATP-dependent reaction is catalyzed by **pyruvate**.

SUMMARY

- Composed of eight reactions
- Four carbon intermediates are regenerated
- Two molecules of CO_2 released (6C ⟶ 4C)
- Most of energy stored as nicotinamide adenine dinudeotide (NADH) and QH_2.

Net reaction for citric acid cycle

Acetyl-CoA + 3NAD$^+$ + Q + GDP (ADP) + P_1 + $2H_2O$ ⟶ HS-CoA + 3NADH + QH_2 + GTP (ATP) + $2CO_2$ + $2H^+$

HIGH-ENERGY COMPOUNDS

In high-energy phosphates, the value of ΔG0' values is higher than that of ATP. The components of this group including ATP are usually anhydrides (e.g. the 1-phosphate of 1,3-bisphosphoglycerate), enolphosphates (e.g. phosphoenolpyruvate) and phosphoguanidines (e.g. creatine phosphate, arginine phosphate). The intermediate position of ATP allows it to play an important role in energy transfer. Other '*high-energy compounds*' are thiol esters involving coenzyme A (e.g. acetyl-CoA), acyl carrier protein, amino acid esters involved in protein synthesis, S-adenosylmethionine (active methionine), UDPGlc (uridine diphosphate glucose) and PRPP (5-phosphoribosyl-1-pyrophosphate).

Significance

High-energy phosphates act as the '***energy currency***' of the cell. ATP is able to act as a donor of high-energy phosphate. Likewise with the necessary enzymes, ADP can accept high-energy phosphate to form ATP from those high-energy compounds. In effect, an ATP/ADP cycle connects those processes that generate ΔP to those processes that utilize ΔP, continuously consuming and regenerating ATP. This occurs at a very rapid rate, since the total ATP/ADP pool is extremely small and sufficient to maintain an active tissue for only a few seconds.

For example, creatine phosphate (also called phosphocreatine), the phosphorylated derivative of creatine found in muscle is a high-energy compound that provides a small, but rapidly mobilized reserve of high-energy phosphates. It can be reversibly transferred to ADP to maintain the intracellular level of ATP during the first few minutes of intense muscular contraction.

ELECTRON TRANSPORT CHAIN

Nicotinamide adenine dinucleotide and flavin adenine dinucleotide can donate electron pairs to a specialized set of proteins that act as an electron conduit to oxygen, the electron transport chain. As the electrons are passed down the chain, they lose much of their free energy. Some of this energy can be captured and stored in the form of a proton gradient that can be used to synthesize ATP from ADP, the remainder of the energy is lost as heat.

Proton Gradient

The term 'proton gradient' means that one side of the membrane (in this case, the intermembrane space side of the mitochondrial inner membrane) has a higher concentration of protons than the other side. Concentration gradients of any kind contain some energy; gradients of charged entities (such as protons) usually involve electrical potential gradients also, which contain energy. The proton gradient generated by the electron transport chain has both concentration and electrical potential terms.

Complexes

Extensive research has located a total of five protein complexes in the mitochondrial inner membrane involved in the electron transport and oxidative phosphorylation pathways:

1. Complexes I, II, III and IV are part of the electron transport chain.
2. Complex V is the enzyme complex that carries out the oxidative phosphorylation reaction, the actual conversion of ADP to ATP.

All of these are large multiprotein complexes.

In addition to the membrane-bound complexes, the electron transport chain requires mobile electron carriers; cytochrome c and coenzyme Q:

1. Coenzyme Q is not a protein, but is a membrane-bound cofactor.
2. Cytochrome c is a small soluble protein located in the intermembrane space.

The overall reaction involves the oxidation of NADH or $FADH_2$ cofactors and results in the reduction of oxygen to water.

The electron transport pathway is often called 'respiratory chain,' because this pathway is the major reason for respiration (= breathing in animals) or for the requirement for oxygen in most organisms.

NADH Dehydrogenase (Complex I)

The first complex contains an iron-sulfurs center and an FMN. Complex I accept electrons from NADH to regenerate NAD, each pair of electrons results in the movement of about 4 H+ from the matrix to the intermembrane space. Complex I donate electrons to coenzyme Q.

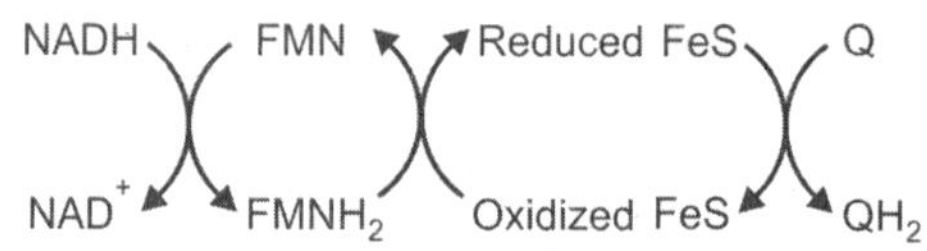

Coenzyme Q

Coenzyme Q is a non-protein electron carrier located in the inner mitochondrial membrane. Coenzyme Q can transfer one or two electrons. Coenzyme Q can accept electrons from complex I and II (and from other proteins), it donates the electrons to complex III.

Succinate Dehydrogenase (Complex II)

Succinate dehydrogenase is one of the enzymes in the TCA cycle. It is the only TCA cycle enzyme embedded in the mitochondrial inner membrane. The conversion of succinate to fumarate results in reduction of the enzyme-bound FAD. The oxidation of the reduced flavin requires the donation of electrons to coenzyme Q. Succinate dehydrogenase does **not** pump protons and therefore any proton gradient formed as a result of the donation of electron to succinate dehydrogenase by succinate occurs only due to later steps in the electron transport pathway.

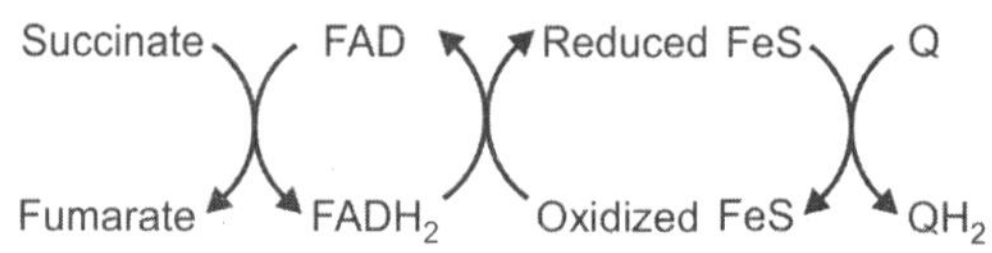

Coenzyme Q-dependent Cytochrome c Reductase (Complex III)

Complex III accepts electrons from coenzyme Q. Complex III is also a proton pump. Complex III contains several heme prosthetic groups. Different heme domains have different absorbance spectra referred to as cytochrome b and cytochrome c1.

Cytochrome c Oxidase (Cytochrome a-a3 Complex) (Complex IV)

Cytochrome c oxidase as the name implies accepts electrons from cytochrome c. Complex IV is the terminal part of the electron chain and transfers electrons directly to oxygen. Like complexes I and III, complex IV is a proton pump (Fig. 6.3).

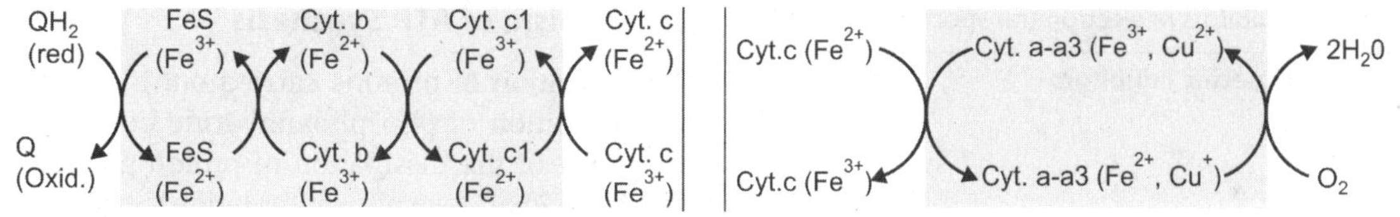

Fig. 6.3: Complex IV (cyt, cytochrome)

F1FO-ATPase = ATP Synthase (Complex V)

The final complex required for the synthesis of ATP is the ATP synthase enzyme complex itself. Complex V uses the proton gradient generated by the proton pumps to synthesize ATP. About 4 H^+ must move down the gradient for each ATP produced.

Summary of electron flow (Fig. 6.4):

- Complex I: NADH ⟶ FMN ⟶ FeS ⟶ CoQ
- Complex II: Succinate ⟶ FAD ⟶ FeS ⟶ CoQ
- Complex III: CoQ ⟶ FeS ⟶ cytochrome b ⟶ cytochrom c1 → cytochrom c
- Complex IV: Cytochrome c ⟶ cytochrome a-a3 ⟶ O_2.

Regulation of the Electron Transport Pathway

The synthesis of ATP by electron transport and oxidative phosphorylation appears to be regulated essentially, exclusively by substrate availability. The pathway cannot proceed without ADP + Pi or NADH and if both are available, then the pathway will result in ATP synthesis.

OXIDATIVE PHOSPHORYLATION

The transfer of electrons down the electron transport chain is energetically favored because of the following reasons:

- NADH is a strong electron donor
- Molecular oxygen is an avid electron acceptor.

However, the flow of electrons from NADH to oxygen does not directly result in ATP synthesis.

CHEMIOSMOTIC HYPOTHESIS

The chemiosmotic hypothesis (also known as the Mitchell hypothesis) explains how the free energy generated by the transport of electrons by the electron transport chain, it is used to produce ATP from ADP + Pi:

1. *Proton pump:* Electron transport is coupled to the phosphorylation of ADP by the transport ('pumping') of protons (H^+) across the inner mitochondrial membrane from the matrix to the intermembrane space at complexes I, III and IV. This process creates:
   a. An electrical gradient (with more positive charges on the outside of the membrane than on the inside).
   b. A pH gradient (the outside of the membrane is at a lower pH than the inside).
   The energy generated by this proton gradient is sufficient to drive ATP synthesis.
2. *ATP synthase:* The enzyme complex ATP synthase (complex V) (F1/Fo ATPase) synthesizes ATP using

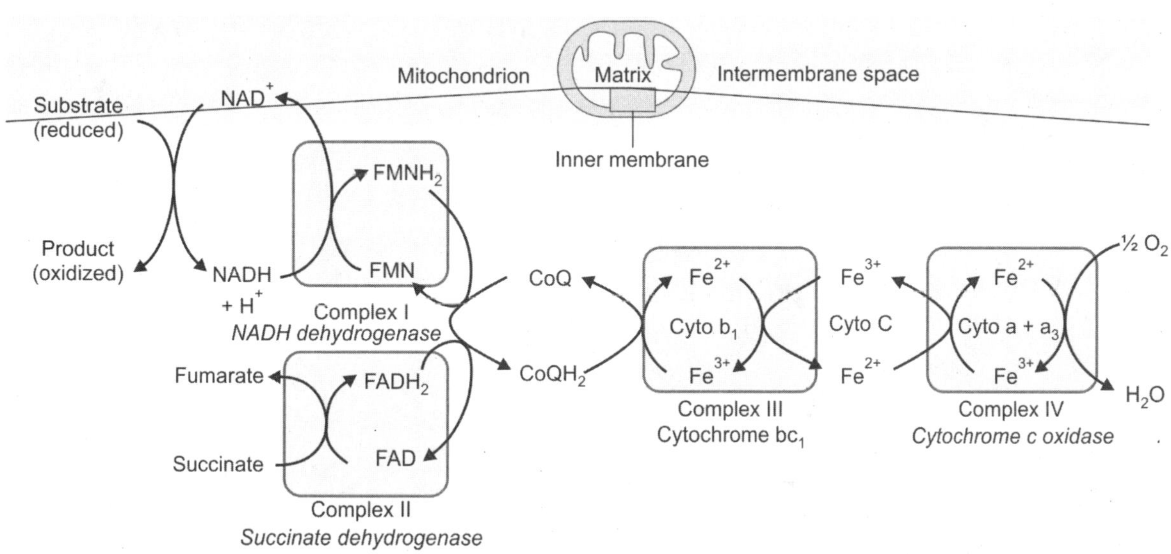

Fig. 6.4: Summary of electron transport chain (FAD, flavin adenine dinucleotide; FMN, flavin mononueleotide; $FMNH_2$, flavin mononueleotide hydroquinone; NADH, nicotinanide adeine dinucleotide).

Box 6.1: Inhibitors of electron transport chain

Complex I to CoQ specific inhibitors
Rotenone
Barbiturates
Chlorpromazine
Complex II to CoQ
Carboxin
Complex III to cytochrome c inhibitors
BAL (British antilewisite)
Naphthoquinone
Antimycin
Complex IV inhibitors
CO
CN-
N3-
H_2S
Between succinate dehydrogenase and CoQ
Carboxin
Malonate
Oxidative phosphorylation inhibitors
Atractyloside
Oligomycin
Ionophores: Valinomycin
Uncouplers
2,4 dinitrophenol
2,4 dinitrocresol
Physiological: Thyroxine

the energy of the proton gradient generated by the electron transport chain.

Mechanism of ATP Synthesis

Translocation of protons carried out by the F0 catalyzes the formation of phosphoanhydride bond of ATP by F1. Coupling of the dissipation of proton gradient with ATP synthesis (oxidative phosphorylation) is through the interaction of F1 and F0.

Inhibitors of Electron Transport Chain

Inhibition of the electron transport chain (ETC) is assessed by the effect of a compound on O_2 consumption. A variety of compounds specifically inhibit the electron transport chain at different points (Box 6.1).

Uncouplers

Uncouplers allow oxidation to proceed, but the energy instead of being trapped by phosphorylation is dissipated as heat. This occurs by removal of the proton gradient.

Uses

In hibernating animals and in newborn infants, the liberation of heat energy is required to maintain body temperature. In brown adipose tissue, thermogenesis is achieved by this process. For example:
- Thermogenin
- Protein in inner mitochondrial membrane of adipocytes
- Alternate pathway for protons.

Chapter 7

Nutrition

Nutrients are the constituents of food, necessary to sustain the normal functions of the body. All energy is provided by three classes of nutrients namely fats, carbohydrates, proteins, and in some diets and ethanol. The intake of these energy-rich molecules is larger than that of the other dietary nutrients. Therefore, they are called macronutrients. Those nutrients needed in lesser amounts, vitamins and minerals are called micronutrients.

VITAMINS

Vitamins are essential organic compounds that the animal organism is not capable of forming itself, although it requires them in small amounts for metabolism. Most vitamins are precursors of coenzymes; in some cases, they are also precursors of hormones or act as antioxidants.

FAT-SOLUBLE VITAMINS

Fat-soluble vitamins are vitamin A, vitamin D, vitamin E and vitamin K. Their general properties include:

1. Their precursors are called provitamins and are found in plants.
2. They are absorbed from gastrointestinal (GI) lumen in the presence of lipids and are emulsified with the bile.
3. They are stored in liver and adipose tissue.
4. Large doses for a long duration cause hypervitaminosis.

Vitamin A

The fat-soluble vitamin A is present only in foods of animal origin. However, its provitamin carotenoids are found in plants. All the compounds with vitamin A activity are referred as retinoids. They include retinol, retinal and retinoic acid.

Absorption of Vitamin A

1. Beta-carotene is cleaved by a dioxygenase to form retinal. The retinal is reduced to retinol by a nicotinamide adenine dinucleotide (NADH) or nicotinamide adenine dinucleotide phosphate (NADPH)-dependent retinal reductase present in the intestinal mucosa. Intestine is the major site of absorption.
2. The absorption is along with other fats and requires bile salts. In biliary tract, obstruction and steatorrhea, vitamin A is reduced.
3. Within the mucosal cell, the retinol is re-esterified with fatty acids, incorporated into chylomicrons and transported to liver. In the liver stellate cells, vitamin A is stored as retinol palmitate.

Transport from Liver to Tissues

The vitamin A from liver is transported to peripheral tissues as trans-retinol by the retinol-binding protein (RBP).

Biochemical Role of Vitamin A

1. Wald's visual cycle: Rhodopsin is a conjugated protein present in rods. It contains 11-cis-retinal. The aldehyde group (of retinal) is linked to amino group of lysine (opsin).

   The primary event in visual cycle, on exposure to light, is the isomerization of 11-cis-retinal to all-trans-retinal (Fig. 7.1). This leads to a conformational change in opsin, which is responsible for the generation of nerve impulse. The all-trans-retinal is immediately isomerized by retinal isomerase (retinal epithelium) to 11-cis-retinal. This combines with opsin to regenerate rhodopsin and complete the visual cycle. However, the conversion of

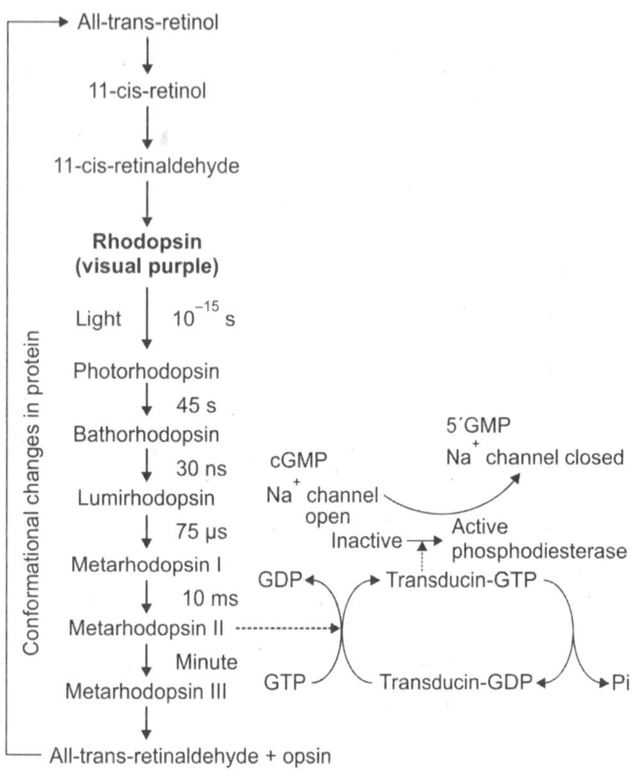

Fig. 7.1: Wald's visual cycle (GDP, guanosine diphosphate; GMP, cyclic guanosine monophosphate; GTP, guanosine triphosphate; pi, inorgamic phosphate).

all-trans-retinal to 11-cis-retinal is incomplete. Therefore, most of the all-trans-retinal is transported to the liver and converted to all-trans-retinol by alcohol. The all-trans-retinol undergoes isomerization to 11-cis-retinol, which is then oxidized to 11-cis-retinal to participate in the visual cycle.

2. Rods and cones: The retina of the eye possesses two types of cells, which are called rods and cones. The rods are in the periphery, while cones are at the center of retina. Rods are involved in dim light vision whereas cones are responsible for bright light and color vision.
3. Dark adaptation time: When a person shifts from a bright light to a dim light, rhodopsin stores are depleted and vision is impaired. However, within a few minutes, known as dark adaptation time, rhodopsin is resynthesized and vision is improved. Dark adaptation time is increased in vitamin A deficient individuals.
4. Color vision:
   a. Cones are responsible for vision in bright light as well as color vision. They contain the photosensitive protein and conopsin.
   b. There are three types of cones, each is characterized by a different conopsin that is maximally sensitive to blue (cyanopsia), green (iodopsin) or red (porphyropsin).
   c. In cone proteins also, 11-cis-retinal is the chromophore. Reduction in number of cones or the cone proteins will lead to color blindness.
5. Other biochemical functions:
   a. Retinol and retinoic acid function almost like steroid hormones. They regulate the protein synthesis and thus are involved in the cell growth and differentiation.
   b. Vitamin A is essential to maintain healthy epithelial tissue. This is due to the fact that retinol and retinoic acid are required to prevent keratin synthesis (responsible for horny surface).
   c. Retinyl phosphate synthesized from retinol is necessary for the synthesis of certain glycoprotein, which is required for growth and mucous secretion.
   d. Retinol and retinoic acid are involved in the synthesis of transferring the iron transport protein.
   e. Vitamin A is considered to be essential for the maintenance of proper immune system to fight against various infections.
   f. Cholesterol synthesis requires vitamin A. Mevalonate, an intermediate in the cholesterol biosynthesis is diverted for the synthesis of coenzyme Q in vitamin A deficiency.
   g. Carotenoids (most important beta-carotene) function as antioxidants and reduce the risk of cancers initiated by free radicals and strong oxidants. Beta-carotene is found to be beneficial to prevent heart attacks. This is also attributed to the antioxidant property.

Recommended Daily Allowance

The recommended daily allowance (RDA) of vitamin A for:

- Children: 400–600 μg/day
- Men: 750–1,000 μg/day
- Women: 750 μg/day
- Pregnancy: 1,000 μg/day.

One international unit is 0.3 mg of retinol. One retinol equivalent to 1 μg of retinol or 6 μg of beta-carotene.

Dietary Sources of Vitamin A

Animal sources include milk, butter, cream, cheese, egg yolk and liver. Fish liver oils (cod liver oil and shark liver oil) are very rich sources of the vitamin A. Vegetable sources contain the yellow pigments of beta-carotene. Carrot contains significant quantity of beta-carotene. Papaya, mango, pumpkins and green leafy vegetables (spinach, amaranth) are other good sources for vitamin A activity. During cooking, the activity is not destroyed.

Deficiency Manifestations

Effect on the eyes

1. Night blindness (nyctalopia): It is one of the earliest symptoms of vitamin A deficiency. The individuals have difficulty to see in dim light, since the dark adaptation time is increased. Prolonged deficiency irreversibly damages a number of visual cells.
2. Xerophthalmia: Severe deficiency of vitamin A leads to xerophthalmia. This is characterized by dryness in conjunctiva and cornea, and keratinization of epithelial cells.
3. In certain areas of conjunctiva, white triangular plaques are seen, known as Bitot's spots (Fig. 7.2).
4. Keratomalacia: If xerophthalmia persists for a long time, corneal ulceration and degeneration occur. This result in the destruction of cornea, a condition referred to as keratomalacia, causing total blindness.

Effect on reproduction

The reproductive system is adversely affected in vitamin A deficiency. Degeneration leads to sterility in males.

Effect on skin and epithelial cells

The skin becomes rough and dry. Keratinization of epithelial cells of GI, urinary tract and respiratory tract is noticed. This leads to increased bacterial infection.

Effect on renal system

Vitamin A deficiency is associated with formation of urinary stones.

Hypervitaminosis

Hypervitaminosis of vitamin A include dermatitis (drying and redness of skin), enlargement of liver, skeletal decalcification, tenderness of long bones, loss of weight, irritability, loss of hair, joint pains, etc.

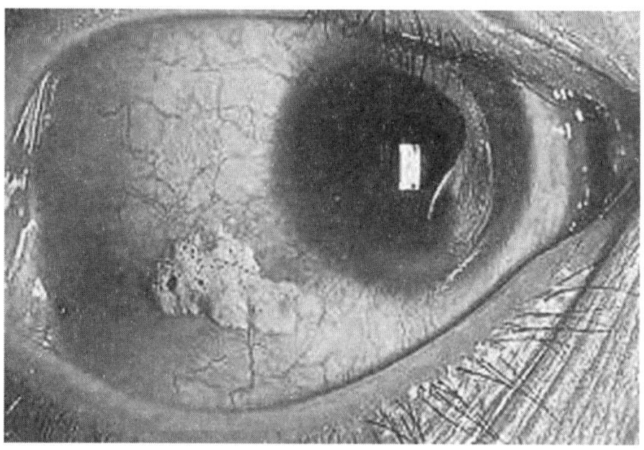

Fig. 7.2: Bitot's spots

> Mnemonic
> Increased vitamin A makes you **'HARD'**:
> - ***H***eadache/Hepatomegaly
> - ***A***norexia/Alopecia
> - ***R***eally painful bones
> - ***D***ry skin/Drowsiness

Vitamin D (Cholecalciferol)

Vitamin D is fat soluble. It resembles steroids in structure and function like a hormone.

Formation of Vitamin D (Fig. 7.3)

Activation of vitamin D:

1. Vitamin D is a prohormone. The cholecalciferol is first transported to liver, where hydroxylation at 25th position occurs, to form 25-hydroxy-cholecalciferol (25-HCC).
2. In plasma, 25-HCC is bound to 'vitamin D-binding protein' (VDBP), an alpha 2-globulin.

   In the kidney, it is further hydroxylated at the first position. It requires cytochrome P450, NADPH and ferrodoxin (an iron-sulfur protein). Thus 1, 25-dihydroxy cholecalciferol (DHCC) is generated. Since it contains three hydroxyl groups at 1, 3 and 25 positions, it is also called calcitriol. The calcitriol thus formed is the active form of vitamin; it is a hormone.

Biochemical Role of Vitamin D

Calcitriol (1, 25-DHCC) is the biologically active form of vitamin D. It regulates plasma levels of calcium and phosphate.

Calcitriol acts at three different levels (intestine, kidney and bone) to maintain plasma calcium (normal 9–11 mg/dL) as follows:

1. Action of calcitriol on the intestine: Calcitriol increases the intestinal absorption of calcium and phosphate. In the intestinal cells, calcitriol binds with a cytosolic receptor to form a calcitriol receptor complex. This complex then approaches the nucleus and interacts with a specific DNA, leading to synthesis of a specific calcium-binding protein. This protein increases the calcium uptake by the intestine. The mechanism of action in calcitriol on the target tissue (intestine) is similar to the action of a steroid hormone.
2. Action of calcitriol on the bone: In the osteoblasts of bone, calcitriol stimulates calcium uptake for deposition as calcium phosphate. Thus calcitriol is essential for bone formation. The bone is an important reservoir of calcium and phosphate. Calcitriol, along with parathyroid hormone,

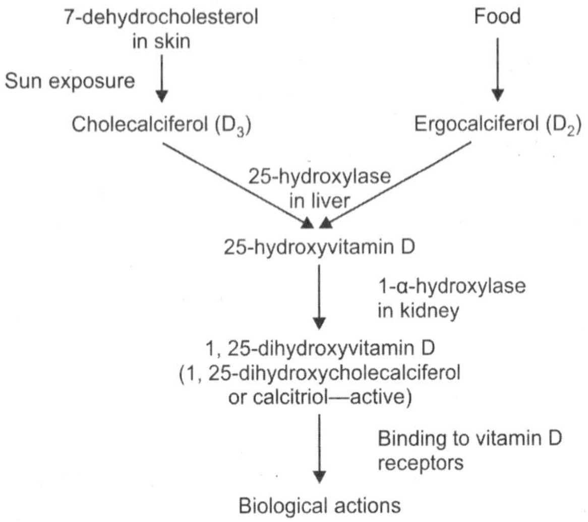

Fig. 7.3: Vitamin D synthesis

increases, the mobilization of calcium and phosphate. This causes elevation in the plasma calcium and phosphate levels.

3. Action of calcitriol on the kidney: Calcitriol is also involved in minimizing the excretion of calcium and phosphate through the kidney by decreasing their excretion and enhancing reabsorption.

Recommended Daily Allowance

Requirement of vitamin D for:

- Children: 10 μg (400 IU)/day
- Adults: 5 μg (200 IU)/day
- Pregnancy, lactation: 10 μg/day
- Above the age of 60: 600 IU/day.

Dietary Sources of Vitamin D

Exposure to sunlight produces cholecalciferol. Moreover fish liver oil, fish and egg yolk are good sources of the vitamin D. Milk contains moderate quantity of the vitamin D.

Deficiency Manifestations of Vitamin D

Vitamin D deficiency is relatively less common, since this vitamin can be synthesized in the body. However, insufficient exposure to sunlight and consumption of diet lacking vitamin D results in its deficiency.

Rickets

Rickets is seen in children. There is insufficient mineralization of bone. Bones become soft and pliable. The bone growth is markedly affected. Plasma calcium and phosphorus are low-normal with alkaline phosphatase (bone isoenzyme) being markedly elevated.

Clinical features

The classical features of rickets are bone deformities. Weight bearing bones are bent (Fig. 7.4).

Clinical manifestations

The clinical manifestations of rickets include bow legs, knock-knee, rickety rosary, bossing of frontal bones and pigeon chest.

An enlargement of the epiphysis at the lower end of ribs and costochondral junction leads to beading of ribs or rickety rosary.

Harrison's sulcus is a transverse depression passing outwards from the costal cartilage to axilla. This is due to the indentation of lower ribs at the site of the attachment of diaphragm.

Different types of rickets

1. The classical vitamin D deficiency—rickets can be cured by giving vitamin D in the diet.
2. The hypophosphatemic rickets mainly result from defective renal tubular reabsorption of phosphate. Supplementation of vitamin D along with phosphate is found to be useful.
3. Vitamin D-resistant rickets is found to be associated with Fanconi syndrome, where the renal tubular reabsorption of bicarbonate, phosphate, glucose and amino acids are also deficient.
4. Renal rickets: In kidney diseases, even if vitamin D is available, calcitriol is not synthesized. These cases will respond to administration of calcitriol.
5. End organ refractoriness to 1, 25-DHCC will also lead to rickets.

Clinical Features of Osteomalacia

1. The bones are softened due to insufficient mineralization and increased osteoporosis. Patients are more prone to get fractures.

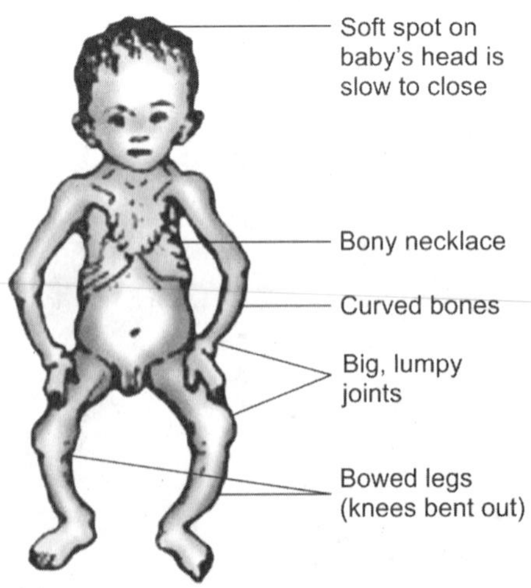

Fig. 7.4: Rickets

2. The abnormalities in biochemical parameters are slightly lower serum calcium and a low serum phosphate.
3. Serum alkaline phosphatase and bone isoenzyme are markedly increased.

Hypervitaminosis D

Doses above 1,500 units per day for very long periods may cause toxicity. Symptoms include weakness, polyuria, intense thirst, difficulty in speaking, hypertension and weight loss. Hypercalcemia leads to calcification of soft tissues (metastatic calcification, otherwise called calcinosis, especially in vascular and renal tissues).

Vitamin E (Tocopherol)

Vitamin E (tocopherol) is a naturally occurring antioxidant. It is essential for normal reproduction in many animals, hence known as antisterility vitamin.

Chemistry

Vitamin E is the name, given to a group of tocopherols and tocotrienols. About eight tocopherols have been identified—α, β, γ, δ, etc. Among these, α-tocopherol is the most active. The tocopherols are derivatives of 6-hydroxychromane (tocol) ring with isoprenoid (3 units) side chain. The antioxidant property is due to the chromane ring.

Biochemical Role of Vitamin E

1. Vitamin E is essential for the membrane structure and integrity of the cell, hence it is regarded as a membrane antioxidant.
2. It prevents the peroxidation of polyunsaturated fatty acids in various tissues and membranes. It protects RBC from hemolysis by oxidizing agents (e.g. H_2O_2).
3. It is closely associated with reproductive functions and prevents sterility.
4. It increases the synthesis of heme by enhancing the activity of enzymes aminolevulinic acid (ALA) synthase and ALA dehydratase.
5. It is required for cellular respiration through electron transport chain.
6. Vitamin E prevents the oxidation of vitamin A and carotene.
7. It is required for proper storage of creatine in skeletal muscle.
8. Vitamin E is needed for optimal absorption of amino acids from the intestine.
9. It is involved in proper synthesis of nucleic acids.
10. Vitamin E protects liver from being damaged by toxic compounds such as carbon tetrachloride.
11. It works in association with vitamins A, C and beta-carotene, to delay the onset of cataract.
12. Vitamin E has been recommended for the prevention of chronic diseases such as cancer and heart diseases.

Vitamin E and Selenium

The element selenium is found in the enzyme glutathione peroxidase that destroys free radicals. Thus, selenium is also involved in antioxidant functions like vitamin E and both of them act synergistically. To a certain extent, selenium can spare the requirement of vitamin E and vice versa.

Recommended Daily Allowance of Vitamin E

Requirement of vitamin E for:

- Man: 10 mg (15 IU)
- Woman: 8 mg (12 IU)
- Vitamin E-supplemented diet is advised for pregnant and lactating women.

Dietary Sources

Many vegetable oils are rich sources of vitamin E. Wheat germ oil, cotton seed oil, peanut oil, corn oil and sunflower oil are the good sources of this vitamin. It is also present in meat, milk, butter and eggs.

Deficiency Manifestations

In many animals, the deficiency is associated with sterility, degenerative changes in muscle; megaloblastic anemia and changes in central nervous system (CNS). Severe symptoms of vitamin E deficiency are not seen in humans except increased fragility of erythrocytes and minor neurological symptoms.

Hypervitaminosis

Among the fat-soluble vitamins (A, D, E and K), vitamin E is the least toxic. No toxic effect has been reported even after ingestion of 300 mg/day.

Vitamin K

Vitamin K is the only fat-soluble vitamin with a specific coenzyme function. It is required for the production of blood-clotting factors, essential for coagulation.

Biochemical Role of Vitamin K

Vitamin K is necessary for coagulation. Factors dependent on vitamin K are factor II (prothrombin); factor VII [serum prothrombin conversion accelerator (SPCA)]; factor IX (Christmas factor); factor X (Stuart-Prower factor).

All these factors are synthesized by the liver as inactive zymogens. They undergo post-translational modification; gamma carboxylation of glutamic acid (GCG) residues. These are the binding sites for calcium ions. The GCG synthesis requires vitamin K as a cofactor.

Vitamin K-dependent gamma carboxylation is also necessary for the functional activity of osteocalcin as well as structural proteins of kidney, lung and spleen. Osteocalcin is synthesized by osteoblasts and seen only in bone. It is a small protein (40–50 amino acids length) that binds tightly to hydroxyapatite crystals of bone. Osteocalcin also contains hydroxyproline, so it is dependent on both vitamins K and C.

Recommended Daily Allowance

Recommended daily allowance is 50–100 mg/day. This is usually available in a normal diet.

Dietary Sources of Vitamin K

Green leafy vegetables are good dietary sources. Even if the diet does not contain the vitamin, intestinal bacterial synthesis will meet the daily requirements, as long as absorption is normal.

Deficiency Manifestations

1. Hemorrhagic disease of the newborn is attributed to vitamin K deficiency. The newborns, especially the premature infants have relative vitamin K deficiency. This is due to lack of hepatic stores and absence of intestinal bacterial flora.
2. It is often advised that premature infants be given prophylactic doses of vitamin K (1 mg menadione).
3. In children and adults, vitamin K deficiency may be manifested as bruising tendency, ecchymotic patches, mucous membrane, hemorrhage, post-traumatic bleeding and internal bleeding.
4. Prolongation of prothrombin time and delayed clotting time are characteristic of vitamin K deficiency.
5. Warfarin and dicoumarol will competitively inhibit the gamma carboxylation due to structural similarity with vitamin K. Hence they are widely used as anticoagulants for therapeutic purposes.
6. Treatment of pregnant women with warfarin can lead to fetal bone abnormalities (fetal warfarin syndrome).

Hypervitaminosis of Vitamin K

Hemolysis, hyperbilirubinemia, kernicterus and brain damage are the manifestations of toxicity. Administration of large quantities of menadione may result in toxicity.

WATER-SOLUBLE VITAMINS

Water-soluble vitamins include vitamin B complex and vitamin C. Their general properties include:

1. Most of them are converted into coenzymes for various metabolic reactions.
2. Due to their water solubility, they cannot be stored to any significant extent.
3. Large doses are passed out in urine and they rarely result in toxicity.

Thiamine (Vitamin B_1)

Vitamin B_1 is also called anti-beriberi factor and antineuritic factor (since it can relieve neuritis).

Chemistry

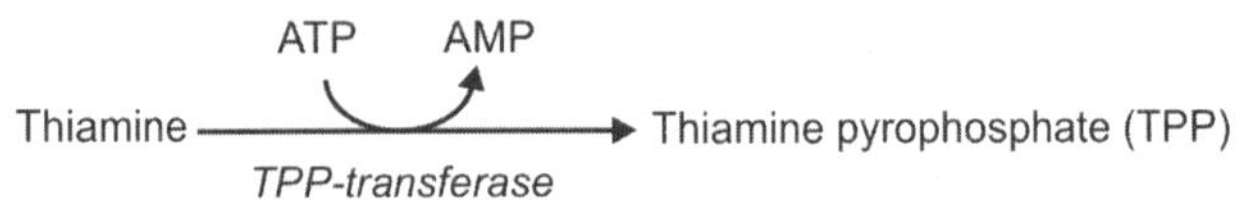

ATP, adenosine triphosphate; AMP, adenosine monophosphate; TPP, thiamine pyrophosphate (TPP).

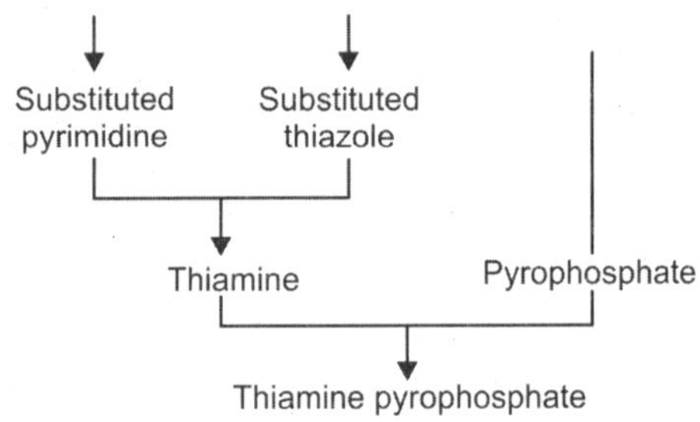

Thiamine contains a pyrimidine ring and a thiazole ring by means of methylene bridge. Alcohol group of thiamine is esterified with 2 moles of phosphate to form its active coenzyme thiamine pyrophosphate.

Biochemical Functions

1. Pyruvate dehydrogenase: The coenzyme form is thiamine pyrophosphate (TPP). It is used in oxidative decarboxylation of alpha-keto acids, e.g. pyruvate dehydrogenase catalyzes the breakdown of pyruvate to acetyl-CoA and carbon dioxide.
2. Alpha-ketoglutarate dehydrogenase: An analogous biochemical reaction that requires TPP is the oxidative decarboxylation of alpha-ketoglutarate to succinyl-CoA and CO_2.
3. Transketolase: The second group of enzymes that use TPP as coenzyme are the transketolases in the hexose monophosphate shunt pathway of glucose.

4. Alpha-keto acid decarboxylase: Thiamine pyrophosphate is required for alpha-keto acid decarboxylase to catalyze oxidative decarboxylation of branched-chain amino acids (valine, leucine isoleucine).
5. Tryptophan pyrrolase: Thiamine is required in tryptophan metabolism for the activity of tryptophan pyrrolase.

Thiamine antagonists: As follows:
- Pyrithiamine
- Oxythiamine.

Recommended Daily Allowance

Recommended daily allowance depends on calorie intake:
- Adult: 1–1.5 mg/day (0.5 mg/1,000 calories of energy)
- Children: 0.7–1.2 mg/day
- Pregnancy and lactation: 2 mg/day.

Dietary Sources

Aleurone layer of cereals (food grains) is a rich source of thiamine. Therefore whole wheat flour and unpolished hand-pound rice have better nutritive value. Yeast is also a very good source. Thiamine is partially destroyed by heat.

Deficiency Manifestations

Beriberi

Deficiency of thiamine leads to beriberi. It is a Sinhalese word, meaning 'weakness'. The early symptoms are anorexia, dyspepsia, heaviness and weakness.

Types of beriberi

1. Wet beriberi: Here cardiovascular manifestations are prominent. Edema of legs, face, trunk and serous cavities are the main features. Death occurs due to heart failure.
2. Dry beriberi: In this condition, CNS manifestations are the major features. Edema is not commonly seen. Muscles become weak. Peripheral neuritis with sensory disturbance leads to complete paralysis.
3. Infantile beriberi: It occurs in infants born to mothers suffering from thiamine deficiency.
4. Wernicke-korsakoff syndrome: It is also called cerebral beriberi. Clinical features are those of encephalopathy:
   - Ophthalmoplegia
   - Nystagmus
   - Cerebellar ataxia—loss of muscle coordination caused by disorders of cerebellum with psychosis.

Polyneuritis

Polyenuritis is common in chronic alcoholics. Alcohol inhibits intestinal absorption of thiamine, leading to thiamine deficiency. Polyneuritis may also be associated with pregnancy and old age. Impairment of conversion of acetate to acetyl-CoA.

$$\text{Pyruvate} \xrightarrow{\text{LDH}} \text{Lactate} \longrightarrow \text{Leading to lactic acidosis}$$

Vitamin B2 (Riboflavin)

Vitamin B2 is also called lactoflavin, ovoflavin, hepatoflavin.

Chemistry

Riboflavin has a dimethyl isoalloxazine ring to which a ribitol is attached.

Coenzyme
- Flavin adenine dinucleotide (FAD)
- Flavin mononucleotide (FMN).

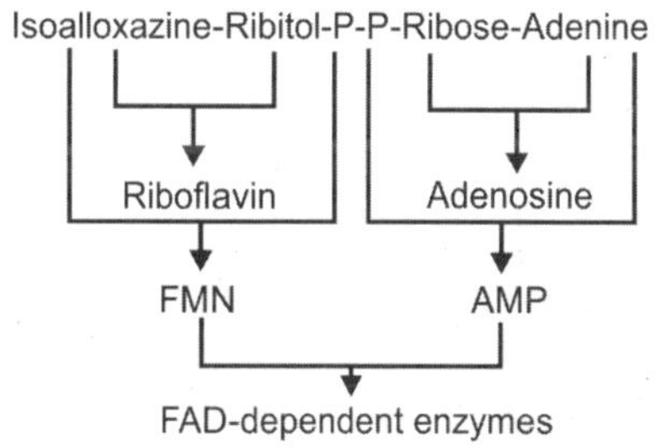

Biochemical Functions

Carbohydrate metabolism
- Pyruvate to acetyl-CoA by pyruvate dehydrogenase
- Alpha-ketoglutarate to succinyl-CoA by alpha-ketoglutarate dehydrogenase
- Succinate to fumarate by succinate dehydrogenase.

Lipid metabolism
- Acyl-CoA to alpha-beta unsaturated acyl-CoA by acyl-CoA dehydrogenase.

Protein metabolism
- Glycine to glyoxylate and ammonia by glycine oxidase
- D-amino acid to alpha-keto acid and ammonia by D-amino acid oxidase.

Purine metabolism
- Xanthine to uric acid by xanthine oxidase.

FMN-dependent enzymes
- L-amino to alpha-keto acid and ammonia by alpha-amino acid oxidase.
- $NAD^+ \longrightarrow FMN \longrightarrow CoQ$. By NADH dehydrogenase.

Riboflavin antagonists
- Dichloro-riboflavin
- Isoriboflavin.

Recommended Daily Allowance

- Adult: 1.5 mg/day
- Pregnancy and lactation: 2–2.5 mg/day.

Dietary Sources

Rich sources are liver, dried yeast, egg and whole milk. Good sources are fish, whole cereals, legumes and green leafy vegetables.

Deficiency Manifestations

Causes

Natural deficiency of riboflavin in man is uncommon, because riboflavin is synthesized by the intestinal flora. Riboflavin deficiency usually accompanies other deficiency diseases such as beriberi, pellagra and kwashiorkor.

Manifestations

Symptoms are confined to skin and mucous membranes:
- Glossitis
- Magenta-colored tongue
- Cheilosis
- Angular stomatitis (inflammation at the corners of mouth)
- Circumcorneal vascularization
- Proliferation of the bulbar conjunctival capillaries.

Vitamin B3 (Niacin)

Vitamin B3 is also called pellagra-preventing factor of Goldberger and nicotinic acid.

Chemistry

Niacin is pyridine-3-carboxylic acid. In tissues, it occurs principally as amide form.

Coenzyme
- Nicotinamide adenine dinucleotide (NAD^+)
- Nicotinamide adenine dinucleotide phosphate ($NADP^+$).

Biochemical Functions

NAD^+-dependent enzymes.

Carbohydrate metabolism include:
1. Lactate dehydrogenase (lactate ⟶ pyruvate).
2. Glyceraldehyde-3-phosphate dehydrogenase (glyceraldehyde-3-phosphate ⟶ 1, 3-bisphosphoglycerate).
3. Pyruvate dehydrogenase (pyruvate ⟶ acetyl CoA).

Lipid metabolism
1. Beta hydroxyacyl-CoA dehydrogenase (beta hydroxyacyl-CoA ⟶ beta-ketoacyl CoA).

$NADP^+$ dependent enzymes
1. Glucose-6-phosphate dehydrogenase in the hexose monophosphate shunt pathway (glucose-6 phosphate ⟶ 6-phosphogluconolactone).
2. Malic enzyme (malate to pyruvate).

NADPH-dependent enzymes
1. Ketoacyl-ACP dehydrogenase (beta-ketoacyl-ACP ⟶ beta-hydroxyacyl-ACP).
2. α,β-unsaturated acyl-ACP ⟶ acyl-ACP.
3. HMG-CoA reductase (HMG-CoA ⟶ mevalonate.
4. Folate reductase (folate ⟶ dihydrofolate ⟶ tetrahydrofolate).
5. Phenylalanine hydroxylase (phenylalanine ⟶ tyrosine).

Recommended Daily Allowance

- Adult: 20 mg/day
- Pregnancy and lactation: 25 mg/day.

Dietary Sources

The richest natural sources of niacin are dried yeast, polished rice, liver, peanut, whole cereals, legumes, meat and fish.

Deficiency Manifestations

Pellagra

Pellagra is characterized by three Ds, which are as follows:
1. Dermatitis: Increased pigmentation around the neck is known as Casal's necklace (Fig. 7.5).
2. Dementia: It is frequently seen in chronic cases. Delirium is common in acute pellagra.
3. Diarrhea: The diarrhea may be mild or severe with blood and mucus.

Vitamin B6 (Pyridoxal Phosphate)

Coenzyme

- Pyridoxine
- Pyridoxal
- Pyridoxamine.

Active form of pyridoxine is pyridoxal phosphate (PLP).

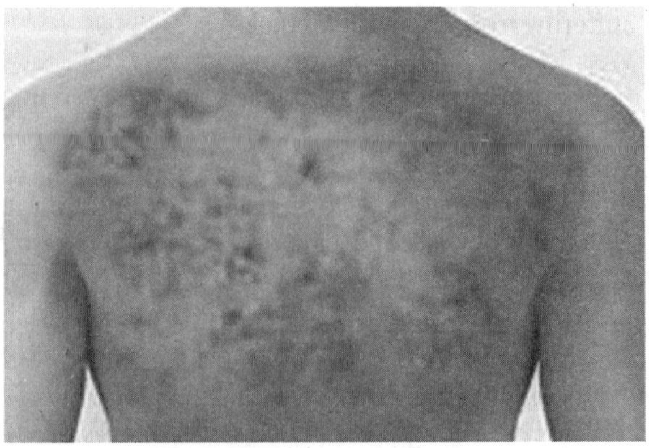

Fig. 7.5: Pellagra

Biochemical Functions

1. Transamination: These reactions are catalyzed by aminotransferases (transaminases), which employ PLP as coenzyme. For example,

Alanine + Alpha-ketoglutarate ⟶ Pyruvate+ glutamic acid
Alanine transaminase

2. Decarboxylation: All decarboxylation reactions of amino acids require PLP as coenzymes. For examples,
   a. Glutamate ⟶ GABA.
   GABA is an inhibitory neurotransmitter and hence in B6 deficiency, especially in children, convulsions may occur.
   b. Histidine ⟶ histamine.
3. Sulfur-containing amino acids: Pyridoxal phosphate plays an important role in methionine and cysteine metabolism.
   Homocysteine + Serine ⟶ Cystathionine (by cystathionine synthase).
   Cystathionine ⟶ Homoserine + Cysteine (by cystathionase).
4. Heme synthesis: Aminolevulinic acid synthase is a PLP-dependent enzyme. This is the rate-limiting step in heme biosynthesis so, in B6 deficiency, anemia may be seen.
5. Production of niacin from tryptophan require PLP.
6. Glycogenolysis: Phosphorylase enzyme (glycogen to glucose-1-phosphate) requires PLP. In fact, more than 70% total PLP content of the body is in muscles, where it is a part of the phosphorylase enzyme.

Recommended Daily Allowance

- Adult: 1–2 mg/day
- Pregnancy and lactation: 2.5 mg/day.

Dietary Sources of Vitamin B6

Rich sources are yeast, polished rice, wheat germs, cereals, legumes (pulses), oil seeds, egg, milk, meat, fish and green leafy vegetables.

Deficiency Manifestations

Neurological manifestations

In vitamin B6 deficiency, PLP-dependent enzymes function poorly. So, serotonin, epinephrine, noradrenalin and GABA are not produced properly. Neurological symptoms are therefore quite common in B6 deficiency. In children, B6 deficiency leads to convulsions due to decreased formation of GABA. The PLP is involved in the synthesis of sphingolipids; so B6 deficiency leads to demyelination of nerves and consequent peripheral neuritis.

Dermatological manifestations

Deficiency of B6 will also affect tryptophan metabolism. Since, niacin is produced from tryptophan, B6 deficiency in turn leads to niacin deficiency, which is manifested as pellagra.

Hematological manifestations

In adults, hypochromic microcytic anemia may occur due to the inhibition of heme biosynthesis. The metabolic disorders, which respond to vitamin B6 therapy are xanthurenic aciduria and homocystinuria.

Vitamin B9 (Folic Acid)

Vitamin B9 is also called liver lactobacillus casei factor, *Streptococcus lactis* resistance (SLR) factor, pteroylglutamic acid (PGA).

Chemistry

The pteridine group with para-aminobenzoic acid (PABA) is pteroic acid. It is then attached to glutamic acid to form pteroylglutamic acid or folic acid.

Coenzyme

Active form is reduced 5, 6, 7, 8-tetrahydrofolic acid (THFA).

The THFA is the carrier of one-carbon groups. One carbon compound is an organic molecule that contains only a single carbon atom. The following groups are one-carbon compounds:

- Formyl (—CH=O)
- Formimino (—CH=NH)
- Methenyl (—CH=)
- Methylene ($—CH_2^-$)
- Hydroxymethyl ($—CH_2OH$)
- Methyl ($—CH_3$).

Folate antagonists:

- Sulfonamides
- Pyrimethamine
- Aminopterin.

Recommended Daily Allowance

- Adult: 200 μg/day
- Pregnancy: 400 μg/day
- Lactation: 300 μg/day.

Dietary Sources

Rich sources of folate are yeast, green vegetables. Moderate sources are cereals, oil seeds and egg.

Deficiency Manifestations

Reduced DNA synthesis

In folate deficiency, THFA is reduced and thymidylate synthase enzyme is inhibited. Hence deoxyuridine monophosphate (dUMP) is not converted to deoxythymidine monophosphate (dTMP). So deoxythymidine triphosphate (dTTP) is not available for DNA synthesis. Thus cell division is arrested.

Macrocytic anemia

1. It is the most characteristic feature of folate deficiency. During erythropoiesis, DNA synthesis is delayed, but protein synthesis is continued. Thus hemoglobin accumulates in RBC precursors leading to immature looking nucleus and macrocytic cells.
2. Reticulocytosis is often seen. These abnormal RBCs are rapidly destroyed. Reduced generation and increased destruction of RBCs result in anemia.
3. Leukopenia and thrombocytopenia are also manifested.

Homocysteinemia

Folic acid deficiency may cause increased homocysteine levels in blood (above 15 μmol/L) with increased risk of coronary artery diseases. It is treated by adequate doses of pyridoxine, vitamins B_{12} and B_9.

Birth defects

Folic acid deficiency during pregnancy causes homocysteinemia and neural tube defects in fetus. Folic acid prevents birth defects malformations such as spina bifida.

Cancer

Bronchial carcinoma and cervical carcinoma.

Mnemonic: Folate deficiency causes:
'A FOLIC DROP'
- *A*lcoholism
- *F*olic acid antagonists
- *O*ral contraceptives
- *L*ow dietary intake
- *I*nfection with Giardia
- *C*eliac sprue
- *D*ilantin
- *R*elative folate deficiency
- *O*ld
- *P*regnant

Vitamin B_{12} (Cobalamin)

Vitamin B_{12} is called antipernicious anemia factor and extrinsic factor of Castle.

Chemistry

Four pyrrole rings coordinated with a cobalt atom is called a corrin ring. The 5th valence of the cobalt is covalently linked to a substituted benzimidazole ring. This is then called cobalamin. The 6th valence of the cobalt is satisfied by any of the following groups namely cyanide, hydroxyl, adenosyl or methyl.

When cyanide is added at the (R) position, the molecule is called cyanocobalamin. When cyanide group is substituted by hydroxyl group, it forms hydroxy, cobalamin.

Absorption of Vitamin B_{12}

Absorption of vitamin B_{12} requires two binding proteins. First is the intrinsic factor (IF) of Castle. The second factor is cobalophilin (Figs 7.6A and B).

Transport and storage

In the blood, methyl B_{12} form is predominant. Transcobalamin, a glycoprotein is the specific carrier. It is stored in the liver cells, as ado-B_{12} form, in combination with transcorrin.

Biochemical Functions

In B_{12} deficiency, methylmalonyl-CoA is excreted in urine (methylmalonic aciduria).

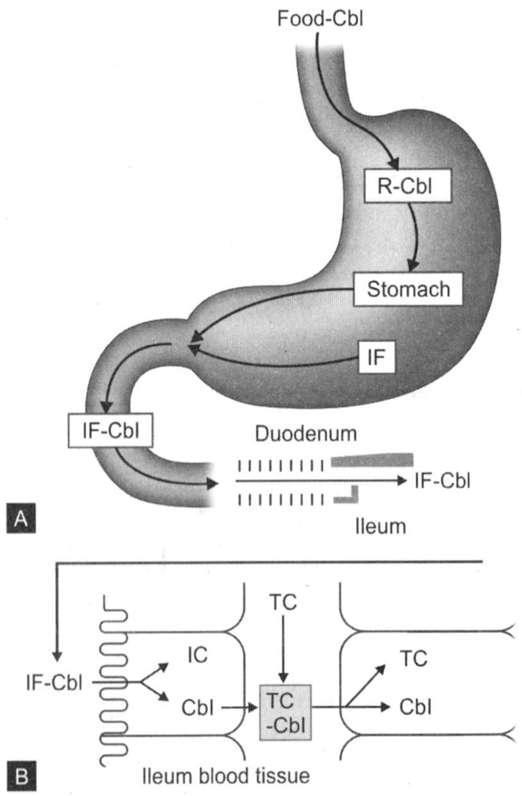

Figs 7.6A and B: Absorption of vitamin B_{12} (R, cobalophilin; Cbl, cobalamin; IF, intrinsic factor; TC, trans cobalamin)

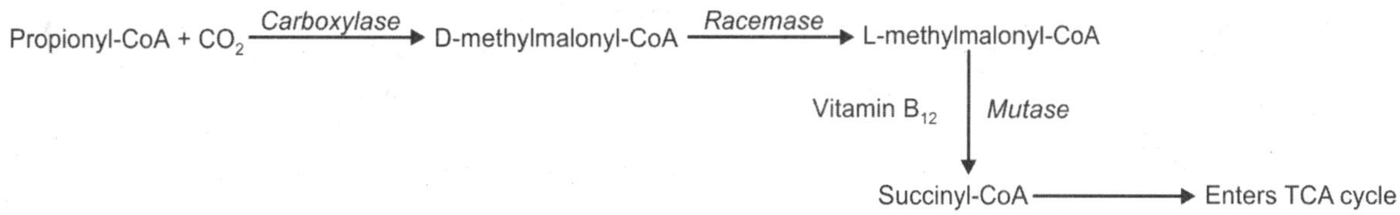

1. Homocysteine Methyltransferase (Fig. 7.7).
2. Methyl folate trap and folate deficiency.
   The production of methyl THFA is an irreversible step. Therefore, the only way for generation of free THFA is step no. 1 in the Figure 7.7. When B_{12} is deficient, this reaction cannot take place. This is called the methyl folate trap, this leads to the associated folic acid scarcity in B_{12} deficiency.

Recommended Daily Allowance

- Adult: 1–2 μg/day
- Pregnancy and lactation: 2 mg/day.

Dietary Sources

Richest source is liver. Curd is a good source.

Causes of B_{12} Deficiency

Nutritional: Nutritional vitamin B_{12} deficiency is very common in India.

Decrease in absorption: Absorptive surface is reduced by gastrectomy, resection of ileum and malabsorption syndromes.

Addisonian pernicious anemia: It is manifested usually in persons over 40 years. It is an autoimmune disease. Antibodies are generated against IF. So, the IF becomes deficient, leading to defective absorption of B_{12}.

Gastric atrophy: Similar atrophy of gastric epithelium leading to deficiency of IF and decreased B_{12} absorption is common in India. In chronic iron deficiency anemia, there is generalized mucosal atrophy.

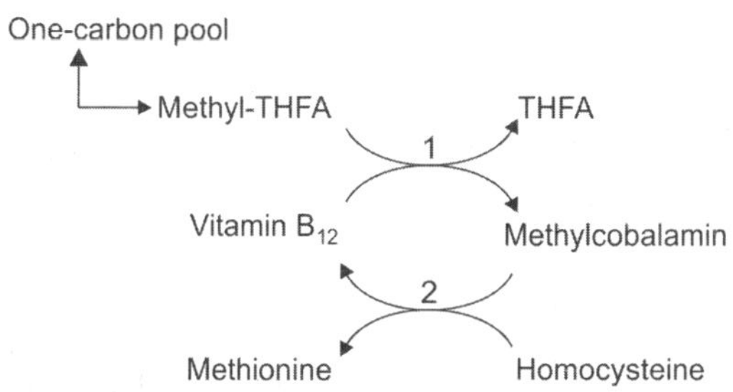

Fig. 7.7: Action of homocysteine methyltransferase (THFA, tetrahydrofolic acid; 1, $-CH_3$; 2, homocysteine methyltransferase)

Pregnancy: Increased requirement of vitamin in pregnancy is another common cause for vitamin B12 deficiency in India.

Fish tapeworm: The fish tapeworm, diphyllobothrium latum has a special affinity to B_{12} causing reduction in available vitamin.

Deficiency Manifestations

Folate trap: Vitamin B_{12} deficiency causes simultaneous folate deficiency due to the folate trap. Therefore all the manifestations of folate deficiency are also seen.

Megaloblastic anemia: In the peripheral blood, megaloblasts and immature RBCs are observed.

Homocysteinemia: In vitamin B_{12} deficiency, homocysteine is accumulated, leading to homocystinuria and myocardial infarction.

Demyelination: In vitamin B_{12} deficiency, nonavailability of active methionine leads to inadequate methylation of phosphatidylethanolamine to phosphatidylcholine. This leads to deficient formation of myelin sheaths of nerves, demyelination and neurological lesions.

Subacute combined degeneration: Damage to nervous system is seen in B_{12} deficiency. There is demyelination affecting cerebral cortex as well as dorsal column and pyramidal tract of spinal cord. Since sensory and motor tracts are affected, it is named as combined degeneration. Symmetrical paresthesia of extremities, alterations of tendon, and deep senses and reflexes, loss of position sense, unsteadiness in gait, positive Romberg's sign (falling when eyes are closed) and positive Babinski's sign (extensor plantar reflex) are seen.

Achlorhydria: Absence of acid in gastric juice is associated with vitamin B_{12} deficiency.

Vitamin C (Ascorbic Acid)

Vitamin C is also called antiscorbutic vitamin.

Chemistry

Vitamin C is easily destroyed by heat, alkali and storage. In the process of cooking, 70% of vitamin C is lost.

The structural formula of ascorbic acid closely resembles that of carbohydrates. The strong reducing property of vitamin C depends on the double-bonded (enediol) carbons.

Only L-ascorbic acid and dehydroascorbic acid have antiscorbutic activity. The D-ascorbic acid has no activity.

Biochemical Functions

Reversible oxidation-reduction

The vitamin can change between ascorbic acid and dehydroascorbic acid. Most of the physiological properties of the vitamin could be explained by this redox system.

$$\text{L-ascorbic acid} \underset{\text{Reduction}}{\overset{\text{Oxidation}}{\rightleftharpoons}} \text{Dehydroascorbic acid}$$

Hydroxylation of proline and lysine

Ascorbic acid is necessary for the post-translational hydroxylation of proline and lysine residue. Hydroxyproline and hydroxylysine are essential for the formation of cross links in the collagen, which gives the tensile strength to the fibers. This process is necessary for the normal production of osteoid, collagen and intercellular cement substance of capillaries.

Tryptophan metabolism

Ascorbic acid is necessary for the hydroxylation of tryptophan to 5-hydroxytryptophan. This is required for the formation of serotonin.

Tyrosine metabolism

Vitamin C helps in the oxidation of para-hydroxyphenyl pyruvate to homogentisic acid.

Iron metabolism

Ascorbic acid enhances the iron absorption from the intestine. Ascorbic acid reduces ferric iron to ferrous state, which is preferentially absorbed.

Hemoglobin metabolism

Vitamin C is useful for reconversion of methemoglobin to hemoglobin (Hb) by methemoglobin reductase.

Folic acid metabolism

Ascorbic acid is helping the enzyme folate reductase to reduce the folic acid to tetrahydrofolic acid. Thus it helps in the maturation of RBC.

Steroid synthesis

Adrenal gland possesses increased level of ascorbic acid, particularly in periods of stress. Vitamin C is necessary for hydroxylation reactions for synthesis of corticosteroids. Vitamin C helps in synthesis of bile acids from cholesterol.

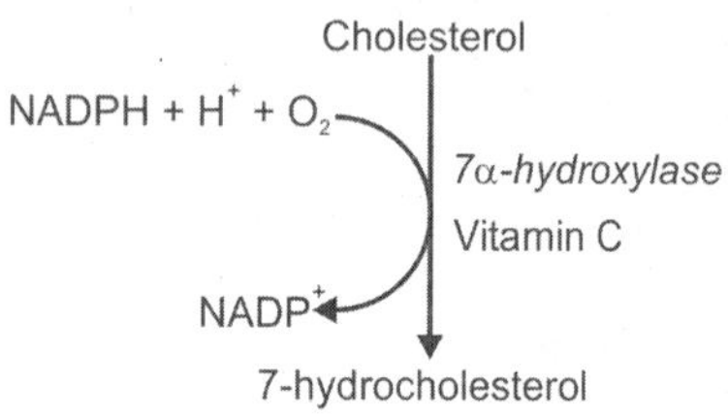

Phagocytosis

Ascorbic acid stimulates phagocytic action of leukocytes and helps in the formation of antibodies.

Antioxidant property

As an antioxidant, it may prevent cancer formation.

Cataract

Vitamin C is concentrated in the lens of eye. Regular intake of ascorbic acid reduces the risk of cataract formation.

Recommended Daily Allowance

- Adult: 75 mg/day
- Pregnancy, lactation and in aged people: 100 mg/day.

Dietary Sources

Rich sources are amla (Indian gooseberry), guava, lime, lemon and green leafy vegetables.

Deficiency Manifestations

Scurvy

Gross deficiency of vitamin C results in scurvy.

Infantile scurvy (Barlow's disease)

In infants between 6 and 12 months of age, (period in which weaning from breast milk), the diet should be supplemented with vitamin C sources. Otherwise, deficiency of vitamin C is seen.

Hemorrhagic tendency

In ascorbic acid deficiency, collagen is abnormal and the intercellular cement substance is brittle. So capillaries are fragile, leading to the tendency to bleed even under minor pressure subcutaneous hemorrhage may be manifested as petechiae (small red or purple spots on skin caused by minor hemorrhage due to broken capillaries) in mild deficiency and as ecchymoses (large purple or black and blue spots produced by extravasation of blood into tissues) or even hematoma in severe conditions.

Internal hemorrhage

In severe cases, hemorrhage may occur in the conjunctiva and retina resulting in epistaxis, hematuria or melena (black colored stools due to oxidation of iron in Hb).

Oral cavity

In severe cases of scurvy, the gum becomes painful, swollen and spongy. The pulp is separated from the dentine and finally teeth are lost. Wound healing may be delayed.

Bones

In the bones, the deficiency results in the failure of the osteoblasts to form the intercellular substance, osteoid. Without the normal ground substance, the deposition of bone is arrested. The resulting scorbutic bone is weak and fractures easily. Painful swelling of joints may prevent locomotion of the patient.

Anemia

Microcytic, hypochromic anemia is seen.

MINERALS

Minerals are essential for the normal growth and maintenance of the body. If the daily requirement is more than 100 mg, they are called major elements or macromineral. If the requirement is less than 100 mg/day, they are known as minor elements or trace elements.

Calcium

Total calcium in the human body is about 1–1.5 kg. About 99% of which is seen in bone and 1% in extracellular fluid.

Sources of Calcium

Milk is a good source of calcium. Egg, fish and vegetables are medium sources for calcium. Cereals contain only small amount of calcium.

Recommended Daily Allowance

Adult: 500 mg/day.
Children: 1,200 mg/day.
Pregnancy and lactation: 1,500 mg/day.

Biological Function

1. Calcification of the growing bones and teeth and maintenance of the mature bones are dependent on adequate dietary intake of calcium and phosphorus.
2. Calcium is an activator for a number of enzymes, e.g. adenylate cyclase, ATPases, protein kinases, etc. Calcium, even in very low concentration, activates phosphorylase kinase through its binding to calmodulin and thus increases the rate of glycogen breakdown. It activates pyruvate dehydrogenase phosphatase, which in turn activates pyruvate dehydrogenase complex to produce acetyl-CoA. Calcium also regulates the enzymes of citric acid cycle at several steps. For example, Ca^{2+} activates isocitrate dehydrogenase and alpha-ketoglutarate dehydrogenase. Thus, Ca^{2+} stimulates the production of ATP.
3. It is essential for clotting of blood.
4. It is required for the contraction of muscles (excitation-contraction coupling).
5. It regulates the permeability of the capillary walls and excitability of the nerve fibers.
6. It is also required for secretion of various hormones and acts as a second messenger.
7. Calcium regulates cell growth and differentiation.

Absorption

Mechanism of absorption of calcium is taking place from the first and second part of duodenum. Calcium is absorbed against a concentration gradient and requires energy. Absorption requires a carrier protein, helped by calcium-dependent ATPase.

Factors causing increased absorption

1. Vitamin D: Calcitriol induces the synthesis of the carrier protein (calbindin) in the intestinal epithelial cells and so facilitates the absorption of calcium.
2. Parathyroid hormone: It increases calcium transport from the intestinal cells.
3. Acidity: It favors calcium absorption.
4. Amino acids: Lysine and arginine increases calcium absorption.

Factors causing decreased absorption

1. Phytic acid: Hexaphosphate of inositol is present in cereals. Fermentation and cooking reduce phytate content.
2. Oxalates: They are present in some leafy vegetables, which cause formation of insoluble calcium oxalates.
3. Malabsorption syndromes: Fatty acid is not absorbed, causing formation of insoluble calcium salt of fatty acid.
4. Phosphate: High-phosphate content will cause precipitation as calcium phosphate. The optimum ratio of calcium to phosphorus, which allows maximum absorption is 1:2 to 2:1 as present in milk.

Calcium Homeostasis

The hormones—calcitriol, parathyroid hormone (PTH) and calcitonin are the major factors that regulate the plasma calcium (homeostasis of Ca) within a narrow range of 9–11 mg/dL (Fig. 7.8).

Calcitriol

The physiologically active form of vitamin D is a hormone, namely calcitriol or 1, 25-dihydroxy cholecalciferol (1, 25 DHCC) (Fig. 7.9).

Parathyroid Hormone

Parathyroid hormone (PTH) is secreted by two pairs of parathyroid glands that are closely associated with thyroid glands. It is originally synthesized as prepro-PTH, which is degraded to pro PTH and, finally to active PTH. The release of PTH from parathyroid glands is under the negative feedback regulation of serum Ca^{2+}.

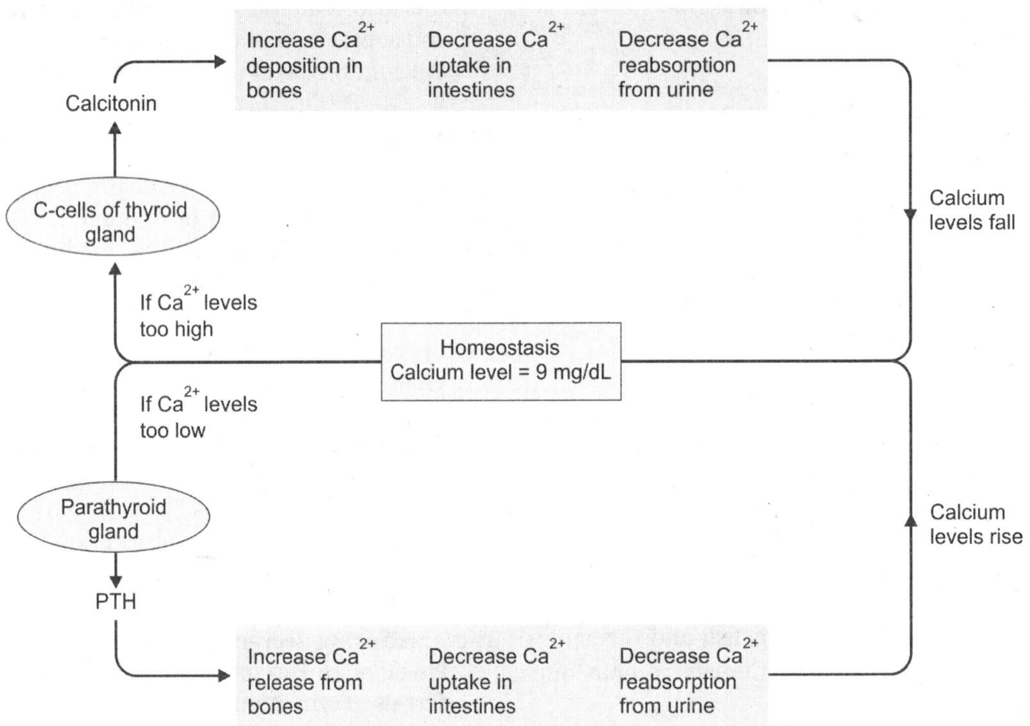

Fig. 7.8: Calcium homeostasis (C-cells, clear cells or parafollicular cells; PTH, parathyroid hormone)

Action on the Bone (Fig. 7.10)

Mechanism of Action of PTH (Fig. 7.11)

Action on the kidney

Parathyroid hormone increases the Ca reabsorption by kidney tubules. This is the most rapid action of PTH to elevate blood Ca levels. PTH promotes the production of calcitriol (1, 25 DHCC) in the kidney by stimulating 1-hydroxylation of 25-hydroxycholecalciferol.

Action on the intestine

The action of PTH on the intestine is indirect. It increases the intestinal absorption of Ca by promoting the synthesis of calcitriol.

Calcitonin

Calcitonin (CT) is a peptide containing 32 amino acids. It is secreted by parafollicular cells of thyroid gland. The action of CT on calcium metabolism is antagonistic to that of PTH (Fig. 7.12).

Plasma Calcium Disease

Hyperparathyroidism causes hypercalcemia. Hypercalcemia may also be caused by:

1. Tumors which cause rapid bone destruction.
2. Tumors secreting a PTH-like substance.
3. Vitamin D poisoning.
4. Excessive ingestion of milk.
5. Excessive intake of alkali by patients with peptic ulcer.

   Signs of hypercalcemia include:

   a. Thirst.

   b. Tiredness.

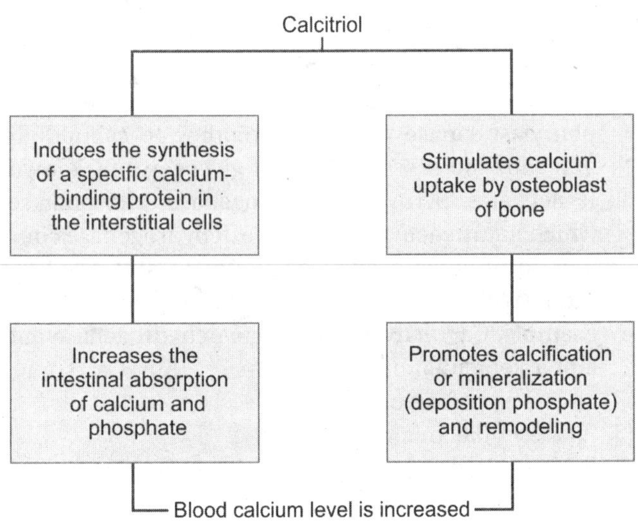

Fig. 7.9: Calcium absorption

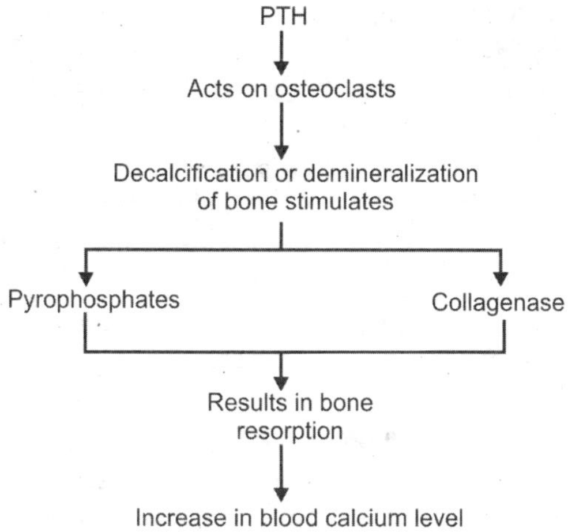

Fig. 7.10: Action on the bone (PTH, parathyroid hormone)

c. Weakness.
d. Mental disturbances, and if severe, then coma and death.

6. Untreated hypercalcemia causes renal damage.

Hypocalcemia is found in:

a. Hypoparathyroidism.
b. Osteomalacia.
c. Rickets.
d. Renal failure.
e. Tetany is a prominent feature.

The outstanding feature of tetany is neuromuscular irritability leading finally to generalized clonic movements especially in children. The muscle hypertonia produces the characteristic attitude of the hand in tetany, the main d'accoucheur. Carpopedal spasm may be accompanied in infants by spasm of the glottis (laryngismus stridulus), cyanosis, tingling feelings and sensations of heat and flushing (paresthesia).

Tapping over the facial nerve in front of the ear produces twitching of the facial muscles (Chvostek's sign), and the motor nerves are unduly excitable to electrical stimulation. Carpal spasm can be induced by inflating a blood pressure cuff around the upper arm to a pressure exceeding the systolic blood pressure maintaining the occlusion for 3 minutes (Trousseau's test).

Iron

Total body content of iron is 3–5 g. Blood contains 14.5 g of hemoglobin per 100 mL.

Requirement of Iron

- Daily allowance of iron for an adult is 20 mg
- Children between 13–15 years need 20–30 mg/day
- Pregnant woman need 40 mg/day.

Sources of Iron

Leafy vegetables, jaggery, meat, liver are good sources. Cooking in iron utensils will improve iron content of the diet. Milk is a poor source of iron.

Biochemical Role of Iron

1. It is involved in the transport of oxygen by hemoglobin and hemoerythrin.
2. It is involved in electron-transfer reactions, including the pathways of oxidative phosphorylation.
3. It is involved in the synthesis of DNA (as an essential component of ribonucleotide reductase).
4. It is involved in the catalysis of oxidation by oxygen and H_2O_2.
5. It is involved in the decomposition of harmful derivatives of oxygen, notably peroxide and superoxide.

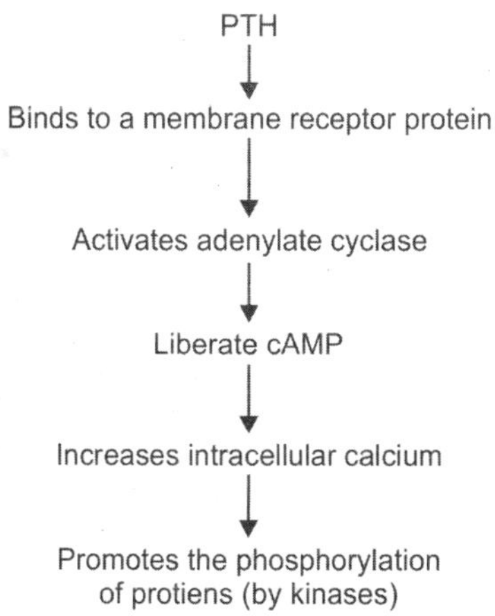

Fig. 7.11: Mechanism of action of parathyroid hormone (PTH)

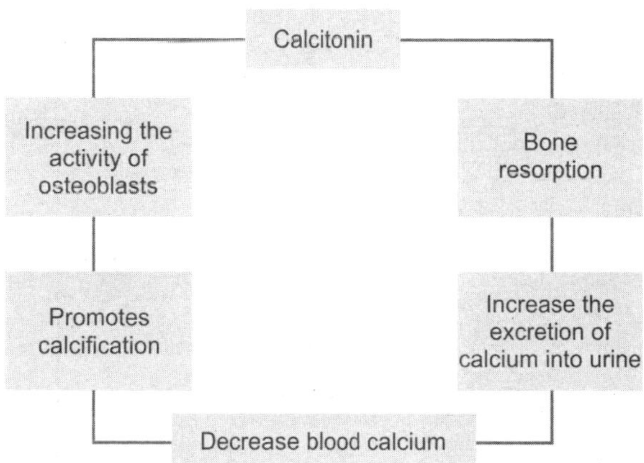

Fig. 7.12: Action of calcitonin

6. Besides, it also plays a very important role in the fixation of nitrogen and hydrogen.

Absorption

Factors affecting iron absorption

1. Intraluminal factors, i.e. dietary iron content, chemical form of dietary iron, dietary constituents, intestinal secretions, intestinal motility, stable chelators, metallic cation competitors, etc.
2. Mucosal factors, i.e. anatomic and histologic, mucosal iron content, etc.
3. Corporeal factors, i.e. body iron concentration, erythropoiesis, iron turnover, etc.

Mechanism of absorption

Granick has proposed 'mucosal block theory' for the absorption of iron (Fig. 7.13). According to it, iron is taken up by tin in the mucosal cell to form ferritin, which then slowly releases iron to transferrin present in the circulating plasma. The amount of iron absorbed is determined by the amount of apoferritin synthesized in gastric mucosal cell and not by the iron present in the lumen, because once the gastric mucosal cell tin gets saturated with iron, it cannot accept more iron. 'Mucosal block theory' is now not considered.

Transport of iron

Iron is transported in the body with a specific iron binding β_1-globulin; transferrin (siderophilin). It performs the functions of selective removal of iron from reticuloendothelial cells and intestinal mucosa and selective delivery of iron to the erythron and placenta. It is a glycoprotein, which binds two atoms of ferric iron. The iron-transferrin complex is very much stable under the physiological conditions.

Abnormal Metabolism of Iron

Iron toxicity

Hemosiderosis: Iron in excess is called hemosiderosis. Hemosiderin pigments are golden brown granules, seen in spleen and liver. Prussian blue reaction is positive for the pigments. Hemosiderosis occurs in persons receiving repeated blood transfusions. This is the commonest cause for hemosiderosis in India.

Primary hemosiderosis: It is also called hereditary hemochromatosis. In these cases, iron absorption is increased and transferrin level in serum is elevated. Excess iron deposits are seen.

Bantu siderosis: Bantu tribe in Africa is prone to hemosiderosis because the staple diet, corn, is low in phosphate content.

Hemochromatosis: When total body iron is higher than 25–30 g, hemosiderosis is manifested. In the liver, hemosiderin deposit leads to death of cells and cirrhosis. Pancreatic cell death leads to diabetes. Deposits under the skin cause yellow-brown discoloration, which is called hemochromatosis. The triad of cirrhosis, hemochromatosis and diabetes is referred to as bronze diabetes.

Copper

Total body content of copper is about 100 mg.

Recommended Daily Allowance

Copper requirement for an adult is 1.5–3 mg/day.

Dietary Sources

Major dietary sources are cereals, meat, liver, nuts and green leafy vegetables. Milk is very poor in copper content.

Absorption and transport of copper in extrahepatic tissue is shown in Figure 7.14.

Physiological Functions

1. It is required in small amounts for the synthesis of normal hemoglobin.

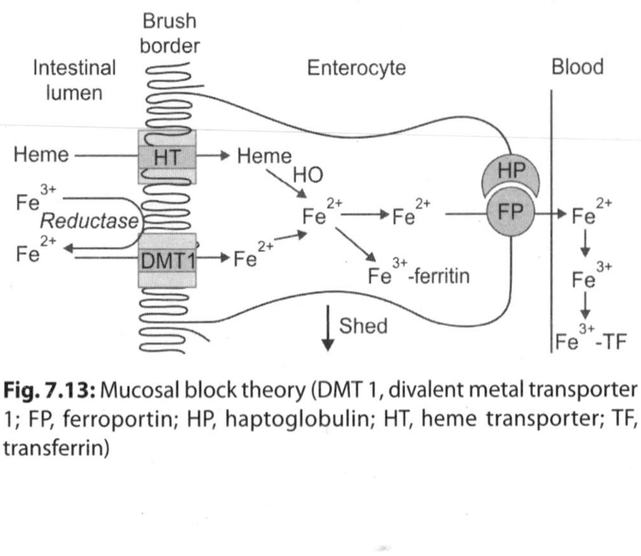

Fig. 7.13: Mucosal block theory (DMT 1, divalent metal transporter 1; FP, ferroportin; HP, haptoglobulin; HT, heme transporter; TF, transferrin)

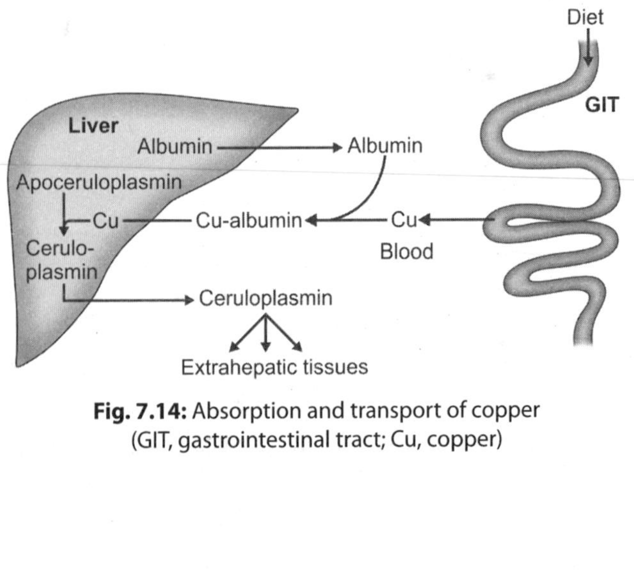

Fig. 7.14: Absorption and transport of copper (GIT, gastrointestinal tract; Cu, copper)

2. It is required for the synthesis of:
    a. Phospholipids.
    b. Melanin.
    c. Collagen.
3. It plays role in the formation of bone.
4. It maintains the integrity of myelin sheath in the nerve fibers.

Copper-containing Enzymes

1. Tyrosinase.
2. Cytochrome oxidase.
3. Ascorbic acid oxidase.
4. Uricase.
5. Monoamine oxidase.
6. Ceruloplasmin (ferroxidase I)—a blue copper-protein complex.
7. Non-ceruloplasmin ferroxidase—a yellow copper-protein complex, etc.

Abnormal Metabolism of Copper

Wilson's disease (hepatolenticular degeneration) is a rare hereditary disorder of copper metabolism, which is due to an autosomal recessive genetic defect.

The basic defect is the mutation in a gene encoding a copper-binding ATPase in cells, which is required for excretion of copper from cells.

Increased copper content in hepatocyte inhibits the incorporation of copper to apoceruloplasmin. So ceruloplasmin level in blood is increased.

Clinical Features

1. Excessive deposition of copper in liver causing hepatic cirrhosis.
2. A visible brown ring (Kayser-Fleischer ring) at the margin of the cornea.
3. Deposits in basal ganglia leads to lenticular degeneration and neurological symptoms.

Menkes disease (kinky hair syndrome) is characterized by skeletal malformations, immunological deficiency, mental retardation and defective thermoregulation.

Normochromic microcytic anemia is caused due to copper deficiency because copper is an integral part of ALA synthase, which is key enzyme in heme synthesis.

Copper deficiency may cause atrophy of myocardium. The elastic tissue of aorta, coronary and pulmonary artery gets deranged. These vessels may rupture, as a result of which end comes into death.

Zinc

Recommended Daily Allowance

Daily intake of about 10–15 mg is sufficient to meet its requirement.

Dietary Sources

Good dietary sources are meat, seafood, eggs, legumes and milk. Colostrum is a very rich source of zinc.

Biological Functions

1. Zinc is a component of several enzymes such as carbonic anhydrase, lactate dehydrogenase, alcohol dehydrogenase, alkaline phosphatase, DNA and RNA polymerases, retinene-retinal reductase, etc.
2. It is an important constituent of insulin. It forms a complex with insulin and helps in its storage and release from the beta cells of the pancreas.
3. It is necessary for maintaining plasma concentration of vitamin A, by stimulating its release from the liver into the blood.
4. It is also present in gustin, a salivary polypeptide, which is necessary for the normal development of taste buds. Thus, zinc is important for taste sensation.
5. It is also an essential component of various regulatory proteins.
6. It has been shown to be essential for normal growth and reproduction.

Abnormal metabolism of zinc

Clinical manifestations of zinc deficiency include:

1. Poor wound healing, loss of appetite, poor growth and alopecia (loss of hair).
2. Impairment of sexual development in children.
3. Impairment in brain functions, DNA synthesis and carbohydrate metabolism.
4. Certain fetal abnormalities during pregnancy besides hypogonadism, dwarfism (stunted growth) and gross skin lesions with severe acrodermatitis.
5. Zinc deficiency has also been shown to affect spermatogenesis, parturition and lactation in experimental animals.

Fluorine

Recommended Daily Allowance

Daily requirement has been defined as 2–3 mg.

Sources

Drinking water is an important source of fluoride in a human diet. One part per million (1 PPM) of fluoride in drinking water supplies nearly 1–2 mg of fluoride/day, which is sufficient to meet the requirement. Tea and sea fishes are also a good sources of fluoride.

Physiological Functions

1. This element is essential for the growth of teeth and bones and is required in minute quantities.
2. Fluoroacetate is a powerful inhibitor of TCA cycle.
3. In combination with vitamin D, it is required for the treatment of bone disease, i.e. osteoporosis, which is characterized by softening of bone as a result of excessive absorption of bone elements.
4. Sodium fluoride acts as a powerful inhibitor of the glycolytic enzyme enolase; therefore, it is used as a blocker of glycolytic pathway while collecting blood samples for the determination of sugar.
5. It forms a protective layer of acid-resistant fluorapatite with hydroxyapatite crystals of the enamel.
6. Fluoride ions inhibit the metabolism of oral bacterial enzymes and also restrict the local production of acids, which are responsible for dental caries.

Abnormal Metabolism of Fluorine

Deficiency disorders

Deficiency of fluoride promotes the development of dental caries in children and osteoporosis in adult particularly in postmenopausal women.

Dental caries is characterized by destruction of tooth enamel as a result of action of microbes (normally present in oral cavity) on food. Breakdown of the enamel exposes dentine and leads to development of caries.

Toxicity

Fluoride toxicity may manifest in two major forms, i.e. as dental fluorosis and skeletal fluorosis, which together constitute endemic fluorosis.

Dental fluorosis: The teeth exhibit fluoride toxicity in the form of mottled enamel. Mottling is characterized by multiple, minute white flecks and yellow-brown spots, which are scattered irregularly over the tooth surface.

Skeletal fluorosis: The clinical features include pain, inflammation and restricted movement of the joints and stiffness of the spine. Further, significantly higher intake of fluoride (more than 3 mg/L in drinking water) results in a severe form of the skeletal fluorosis called `genu valgum' (knock knee syndrome) (Fig. 7.15).

Selenium

Recommended Daily Allowance

Requirement is 50–100 μg/day. Normal serum level is also 50–100 μg/dL.

Physiological Functions

1. It is a constituent of glutathione peroxidase, which catalyzes the breakdown of H_2O_2 in RBCs. Deficiency of selenium in human beings is not yet well established.
2. Tocopherol sparing action: Selenium has got close metabolic relationship with vitamin E. It reduces the requirement of vitamin E in more than one way:
   a. Selenium-containing glutathione peroxidase destroys acylhydroperoxides, thus lowers the need for antioxidant action of vitamin E in preventing peroxidative damage.
   b. Selenium-May probably help in retaining vitamin E in lipoproteins.
3. It is involved in the mitochondrial ATP synthesis, ubiquinone synthesis and immune mechanisms.
4. It has been reported to be a cancer-preventing agent.

Abnormal Metabolism of Selenium

Selenium deficiency is characterized by multifocal myocardial necrosis, cardiac arrhythmias and cardiac enlargement. Selenium is known to cure the disease. Isolated selenium deficiency causes liver necrosis, cirrhosis, cardiomyopathy and muscular dystrophy.

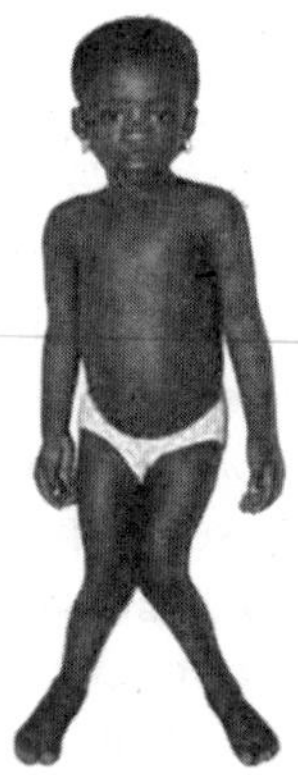

Fig. 7.15: Genu valgum

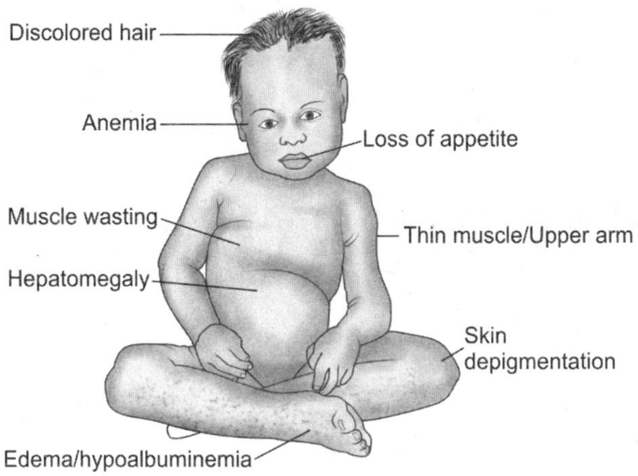

Fig. 7.16: Kwashiorkor

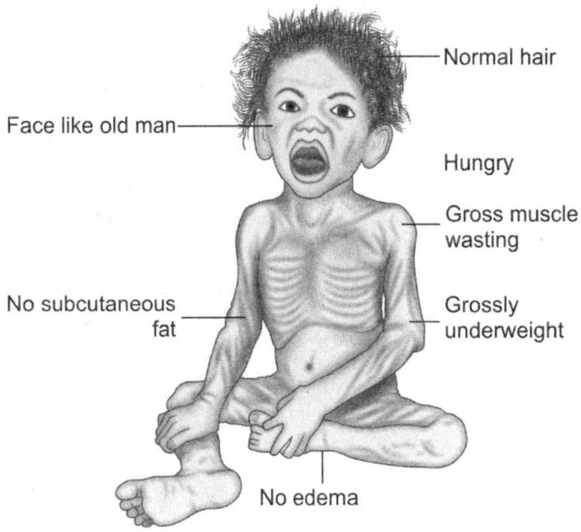

Fig. 7.17: Marasmus

Table 7.1: Comparison between kwashiorkor and marasmus

Sl No	Kwashiorkor	Marasmus
1.	Occurs in the postweaning period (1–3 year)	Occurs due to early weaning (< 1 year)
2.	Deficiency of dietary proteins	Deficiency of dietary proteins plus energy
3.	Rapid/Acute onset	Slow/Chronic development
4.	Moderate weight loss; child is 60%–80% weight for age	Severe weight loss; child is < 60% weight for age
5.	Moderate muscle wasting with retention of some body fat	Severe muscle wasting with practically no body fat
6.	Edema is a conspicuous feature	No edema
7.	Enlarged and fatty liver	Liver is normal
8.	Face reflects irritability and misery	Face shows apathy and anxiety
9.	Loss of appetite	Good appetite possible
10.	Hair shows color changes (flag sign) and becomes straight	Hair is sparse, thin and dry
11.	Skin may develop lesions	Skin is dry, thin and easily wrinkled

Selenium toxicity is called selenosis. The toxic symptoms include hair loss, falling of nails, diarrhea, weight loss and garlicky odor in breath.

PROTEIN ENERGY MALNUTRITION

Protein energy malnutrition (PEM) is one of the largest public health problems of the country. As the name suggests, this condition is a deficiency of protein and calories in the diet. Strictly speaking, it is not one disease, but a spectrum of conditions arising from an inadequate diet. Although it affects people of all ages, the results are most dramatic in childhood due to the highest requirement in that period.

Protein energy malnutrition is a general term, which includes two different types of nutritional deficiencies:

1. Kwashiorkor (Fig. 7.16).
2. Marasmus (Fig. 7.17).

The difference between kwashiorkar and maraemus is given in Table 7.1.

Chapter

8

Tissue Biochemistry

HEME SYNTHESIS

Heme is the most important porphyrin containing compound. It is primarily synthesized in the liver and the erythrocyte-producing cells of bone marrow (erythroid cells). However, mature erythrocytes lacking mitochondria are a notable exception.

Structure of Heme

1. Heme is a derivative of the porphyrin. Porphyrins are cyclic compounds formed by fusion of four pyrrole rings linked by methenyl (=CH—) bridges.
2. Since an atom of iron is present, heme is a ferroprotoporphyrin. The pyrrole rings are named as I, II, III, IV and the bridges as alpha (α), beta (β), gamma (γ) and delta (δ). The possible areas of substitution are denoted as 1–8 (Fig. 8.1).

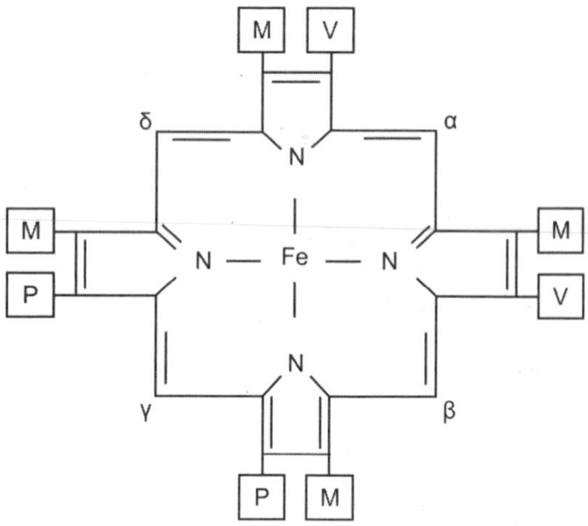

Fig. 8.1: Structure of heme

3. Type III is the most predominant in biological systems. It is also called series 9.

Biosynthesis of Heme

Heme can be synthesized by almost all the tissues in the body. Heme is synthesized in the normoblasts, but not in the matured erythrocytes. The pathway is partly cytoplasmic and partly mitochondrial.

Step 1: Formation of δ-aminolevulinate Acid

Glycine, a non-essential amino acid and succinyl-CoA, an intermediate in the citric acid cycle are the starting materials for porphyrin synthesis. Glycine combines with succinyl-CoA to form delta-aminolevulinate (ALA). This reaction catalyzed by a pyridoxal phosphate-dependent δ-aminolevulinate synthase occurs in the mitochondria. It is a rate-controlling step in porphyrin synthesis.

Step 2: Synthesis of Porphobilinogen

Two molecules of δ-aminolevulinate condense to form porphobilinogen (PBG) in the cytosol. This reaction is catalyzed by a Zn-containing enzyme, ALA dehydrogenase. It is sensitive to inhibition by heavy metals such as lead.

Step 3: Formation of Uroprophyrinogen

Condensation of four molecules of the PBG results in the formation of the first porphyrin of the pathway, namely uroporphyrinogen (UPG). The enzyme for this reaction is PBG deaminase [otherwise called uroporphyrin I synthase or hydroxymethylbilane (HMB) synthase]. HMB molecule will cyclize spontaneously to form uroporphyrinogen I. It is converted to uroporphyrinogen III by the enzyme uroporphyrinogen III synthase.

Step 4: Synthesis of Coproporphyrinogen

The UPG-III is next converted to coproporphyrinogen (CPG-III) by decarboxylation. Four molecules of CO_2 are eliminated by uroporphyrinogen decarboxylase.

Step 5: Synthesis of Protoporphyrinogen

Further metabolism takes place in the mitochondria. CPG is oxidized to protoporphyrinogen (PPG-III) by coproporphyrinogen oxidase. This enzyme specifically acts only on type III series.

Step 6: Generation of Protoporphyrin

The protoporphyrinogen-III is oxidized by the enzyme protoporphyrinogen oxidase to protoporphyrin-III (PP-III) in the mitochondria. The oxidation requires molecular oxygen.

Step 7: Generation of Heme

The incorporation of ferrous ion (Fe^{2+}) into protoporphyrin-IX is catalyzed by the enzyme heme synthetase (ferrochelatase). This enzyme can be inhibited by lead (Fig. 8.2).

Regulation of Heme Synthesis

1. The ALA synthase is regulated by repression mechanism. Heme inhibits the synthesis of ALA synthase by acting as a co-repressor.
2. The ALA synthase is also allosterically inhibited by hematin. When there is excess of free heme, the Fe^{2+} is oxidized to Fe^{3+} (ferric), thus forming hematin.
3. The compartmentalization of the enzymes of heme synthesis makes the regulation easier for the regulation. The rate-limiting enzyme is in the mitochondria. Some steps take place inside mitochondria, while rest occurs in cytoplasm.
4. Drugs like barbiturates induce heme synthesis. Barbiturates require the heme-containing cytochrome p^{450} for their metabolism.
5. The steps catalyzed by ferrochelatase and ALA dehydratase are inhibited by lead.
6. Isonicotinic acid hydrazide (INH) that decreases the availability of pyridoxal phosphate may also affect heme synthesis.
7. High cellular concentration of glucose prevents induction of ALA synthase.

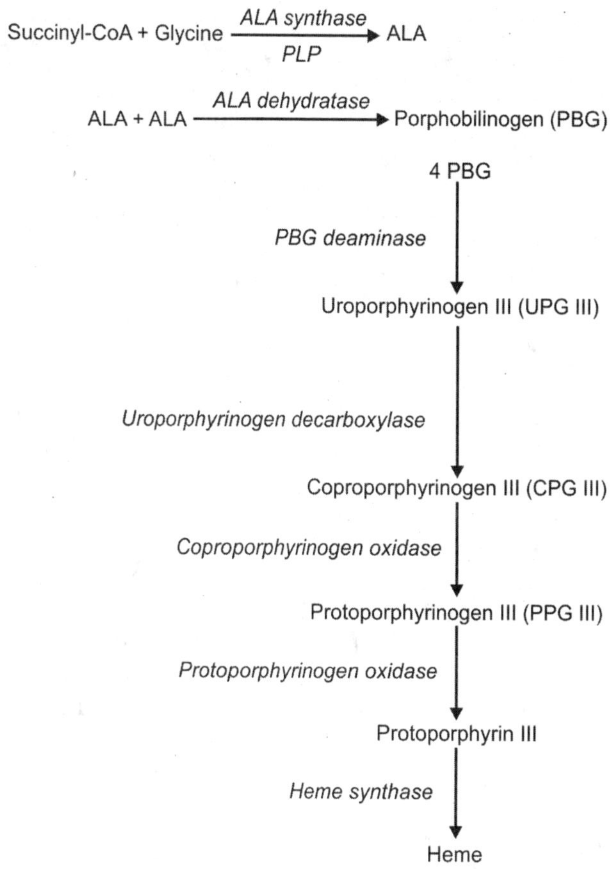

Fig. 8.2: Biosynthesis of heme

Disorders of Heme Synthesis

Porphyrias

Porphyrias are the metabolic disorders of heme synthesis characterized by the increased excretion of porphyrins or porphyrin precursors. Porphyrias are either inherited or acquired. They are broadly classified into two categories (Table 8.1):

- Erythropoietic: Enzyme deficiency occurs in the erythrocytes
- Hepatic: Enzyme defect lies in the liver.

Acute intermittent porphyria

Acute intermittent porphyria is characterized by increased excretion of porphobilinogen and 8-aminolevulinate. The urine gets darkened on exposure to air due to the conversion of porphobilinogen to porphobilin and porphyria. The other characteristic features of acute intermittent porphyria are as follows:

1. The symptoms include abdominal pain, vomiting and cardiovascular abnormalities. The neuropsychiatric

Table 8.1: Porphyrias

Types	Deficient enzyme	Features
Hepatic		
Acute intermittent porphyria	Uroporphyrinogen synthase (PBG deaminase)	Abdominal pain, neuropsychiatric symptoms
Porphyria cutanea tarda	Uroporphyrinogen de-arboxylase	Photosensitivity
Hereditary coproporphyria	Coproporphyrinogen oxidase	Abdominal pain
Erythropoietic		
Congenital erythropoietic porphyria	Uroporphyrinogen IIIco-synthase	Photosensitivity
Protoporphyria	Ferrochelatase	Photosensitivity

disturbances observed in these patients are believed to be due to reduced activity of tryptophan pyrrolase, resulting in accumulation of tryptophan and serotonin.

2. The symptoms are more severe after administration of drugs (e.g. barbiturates) that induce the synthesis of cytochrome P^{450}. This is due to the increased activity of ALA synthase causing accumulation of PBG and ALA.
3. These patients are not photosensitive since the enzyme defect occurs prior to the formation of uroporphyrinogen.
4. Acute intermittent porphyria is treated by administration of hematin, which inhibits the enzyme ALA synthase and the accumulation of porphobilinogen.

Acute intermittent porphyria symptoms (5 P's):
- *P*ain in abdomen
- *P*olyneuropathy
- *P*sychological abnormalities
- *P*ink urine
- *P*recipitated by drugs (e.g. barbiturates, oral contraceptives and sulfa drugs)

Congenital erythropoietic porphyria

1. Congenital erythropoietic porphyria is a rare congenital disorder caused by autosomal recessive mode of inheritance, mostly confined to erythropoietic tissues.
2. The individuals excrete uroporphyrinogen I and coproporphyrinogen I, which oxidize respectively to uroporphyrin I and coproporphyrin I (red pigments).
3. The patients are photosensitive (itching and burning of skin when exposed to visible light) due to the abnormal prophyrins that accumulate.
4. Increased hemolysis is also observed in the individuals affected by this disorder.

Porphyria cutanea tarda

Porphyria cutanea tarda is also known as cutaneous hepatic porphyria and is the most common porphyria, usually associated with liver damage caused by alcohol overconsumption or iron overload. Cutaneous photosensitivity is the most important clinical manifestation of these patients.

HEME CATABOLISM

In heme catabolism, heme oxygenase is a complex microsomal enzyme namely heme oxygenase utilizes NADPH and O_2, and cleaves the methenyl bridges between the two pyrrole rings to form biliverdin. Simultaneously, ferrous ion (Fe^{2+}) is oxidized to ferric form (Fe^{3+}) and released. The products of heme oxygenase reaction are biliverdin (a green pigment), Fe^{3+} and carbon monoxide (CO). Heme promotes the activity of this enzyme.

Generation of Bilirubin

Biliverdin reductase: Biliverdin's methenyl bridges are reduced to methylene group to form bilirubin (yellow pigment). This reaction is catalyzed by an NADPH-dependent soluble enzyme, biliverdin reductase. 1 g of hemoglobin on degradation finally yields about 35 mg bilirubin. Approximately, 250–350 mg of bilirubin is daily produced in human adults. The term bile pigments are used to collectively represent bilirubin and its derivatives.

Transport of Bilirubin to Liver

Bilirubin is lipophilic and therefore insoluble in aqueous solution. Bilirubin is transported in the plasma in a bound (noncovalently) form to albumin. Albumin has two binding sites for bilirubin, a high-affinity site and a low-affinity site. As the albumin-bilirubin complex enters the liver, bilirubin dissociates and is taken up by sinusoidal surface of the hepatocytes by a carrier-mediated active transport.

Conjugation

In the liver, bilirubin is conjugated with two molecules of glucuronate supplied by UDP-glucuronate. This reaction, catalyzed by bilirubin glucuronyltransferase (of smooth endoplasmic reticulum) results in the formation of a water-soluble bilirubin diglucuronide. The enzyme bilirubin glucuronyltransferase can be induced by a number of drugs (e.g. phenobarbital).

Excretion of Bilirubin into Bile

Conjugated bilirubin is excreted into the bile canaliculi against a concentration gradient, which then enters the bile. The transport of bilirubin diglucuronide is an active, energy-dependent and rate-limiting process. This step is easily susceptible to any impairment in liver function.

Fate of Bilirubin

Bilirubin glucuronides are hydrolyzed in the intestine by specific bacterial enzymes namely P-glucuronidases to liberate bilirubin. The latter is then converted to urobilinogen (colorless compound), a small part of which may be reabsorbed into the circulation. Urobilinogen can be converted to urobilin (a yellow color compound) in the kidney and excreted. The characteristic color of urine is due to urobilin. A major part of urobilinogen is converted by bacteria to stercobilin, which is excreted along with feces. The characteristic brown color of feces is due to stercobilin.

Enterohepatic Circulation

About 20% of the urobilinogen (UBG) is reabsorbed from the intestine and returned to the liver by portal blood. The UBG is again re-excreted (enterohepatic circulation). Since the UBG is passed through blood, a small fraction is excreted in urine (less than 4 mg/day).

Plasma Bilirubin

Normal plasma bilirubin level ranges from 0.2 to 0.8 mg/dL. The unconjugated bilirubin is about 0.2–0.6 mg/dL, while conjugated bilirubin is only 0–0.2 mg/dL. If the plasma bilirubin level exceeds 1 mg/dL, the condition is called hyperbilirubinemia. When the bilirubin level exceeds 2 mg/dL, it diffuses into tissues producing yellowish discoloration of sclera, conjunctiva, skin and mucous membrane resulting in jaundice.

van den Bergh Test for Bilirubin

1. Bilirubin reacts with diazo reagent (diazotized sulfanilic acid) to produce colored azo pigment.
2. At pH 5, the pigment is purple in color.
3. Conjugated bilirubin, being water soluble gives the color immediately; hence called direct reaction.
4. Free bilirubin is water insoluble. It has to be extracted first with alcohol, when the reaction becomes positive; hence called indirect reaction.

Hyperbilirubinemia

Congenital Hyperbilirubinemias

Congenital hyperbilirubinemias result from abnormal uptake, conjugation or excretion of bilirubin due to inherited defects.

Crigler-najjar syndrome type I: This is also known as congenital (non-hemolytic jaundice). It is a rare disorder and is due to a defect in the hepatic enzyme UDP-glucuronyltransferase. Generally, the children die within first 2 years of life.

Crigler-najjar syndrome type II: This is again a rare hereditary disorder due to a less severe defect in the bilirubin conjugation. It is believed that hepatic UDP-glucuronyltransferase that catalyzes the addition of second glucuronyl group is defective. The serum bilirubin concentration is usually less than 20 mg/dL and this is less dangerous than type I.

Gilbert's disease: This is not a single disease. It includes:

- A defect in the uptake of bilirubin by liver
- An impairment in conjugation due to reduced activity of UDP-glucuronyltransferase
- Decreased hepatic clearance of bilirubin.

Dubin-johnson syndrome: It is an autosomal recessive trait leading to defective excretion of conjugated bilirubin; so conjugated bilirubin in blood is increased. The disease results from the defective adenosine triphosphate (ATP)-dependent organic anion transport in bile canaliculi. The bilirubin gets deposited in the liver and the liver appears black. The condition is referred to as black liver jaundice.

Acquired Hyperbilirubinemias

Jaundice: It is a clinical condition characterized by yellowish discolorization of skin and mucous membrane. It is caused by elevated serum bilirubin level more than 3 mg/dL. On pathological basis, jaundice is classified into-three groups:

1. Hemolytic jaundice or prehepatic jaundice.
2. Hepatocellular jaundice or hepatic jaundice.
2. Obstructive jaundice or posthepatic jaundice.

Hemolytic jaundice

Hemolytic diseases of the newborn

This condition results from incompatibility between maternal and fetal blood groups. Rh +ve fetus may produce antibodies in Rh -ve mother. In Rh incompatibility, the first child often escapes. But in the second pregnancy, the Rh antibodies will pass from mother to the fetus. They would start destroying fetal red cells even before birth.

Sometimes the child is born with severe hemolytic disease often referred to as erythroblastosis fetalis.

When the blood level is more than 20 mg/dL the capacity of albumin to bind bilirubin is exceeded. In young children before the age of 1 year, the blood-brain barrier is not fully matured and therefore free bilirubin enters the brain. It is deposited in brain leading to mental retardation, fits toxic encephalitis and spasticity. This condition is known as kernicterus.

Hemolytic diseases of adults

This condition is seen in increased rate of hemolysis. The characteristic features are increase in unconjugated bilirubin in blood.

Hepatocellular jaundice

1. Most common cause is viral hepatitis, caused by hepatitis viruses. Conjugation in liver is decreased and hence free bilirubin is increased in circulation. However, inflammatory edema of cell often compresses intracellular canaliculi at the site of bile formation and this produces an element of obstruction. Unconjugated bilirubin level also increases. Bilirubinuria also occurs.
2. Dark-colored urine due to excessive excretion of bilirubin and urobilinogen.
3. Patient pass pale, clay-colored stools due to the absence of stercobilinogen.
4. Affected one experience nausea and anorexia (loss of appetite).
5. Increased activities of serum glutamic-pyruvic transaminase (SGPT) and serum glutamic oxaloacetic transaminase (SGOT) released in to circulation due to damage to hepatocytes.

Obstructive jaundice

1. Conjugated bilirubin is increased in blood and it is excreted in urine. If there is complete obstruction, UBG will be decreased in urine or even absent.
2. In total obstruction of biliary tree, the bile does not enter the intestine. Since no pigments are entering into the gut, the feces become clay colored.
3. The common causes of obstructive jaundice are: Intrahepatic cholestasis and extrahepatic obstruction.
4. Serum alkaline phosphatase is elevated.
5. Dark-colored urine due to elevated excretion of bilirubin.
6. Feces contain excess fat due to impaired fat digestion.
7. Patient experience nausea and vomiting.

Some other important types of jaundice are given below.

Physiological jaundice

Physiological jaundice is also called as neonatal hyperbilirubinemia. In all newborn infants after the 2nd day of life mild jaundice is present. This transient hyperbilirubinemia is due to an accelerated rate of destruction of RBCs and also because of immature hepatic system of conjugation of bilirubin.

Breast milk jaundice

Prolongation of jaundice in mother may increase an estrogen derivative in blood, which will transfer to the infant through breast milk. This will inhibit glucuronyltransferase system.

HEMOGLOBIN

Hemoglobin (Hb) is the red blood pigment, exclusively found in erythrocytes. The normal concentration of Hb in blood in males is 14–16 g/dL and in females 13–15 g/dL. Hemoglobin performs two important biological functions concerned with respiration:

1. Delivery of O_2 from the lungs to the tissues.
2. Transport of CO_2 and protons from tissues to lungs for excretion.

Structure of Hemoglobin

The fetal Hb (HbF) is made up of two alpha and two gamma chains. Adult Hb (HbA) has two alpha chains and two beta chains. HbA_2 has two alpha and two delta chains.

Normal adult blood contains 97% HbA, about 2% HbA_2 and about 1% HbF.

There are four heme residues per Hb molecule, one for each subunit in Hb. The iron atom of heme occupies the central position of the porphyrin ring. The reduced state is called ferrous (Fe^{2+}) and the oxidized state is ferric (Fe^{3+}). In hemoglobin, iron remains in the ferrous state.

Transport of Oxygen by Hemoglobin

Hemoglobin has all requirements of an ideal respiratory pigment:

- It can transport large quantities of oxygen
- It has great solubility
- It can take up and release oxygen at appropriate partial pressures
- It is a powerful buffer
- Each molecule of hemoglobin can bind with four molecules of O_2.

Oxygen Dissociation Curve

The binding ability of hemoglobin with O_2 at different partial pressures of oxygen (pO_2) can be measured by a graphic representation known as O_2 dissociation curve. The curves obtained for hemoglobin and myoglobin are depicted in Figure 8.3.

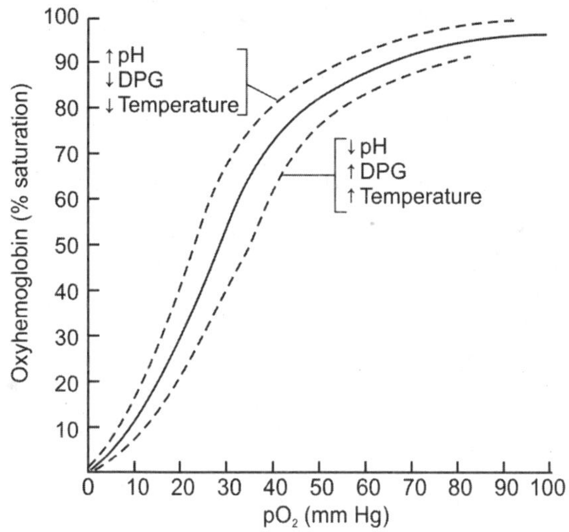

Fig. 8.3: Oxygen dissociation curve (ODC) (DPG, diphosphoglycerate)

It is evident from the graph that myoglobin has much higher affinity for O_2 than hemoglobin. Hence O_2 is bound more tightly with myoglobin than with hemoglobin. Further, pO_2 needed for half saturation (50% binding) of myoglobin is about 1 mm Hg compared to about 26 mm Hg for hemoglobin.

> **Hemoglobin binding curve: Causes of shift to right**
> '**CADET**, face right!'
> - ***C**O_2*
> - ***A**cid*
> - 2,3-***D**PG*
> - ***E**xercise*
> - ***T**emperature*

Heme-Heme Interaction and Cooperativity

The oxygen dissociation curve for hemoglobin is sigmoidal in shape, it is due to the allosteric effect or cooperativity. This indicates that the binding of oxygen to one heme increases the binding of oxygen to other hemes. Thus, the affinity of Hb for the last O_2 is about 100 times greater than the binding of the first O_2 to Hb. This phenomenon is referred to as cooperative binding of O_2 to Hb or simply heme-heme interaction. On the other hand, release of O_2 from one heme facilitates the release of O_2 from others.

The binding of oxygen to one heme residue increases the affinity of remaining heme residues for oxygen (homotropic interaction). This is called positive cooperativity. Binding of 2,3-bisphosphoglycerate (BPG) at a site other than the oxygen binding site, lowers the affinity for oxygen (heterotropic interaction). The quaternary structure of oxyHb is described as R (relaxed) form and that of deoxyHb is T (tight) form.

Effect of pH and pCO_2

When the pCO_2 is elevated, the H^+ concentration increases and pH falls. In the tissues, the pCO_2 is high and pH is low due to the formation of metabolic acids like lactate. Then, the affinity of hemoglobin for O_2 is decreased (the ODC is shifted to the right) and so more O_2 is released to the tissues. In the lungs, the opposite reaction is found, where the pCO_2 is low, pH is high and pO_2 is significantly elevated.

Bohr Effect

The binding of oxygen to hemoglobin decreases with increasing H^+ concentration (lower pH) or when the hemoglobin is exposed to increased partial pressure of CO_2 (pCO_2). This phenomenon is known as Bohr effect. It is due to a change in the binding affinity of oxygen to hemoglobin. Bohr effect causes a shift in the ODC to the right. Bohr effect is primarily responsible for the release of O_2 from the oxyhemoglobin to the tissue. This is because of increased pCO_2 and decreased pH in the actively metabolizing cells.

Chloride Shift

When CO_2 is taken up, the HCO_3 concentration within the cell increases. This would diffuse out into the plasma. Simultaneously, chloride ions from the plasma would enter in the cell to establish electrical neutrality. This is called chloride shift or Hamburger effect. When the blood reaches the lungs, the reverse reaction takes place.

Effect of Temperature

The term p50 means, the pO_2 at which Hb is half saturated (50%) with O_2. The p50 of normal Hb at 37°C is 26 mm Hg. Metabolic demand is low when there is relative hypothermia.

Effect of 2,3-Bisphosphoglycerate

The 2,3-BPG preferentially binds to deoxyHb and stabilizes the T conformation. When the T form reverts to the R conformation, the 2,3-BPG is ejected. During oxygenation, BPG is released. The high-oxygen affinity of fetal blood (HbF) is due to the inability of gamma chains to bind 2,3-BPG.

Transport of Carbon Dioxide

Hemoglobin actively participates in the transport of CO_2 from the tissues to the lungs. About 15% of CO_2 carried in blood directly binds with Hb. The rest of the tissue CO_2 is transported as bicarbonate (HCO_3).

Carbon dioxide molecules are bound to the uncharged amino acids of hemoglobin to form carbamyl hemoglobin as shown below.

$$Hb\text{-}NH_2 + CO_2 \longrightarrow Hb\text{-}NH\text{-}COO^- + H^+$$

As the CO_2 enters the blood from tissues, the enzyme carbonic anhydrase present in erythrocytes catalyzes the formation of carbonic acid (H_2CO_3). Bicarbonate (HCO_3) and proton (H^+) are released on dissociation of carbonic acid. Hemoglobin acts as a buffer and immediately binds with protons.

Haldane effect

In isohydric transport of CO_2 minimum change in pH occurs. The H^+ ions are buffered by deoxyHb and this is called Haldane effect.

Effect of 2,3-BPG

The 2,3-BPG is the most abundant organic phosphate in the erythrocytes. Its molar concentration is approximately equivalent to that of hemoglobin. 2,3-BPG is produced in the erythrocytes from an intermediate (1, 3-bisphosphoglycerate) of glycolysis. This short pathway referred to as Rapaport-Leubering cycle is described in carbohydrate metabolism.

The 2,3-BPG regulates the binding of O_2 to hemoglobin. It specifically binds to deoxyhemoglobin (and not to oxyhemoglobin) and decreases the O_2 affinity to Hb. The reduced affinity of O_2 to Hb facilitates the release of O_2 at the partial pressure found in the tissues. This 2,3-BPG shifts the oxygen dissociation curve to the right.

Clinical correlation

1. In hypoxia: The concentration of 2,3-BPG in erythrocytes is elevated in chronic hypoxic conditions associated with difficulty in O_2 supply. These include adaptation to high altitude, obstructive pulmonary edema.
2. In anemia: The 2,3-BPG levels are increased in severe anemia in order to cope up with the oxygen demands of the body. This is an adaptation to supply as much O_2 as possible to the tissue, despite the low hemoglobin levels.
3. In blood transfusion: Storage of blood in acid citrate-dextrose medium results in the decreased concentration of 2,3-BPG. Such blood when transfused fails to supply O_2 to the tissues immediately.
4. Fetal hemoglobin: The binding of 2,3-BPG to fetal hemoglobin is very weak. Therefore, HbF has higher affinity for O_2 compared to adult hemoglobin. This may be needed for the transfer of oxygen from the maternal blood to the fetus.

Hemoglobin Derivatives

Fetal Hemoglobin (HbF)

- HbF has two alpha chains and two gamma chains. Gamma chain has 146 amino acids
- HbF shows increased solubility and slower electrophoretic mobility
- HbF has decreased interaction with 2,3-BPG
- The synthesis of HbF starts by 7th week of gestation.

Methemoglobin (MetHb)

For the biological function of hemoglobin to carry oxygen, the iron should remain in the ferrous (Fe^{2+}) state. Hemoglobin (with Fe^{2+}) can be oxidized to methemoglobin (with Fe^{3+}). The oxidation of hemoglobin to methemoglobin (metHb) may be caused in the living system by hydrogen peroxide (H_2O_2), free radicals and drugs. The methemoglobin (with Fe^{3+}) is unable to bind to O_2. Instead, a water molecule occupies the oxygen site in the heme of metHb.

Carboxyhemoglobin (COHb)

Carbon monoxide (CO) is a toxic compound (an industrial pollutant) that can bind with Hb in the same manner as O_2 binds. CO has about 200 times more affinity than O_2 for binding with Hb. Clinical manifestations of CO toxicity are observed, when the COHb concentration exceeds 20%. The symptoms include headache, nausea, breathlessness and vomiting.

Abnormal Hemoglobins

Abnormal hemoglobins are the resultant of mutations in the genes that code for alpha or beta chains of hemoglobin.

Hemoglobin S (HbS) or Sickle Cell Hemoglobin

Sickle cell anemia (HbS) is the most common form of abnormal hemoglobins. It is so named because the erythrocytes of these patients adapt a sickle shape. In HbS, glutamate at sixth position of beta chain is replaced by valine (Glu Val):

1. Homozygous and heterozygous HbS: Sickle cell anemia is said to be homozygous, if caused by inheritance of two mutant genes (one from each parent) that code for beta chains. In case of heterozygous HbS, only one gene is affected while the other is normal. The erythrocytes of heterozygotes contain both HbS and HbA and the disease is referred to as sickle cell trait, which is more common in blacks. The individuals of sickle cell trait lead a normal life and do not usually show clinical symptoms. This is in contrast to homozygous sickle cell anemia.
2. Sickle cell anemia is characterized by: Lifelong hemolytic anemia, tissue damage and pain, increased susceptibility to infection and premature death.

3. Sickle cell trait (heterozygous state with about 40% HbS) provides resistance to malaria, which is a major cause of death in tropical areas. Malaria is a parasitic disease caused by *Plasmodium falciparum* in Africa. The malarial parasite spends a part of its life cycle in erythrocytes. Increased lysis of sickled cells (shorter life span of erythrocytes) interrupts the parasite cycle.

Diagnosis of Sickle Cell Anemia

Sickling test: This is a simple microscopic examination of blood smear prepared by adding reducing agents such as sodium dithionite. Sickled erythrocytes can be detected under the microscope.

Electrophoresis: When subjected to electrophoresis in alkaline medium (pH 8.6), sickle cell hemoglobin (HbS) moves slowly towards anode (positive electrode) than does adult hemoglobin. The slow mobility of HbS is due to less negative charge.

Thalassemias

Thalassemias are a group of hereditary hemolytic disorders characterized by impairment/imbalance in the synthesis of globin chains of Hb. Thalassemia mostly occurs in the regions surrounding the Mediterranean sea, hence the name. Thalassemias are characterized by a defect in the production of alpha- or beta-globin chain.

Thalassemias occur due to a variety of molecular defects such as gene deletion or substitution, underproduction or instability of mRNA, defect in the initiation of chain synthesis, premature chain termination.

Alpha Thalassemia

Alpha thalassemias are caused by a decreased synthesis or total absence of alpha-globin chain of Hb. The salient features of different alpha thalassemias are:

- Silent carrier state
- Alpha thalassemia trait
- Hemoglobin H disease
- Hydrops fetalis.

Beta Thalassemia

Decreased synthesis or total lack of the formation of beta-globin chain causes beta thalassemias. The production of alpha-globin chain continues to be normal leading to the formation of a globin tetramer that precipitate. This causes premature death of erythrocytes. There are mainly two types of beta thalassemias:

1. Beta thalassemia minor: This is an heterozygous state with a defect in only one of the two beta-globin gene pairs on chromosome 11. This disorder also known as beta thalassemia trait is usually asymptomatic, since the individuals can make some amount of beta globin from the affected gene.
2. Beta thalassemia major: This is a homozygous state with a defect in both the genes responsible for beta-globin synthesis. The infants born with beta thalassemia major are healthy at birth since beta globin is not synthesized during the fetal development. They become severely anemic and die within 1–2 years.

MYOGLOBIN

1. Myoglobin (Mb) is seen in muscles.
2. Myoglobin is a single polypeptide chain.
3. One of Mb can combine with one molecule of oxygen.
4. Myoglobin has higher affinity for oxygen than that of Hb.
5. Myoglobin has a high oxygen affinity, while Bohr effect and 2,3-BPG effect are absent.
6. Severe crush injury causes release of Mb from the damaged muscles. Being a small molecular weight protein, Mb is excreted through urine (myoglobinuria). Urine color becomes dark red.
7. Myoglobin will be released from myocardium during myocardial infarction (MI) and is seen in serum. Serum myoglobin estimation is useful in early detection of myocardial infarction.

IMMUNOCHEMISTRY

Immunology is one of the rapidly advancing branches of medical science. Three salient features of immunological reactions are: Recognition of self from non-self or foreign substances, specificity of the reactions and memory of the response.

IMMUNITY

The ability of the body to detect and respond appropriately to the invading microorganisms and other foreign materials that have managed to penetrate the body is called immunity. Based on the time of development of immunity, it is classified into innate and acquired/adaptive immunity; whereas based on the mode of development it is classified into active and passive immunity.

Types of Immunity

Based on the development, immunity can be divided into innate and acquired immunity (Table 8.2).

Table 8.2: Types of immunity

Innate immunity	Acquired immunity
By virtue of genetic makeup of an individual	Acquired as the individual grows up
No prior antigenic stimulus is required	Prior antigenic stimulation is required
Present since birth, hence no lag phase	Define lag phase following antigenic challenge

Acquired Immunity

Acquired immunity is developed during the life time of an individual. Classification is shown in Table 8.3.

Table 8.3: Classification of acquired immunity

Active immunity	Passive immunity
Produced actively by host immune system	Received passively by host
Requires antigenic challenge	Introduction of ready-made antibodies
Effective and durable	Less effective and transient
Lag phase is required to generate immune response	No lag phase
Immunological memory present	No immunological memory present
Not applicable in immunocompromised host	Applicable in immunocompromised host

Mechanism of Immunity

Foreign cells are destroyed or removed either by cell-mediated immunity or by humoral immunity.

Cell-mediated Immunity

1. Cell-mediated immunity is mediated by T lymphocytes.
2. Immunity against infections: T cells mediate effective immunity against bacteria, viruses and almost all parasites.
3. Rejection of allograft: When an organ is transplanted from one person to another it is called allograft. Body tries to reject such transplanted organs, mainly by T cell-mediated mechanism.
4. Helper function: T-helper (TH) cells are necessary for optimal antibody production by plasma cells and for generation of cytotoxic T cells. They are selectively destroyed in AIDS.
5. Tumor cell destruction: Although other mechanisms are also involved in killing tumor cells, T cell activity is the predominant one.

Humoral Immunity

1. Humoral immunity mediated by B lymphocytes.
2. Antibodies are produced by plasma cells, which are derived from B lymphocytes. These are immunoglobulins.
3. The antigen-antibody reaction leads to activation of complement system, which destroys the foreign cells.

IMMUNOGLOBULINS

Immunoglobulins (Ig) form a related, but enormously diverse group of proteins (globulins) with 'antibodies activity'. These are synthesized and secreted by mature B lymphocytes called plasma cells, in response to invasion by an antigen.

Salient Features of Immunoglobulins

1. Immunoglobulin is a Y-shaped molecule having two arms and a stem.
2. It has a quaternary structure with four polypeptide chains, which are bound by disulfide (-S-S-) linkages.
3. They comprise of two small subunits called light (L) chains and two large subunits called heavy (H) chains.
4. Each subunit has a variable region towards the N-terminal end and constant region(s) towards the C-terminal end.
5. The two arms are called the Fab fragments (antigen-binding fragments), whereas the stem is called the Fc fragment (crystallizable fragment).
6. The arms and the stem are linked together by a flexible region called hinge region.

Classification of Immunoglobulin

Humans have five classes of immunoglobulins, namely IgG, IgA, IgM, IgD and IgE.

Immunoglobulin G

1. Immunoglobulin G (IgG) is the most abundant (75%–80%) class of immunoglobulins.
2. IgG is composed of a single Y-shaped unit (monomer) (Fig. 8.4).
3. It can traverse blood vessels readily.
4. IgG is the only immunoglobulin that can cross the placenta and transfer the mother's immunity to the developing fetus (passive immunity).
5. IgG triggers destruction mediated by complement system.

Immunoglobulin A

1. Immunoglobulin A (IgA) occurs as a single (monomer—serum IgA) or double unit (dimer—secretory IgA) held together by J chain.

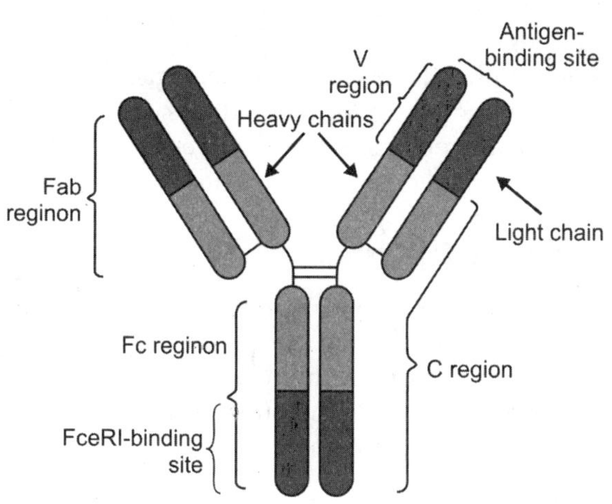

Fig. 8.4: Immunoglobulin (Fab, fragment antigen binding; Fc, fraction crystallizable; FceRI, receptor for Fc region of IgE; C, constant; V, variable).

2. It is mostly found in tears, sweat, milk and the walls of intestine.
3. IgA is the most predominant antibody in colostrum.
4. The IgA molecules bind with bacterial antigens present on the body surfaces and remove them. In this way, IgA prevents the foreign substances from entering the body cells.

Immunoglobulin M

1. Immunoglobulin M (IgM) is the largest immunoglobulin composed of five Y-shaped units held together by J chain (pentamer).
2. Due to its large size, IgM cannot traverse blood vessels, hence it is restricted to the bloodstream.
3. IgM is the first antibody produced in response to antigen and is the most effective against invading microorganisms.

Immunoglobulin D

1. Immunoglobulin D (IgD) is composed of a single Y-shaped unit and is present in a low concentration in the circulation.
2. IgD molecules are present on the surface of B cells.
3. It may function as B-cell receptor.

Immunoglobulin E

1. Immunoglobulin E (IgE) is a single Y-shaped monomer.
2. It is normally present in minute concentration in blood.
3. IgE levels are elevated in individuals with allergies as it is associated with the body's allergic responses.
4. The IgE molecules tightly bind with mast cells, which release histamine and cause allergy.

Multiple Myeloma

Multiple myeloma is due to the malignancy of a single clone of plasma cells in the bone marrow and results in overproduction of abnormal immunoglobulins, mostly IgG and in some cases IgA or IgM. In patients of multiple myeloma, the synthesis of normal immunoglobulins is diminished causing depressed immunity. Hence, recurrent infections are common in these patients.

Electrophoretic Pattern

There is a sharp and distinct band (M band for myeloma globulin) between beta- and gamma-globulins. M band almost replaces the gamma globulin band due to the diminished synthesis of normal gamma-globulins.

Bence-Jones Proteins

Bence-Jones proteins are the light chains of immunoglobulins that are synthesized in excess. About 20% of the patients of multiple myeloma, Bence-Jones proteins are excreted in urine, which often damages the renal tubules. The presence of Bence-Jones proteins in urine can be detected by specific tests:

1. Electrophoresis of concentrated urine is the best test to detect Bence-Jones proteins in urine.
2. The classical heat test involves the precipitation of Bence-Jones protein, when slightly acidified urine is heated to 40°C–50°C. This precipitate redissolves on further heating of urine to boiling point. It reappears again on cooling urine to about 70°C.
3. Bradshaw's test involves layering of urine on concentrated HCl that forms a white ring of precipitate, if Bence-Jones proteins are present.

Amyloidosis

Amyloidosis is characterized by the deposits of light chain fragments in the tissue (liver, kidney, intestine) of multiple myeloma patients.

Clinical Correlation

Amyloidosis occurs by the deposition of fragments of various plasma proteins in tissues, amyloidosis is the accumulation of various insoluble fibrillar proteins between the cells of tissues to an extent that affects function. The fibrils generally represent proteolytic fragments of various plasma proteins and possess a beta-pleated sheet structure.

ACID-BASE BALANCE

Acids and Bases

According to Bronsted, acids are substances that are capable of donating protons and bases are those that accept protons. Acids are proton donors and bases are proton acceptors.

Henderson-Hasselbalch equation:

$$pH = pK_a + \log [base]/[acid]$$

or

$$pH = pK_a + \log [salt]/[acid]$$

MAINTENANCE OF BLOOD pH

The body has developed three lines of defense to regulate the body's acid-base balance and maintain the blood pH:

- Blood buffers
- Respiratory mechanism
- Renal mechanism.

BUFFERS OF THE BODY FLUIDS

A buffer may be defined as a solution of a weak acid and its salt with a strong base and it resists the change in pH by the addition of acid or alkali and the buffering capacity is dependent on the absolute concentration of salt and acid. The blood contains three buffer systems:

- Bicarbonate buffer
- Phosphate buffer
- Protein buffer.

Bicarbonate Buffer System

The most important buffer system in plasma is the bicarbonate-carbonic acid system ($NaHCO_3/H_2CO_3$). The base constituent, bicarbonate ion (HCO_3^-) is regulated by the kidney (metabolic component). The acid part, carbonic acid (H_2CO_3) is under respiratory regulation (respiratory component).

The normal bicarbonate level of plasma is 24 mmol/L. The normal pCO_2 of arterial blood is 40 mm Hg. Hence, normal carbonic acid concentration in blood is 1.2 mmol/L. The pK_a for carbonic acid is 6.1.

$$H_2CO_3 \longleftrightarrow H^+ + HCO_3^-$$

Substituting these values in the Henderson-Hasselbalchs equation:

$$pH = pKa + \log [HCO_3^-]/[H_2CO_3]$$

$$pH = 6.1 + \log 24/1.2 = 6.1 + \log 20 = 7.4$$

The ratio of HCO_3^- : H_2CO_3 at pH 7.4 is 20 under normal conditions.

The bicarbonate carbonic acid buffer system is most important for the following reasons:

1. Presence of bicarbonate in relatively high concentrations.
2. The components are under physiological control, CO_2 by lungs and bicarbonate by kidneys.

Bicarbonate represents the alkali reserve and it has to be sufficiently high to meet the acid load.

Phosphate Buffer System

Phosphate buffer system is mainly an intracellular buffer. Its concentration in plasma is very low. Sodium dihydrogen phosphate and disodium hydrogen phosphate (NaH_2PO_4-Na_2HPO_4) constitute the phosphate buffer, with pKa of 6.8 close to blood pH 7.4.

Protein Buffer System

The plasma proteins and hemoglobin together constitute the protein buffer system of the blood. The buffering capacity of proteins is dependent on the pKa of ionizable groups of amino acids. Hemoglobin of red blood cell (RBC) is also an important buffer.

RESPIRATORY REGULATION OF pH

Respiratory system provides a rapid mechanism for the maintenance of acid-base balance. This is achieved by regulating the concentration of H_2CO_3 in the blood.

$$H_2CO_3 \xleftrightarrow{\textit{Carbonic anhydrase}} CO_2 + H_2O$$

The large volumes of CO_2 produced by the cellular metabolic activity endanger the acid-base equilibrium of the body. But in normal circumstances, all of this CO_2 is eliminated from the body in expired air via the lungs.

Hemoglobin as a Buffer

Hemoglobin of RBCs is also important in the respiratory regulation of pH. At tissue level Hb binds to H^+, helps to transport CO_2 as HCO_3^- (isohydric transport). In the lungs, Hb combines with O_2, H^+ ions are removed, which combine with HCO_3^- to form H_2CO_3.

RENAL REGULATION OF pH

Normal urine has pH around 6; this pH is lower than that of extracellular fluid (pH = 7.4). This is called acidification of urine. The pH of the urine may vary from as low as 4.5 to as high as 9.8. The major mechanisms for regulation of pH are:

- Excretion of H^+
- Reabsorption of bicarbonate (recovery of bicarbonate)
- Excretion of titratable acid
- Excretion of NH_4^+ (ammonium ions).

Excretion of H^+, Generation of Bicarbonate

Excretion of H^+ occurs in the proximal convoluted tubules of the nephron. There is net excretion of hydrogen ions and net generation of bicarbonate. So this mechanism serves to increase the alkali reserve (Fig. 8.5).

Reabsorption of Bicarbonate

Reabosorption of bicarbonate is mainly a mechanism to conserve base. There is no net excretion of H^+. Bicarbonate is filtered by the glomerulus. This is completely reabsorbed by the proximal convoluted tubule, so that the urine is normally bicarbonate free. The net effect of these processes is the reabsorption of filtered bicarbonate, which is mediated by the sodium-hydrogen exchanger. But this mechanism prevents the loss of bicarbonate through urine (Fig. 8.6).

Excretion of H^+ as Titratable Acid

In the distal convoluted tubules, net acid excretion occurs. Hydrogen ions are secreted by the distal tubules and collecting ducts by hydrogen ion-ATPase located in the apical cell membrane. The hydrogen ions are generated in the tubular cell by a reaction catalyzed by carbonic anhydrase. The bicarbonate generated within the cell passes into plasma (Fig. 8.7). The major titratable acid present in the urine is sodium acid phosphate. The acid and basic phosphate pair is considered as the urinary buffer. The maximum limit of acidification is pH 4.5. This process is inhibited by carbonic anhydrase inhibitors like acetazolamide.

Excretion of Ammonium Ions

Excretion of ammonium ions occur at the distal convoluted tubules. This would help to excrete H^+ and reabsorb HCO_3.

This mechanism also helps to trap hydrogen ions in the urine, so that large quantity of acid may be excreted with minor changes in pH. The excretion of ammonia helps

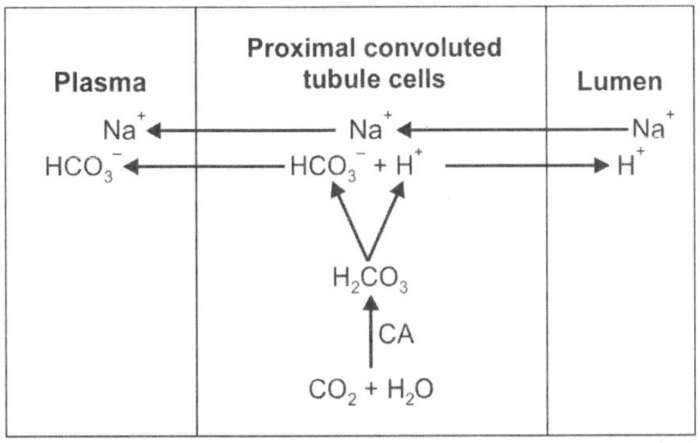

Fig. 8.5: Excretion of hydrogen ion (CA, carbonic anhydrase; HCO_3, bicarbonate; H_2CO_3, carbonic acid)

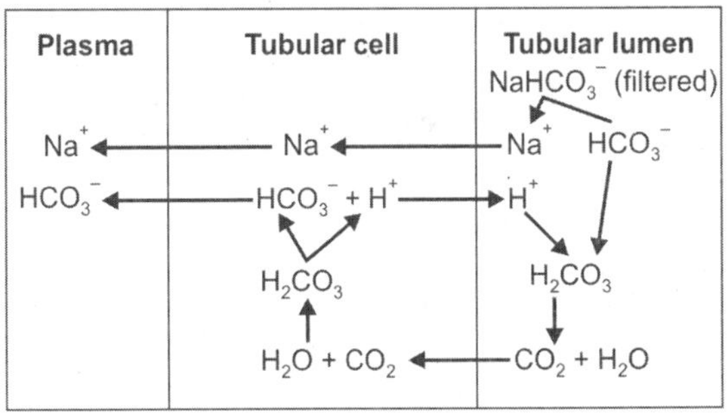

Fig. 8.6: Reabsorption of bicarbonate (HCO_3, bicarbonate; $NAHCO_3$, sodium bicarbonate)

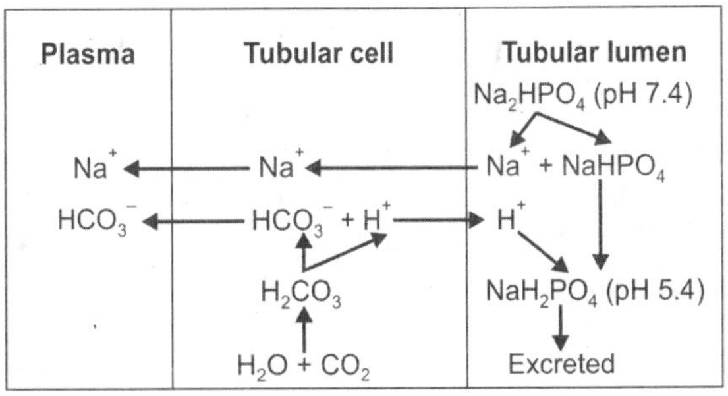

Fig. 8.7: Excretion of H^+ as titratable acid (HCO_3, bicarbonate; H_2CO_3, carbonic acid; Na_2HPO_4, disodium phosphote)

in the elimination of hydrogen ions without appreciable change in the pH of the urine (Fig. 8.8).

DISTURBANCES IN ACID-BASE BALANCE

The acid-base disorders are mainly classified as:

1. Acidosis (fall in pH).
   a. Respiratory acidosis: Primary excess of carbonic acid.
   b. Metabolic acidosis: Primary deficit of bicarbonate.
2. Alkalosis (rise in pH):
   a. Respiratory alkalosis: Primary deficit of carbonic acid.
   b. Metabolic alkalosis: Primary excess of bicarbonate.

Anion Gap

Anion gap is defined as the difference between the total concentration of measured cations (Na^+ and K^+) and thatof measured anions (Cl^- and HCO_3^-). The anion gap (A^-) in fact represents the unmeasured anions in the plasma. Normally, this is about 12 mmol/L.

Metabolic Acidosis

The primary defect in metabolic acidosis is a reduction in bicarbonate concentration, which leads to a fall in blood pH. When there is excess acid production, the bicarbonate is used up for buffering. Depending on the cause, the anion gap is altered.

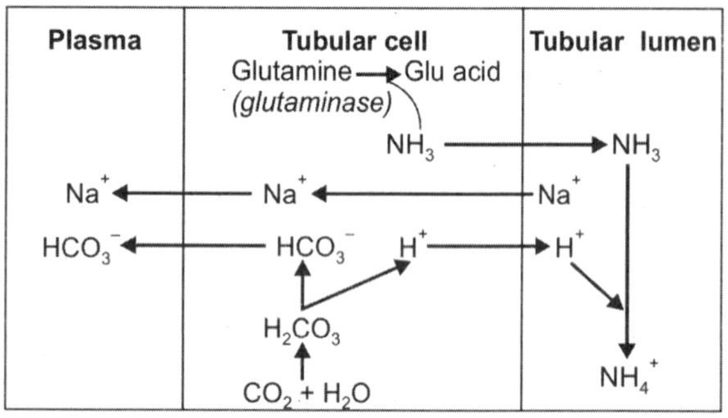

Fig. 8.8: Excretion of ammonium ions (HCO_3, bicarbonate; H_2CO_3, carbonic acid; NH_3, ammonia; NH_4^+, ammonium ion)

High Anion Gap Metabolic Acidosis

A value between 15 and 20 is accepted as reliable index of accumulation of acid anions in metabolic acidosis. The gap is artificially increased, when the cations are decreased (hypokalemia, hypocalcemia, hypomagnesemia). It is artificially altered when there is hypoalbuminemia (decrease in negatively charged protein), hypergammaglobulinemia (increase in positively charged protein):

1. Renal failure: The excretion of H^+ as well as generation of bicarbonate are both deficient. The anion gap increases due to accumulation of other buffer anions.
2. Diabetic ketoacidosis: Increased production and accumulation of organic acids causes an elevation in the anion gap.
3. Lactic acidosis: Normal lactic acid content in plasma is less than 2 mmol/L. It is increased in tissue hypoxia, circulatory failure and intake of biguanides. Lactic acidosis causes a raised anion gap.

Normal Anion Gap Metabolic Acidosis

When there is a loss of both anions and cations, the anion gap is normal, but acidosis may prevail:

1. Diarrhea: Loss of intestinal secretions lead to acidosis. Bicarbonate, sodium and potassium are lost.
2. Hyperchloremic acidosis may occur in renal tubular acidosis, acetazolamide (carbonic anhydrase inhibitor) therapy and ureteric transplantation into large gut (done for bladder carcinoma).
3. Urine anion gap (UAG) is useful to estimate the ammonium excretion.

Decreased Anion Gap

- Hypoalbuminemia
- Multiple myeloma (paraproteinemia)
- Bromide intoxication
- Hypercalcemia.

Osmolal Gap

Osmolal gap is the difference between the measured plasma osmolality and the calculated osmolality, which can be calculated as:

$2 \times [Na] + [glucose] + [urea]$

The normal osmolal gap is < 10 mOsm.

Acute poisoning should be considered in patients with a raised anion gap metabolic acidosis and an increased plasma osmolal gap.

Compensation of Metabolic Acidosis

The acute metabolic acidosis is usually compensated by hyperventilation of lungs. This leads to an increased elimination of CO_2 from the body. Respiratory compensation is only short lived. Renal compensation sets in within 3–4 days and the H^+ ions are excreted as NH_4^+ ions.

Clinical Correlation

1. Respiratory response to metabolic acidosis is to hyperventilate. So, there is marked increase in respiratory rate and depth of respiration, this is called Kussmaul respiration.
2. The acidosis is said to be dangerous, when pH is less than 7.2 and serum bicarbonate isless than 10 mmol/L.
3. Treatment is to stop the production of acid. In ketoacidosis, treatment is to give intravenous fluids, insulin and potassium replacement. Oxygen is given in patient with lactic acidosis.

Metabolic Alkalosis

The primary abnormality in respiratory alkalosis is a increase in HCO_3^- concentration:

1. Loss of acid may result from severe vomiting or gastric aspiration leading to loss of chloride and acid. Therefore, hypochloremic alkalosis results.
2. Hyperaldosteronism causes retention of sodium and loss of potassium (Cushing's syndrome).
3. Hypokalemia is closely related to metabolic alkalosis.

The respiratory mechanism initiates the compensation by hypoventilation to retain CO_2. This is slowly taken over by renal mechanism, which excretes more HCO_3^- and retains H^+.

Respiratory Acidosis

The primary defect in respiratory acidosis is due to a retention of CO_2 (H_2CO_3):

1. Acute respiratory acidosis may result from bronchopneumonia or status asthmatic.

2. Depression of respiratory center due to overdose of sedatives or narcotics may also lead to hypercapnia.
3. Chronic obstructive lung disease will lead to chronic respiratory acidosis.

The renal mechanism comes for the rescue to compensate respiratory acidosis. More HCO_3 is generated and retained by the kidneys, which add up to the alkali reserve of the body.

Respiratory Alkalosis

The primary abnormality in this is a decrease in H_2CO_3 concentration. It is due to prolonged hyperventilation. Hyperventilation is observed in hysteria, hypoxia and raised intracranial pressure, salicylic poisoning, etc.

The renal mechanism tries to compensate by increasing urinary excretion of HCO_3^-. Clinically, hyperventilation, muscle cramps, tingling and paraesthesia are seen. Causes of acid-base disturbances are given in Table 8.4.

Table 8.4: Disturbances in acid-base balance

Acidosis	Alkalosis
Respiratory acidosis	**Respiratory alkalosis**
Pneumonia	High altitude
Bronchitis	Hyperventilation
Asthma	Hysteria
COPD*	Septicemia
Pneumothorax	Meningitis
Narcotics	Congestive cardiac failure
CNS† trauma	
Metabolic acidosis	**Metabolic alkalosis**
Diabetic ketosis	Severe vomiting
Lactic acidosis	Cushing's syndrome
Renal failure	Diuretic therapy
Diarrhea	
Renal tubularacidosis	
Addison's disease	

*COPD, chronic obstructive pulmonary disease; †CNS,central nervous system.

PLASMA PROTEINS

Plasma contains over 300 proteins. Albumin, globulins and fibrinogen are the major plasma proteins, all are synthesized in the liver (except gamma-globulins). Others include apolipoproteins, protein hormones (such as insulin, prolactin, etc.), enzymes and coagulation proteins.

Total protein concentration varies from 6.3 to 8.0 g/dL out of which albumin constitutes 3.7–5.3 g/dL. Globulins constitute 1.8–3.7 g/dL. Thus, albumin: globulin ratio (A/G ratio) is 1.2–2.0:1.

The A/G ratio is lowered either due to decrease in albumin or increase in globulins, as found in the following conditions:

1. Decreased synthesis of albumin by liver—usually found in liver diseases and severe protein malnutrition.
2. Excretion of albumin into urine in kidney damage.
3. Increased production of globulins associated with chronic infections, multiple myelomas, etc.

Albumin

Albumin is the major constituent (60%) of plasma proteins with a concentration of 3.5–5.0 g/dL. Human albumin has a molecular weight of 69,000.

Synthesis

Albumin is synthesized by hepatocytes; therefore estimation of albumin is a liver function test.

Functions

1. Colloidal-osmotic pressure of plasma: Due to its high concentration and low molecular weight, albumin contributes to 75%–80% of the total plasma osmotic pressure (25 mm Hg). Thus, albumin plays a predominant role in maintaining blood volume and body fluid distribution. Decrease in plasma albumin level results in a fall in osmotic pressure, leading to enhanced fluid retention in tissue spaces, causing edema. The edema observed in kwashiorkor, a disorder of protein-energy malnutrition, is attributed to a drastic reduction in plasma albumin level.
2. Transport function: Albumin is the carrier of various hydrophobic substances in the blood:
   a. Bilirubin and non-esterified fatty acids are specifically transported by albumin.
   b. Drugs (sulfa, aspirin, salicylate, dicoumarol, phenytoin).
   c. Hormones: Steroid hormones, thyroxine.
   d. Metals: Albumin transports copper. Calcium and heavy metals are non-specifically carried by albumin.
3. Buffering action: Because of its high concentration in blood, albumin has maximum buffering capacity. Albumin has a total of 16 histidine residues, which contribute to this buffering action.
4. Nutritional function: Albumin may be considered as the transport form of essential amino acids from liver to extrahepatic cells. Human albumin is clinically useful in treatment of liver diseases, hemorrhage, shock and burns.

Clinical Correlation

1. Albumin, binding to certain compounds in the plasma, prevents them from crossing the blood-brain

barrier, e.g. albumin-bilirubin complex, albumin-free fatty acid complex.
2. Hypoalbuminemia (lowered plasma albumin) is observed in malnutrition, nephrotic syndrome and cirrhosis of liver.
3. Albumin is excreted into urine (albuminuria) in nephrotic syndrome and in certain inflammatory conditions of urinary tract. Microalbuminuria (30–300 mg/day) is clinically important for predicting the future risk of renal diseases.
4. Albumin is therapeutically useful for the treatment of burns and hemorrhage.

Globulin

Globulins constitute several proteins that are separated into four distinct bands (alpha1, alpha2, beta and gamma-globulins) on electrophoresis. Globulins, in general, are bigger in size than albumin. They perform a variety of functions, which include transport and immunity.

Hypergammaglobulinemias

Low albumin level: When albumin level is decreased, body tries to compensate by increasing the production of globulins from reticuloendothelial system:
1. Chronic infections: Gamma-globulins are increased, but the increase is smooth and wide based.
2. Multiple myeloma.

TRANSPORT PROTEINS

Blood is a watery medium, so lipids and lipid-soluble substances will not easily dissolve in the aqueous medium of blood. Hence, such molecules are carried by specific carrier proteins, which are given in Table 8.5.

Table 8.5: Transport proteins

Transport proteins	Compound bound or transported
Albumin	Bilirubin, free fatty acids, calcium and drugs
Prealbumin or transthy-retin thyroxine-binding prealbumin (TBPA)	Thyroid hormones, thyroxine (T_4) and triiodothyronine (T_3)
Retinol-binding protein (RBP)	Vitamin A
Thyroxine-binding globulin (TBG)	Thyroxine and triiodothyronine
Transcortin or cortisol-binding globulin (CBG)	Cortisol and corticosterone
Haptoglobin	Hemoglobin
Hemopexin	Heme
Transferrin	Iron

ACUTE PHASE PROTEINS

C-reactive Protein

The C-reactive protein (CRP) is so named because it reacts with C-polysaccharide of capsule of pneumococci. The CRP is a beta-globulin. It is synthesized in liver. It can stimulate complement activity and macrophage phagocytosis. When the inflammation has subsided, CRP quickly falls, followed later by erythrocyte sedimentation rate (ESR). The CRP level, especially high sensitivity C-reactive protein level in blood has a positive correlation in predicting the risk of coronary artery diseases.

Ceruloplasmin

Ceruloplasmin is a blue-colored, alpha2 copper—containing a2-globulin. Its plasma concentration is about 30 mg/dL. Ceruloplasmin binds with almost 90% of plasma copper (6 atoms of Cu bind to a molecule). This binding is rather tight and as a result, copper from ceruloplasmin is not readily released to the tissues. Albumin carrying only 10% of plasma copper is the major supplier of copper to the tissues. Ceruloplasmin possesses oxidase activity and it is associated with Wilson's disease.

Alpha-1 Antitrypsin (AAT)

The AAT is otherwise called alpha-antiproteinase or protease inhibitor. It inhibits all serine proteases (proteolytic enzymes having a serine at their active center) such as plasmin, thrombin, trypsin, chymotrypsin, elastase and cathepsin. Serine protease inhibitors are abbreviated as serpins.

The AAT is synthesized in liver. It is a glycoprotein with a molecular weight of 50 kDa. It forms the bulk of molecules in serum having alpha-1 mobility.

The AAT deficiency causes the following conditions.

Emphysema: The total activity of AAT is reduced in these individuals. Bacterial infections in lung attract macrophages, which release elastase. In the AAT deficiency, unopposed action of elastase will cause damage to lung tissue leading to emphysema.

Chapter

9

Molecular Biology

Nucleotides are the monomer units or building blocks of nucleic acids, which serve multiple additional functions. They form a part of many coenzymes and serve as donors of phosphoryl groups, e.g. adenosine triphosphate (ATP), guanosine triphosphate (GTP), of sugars, e.g. uridine diphosphate (UDP), guanosine diphosphate (GDP) sugars, or of lipid, e.g. cytidine diphosphate (CDP) diacylglycerol. Regulatory nucleotides include the second messengers cyclic adenosine monophosphate (cAMP) and cyclic guanosine monophosphate (cGMP), the control by adenosine diphosphate (ADP) of oxidative phosphorylation, and allosteric regulation of enzyme activity by adenosine triphosphate (ATP), adenosine monophosphate (AMP) and cytidine triphosphate (CTP).

PURINE AND PYRIMIDINE METABOLISM

Nucleotides are precursors of the nucleic acids, deoxyribonucleic acid (DNA) and ribonucleic acid (RNA). Purine and pyrimidine nucleotides are synthesized in vivo at rates consistent with physiologic need. Intracellular mechanisms sense and regulate the pool sizes of nucleotide triphosphates (NTPs), which rise during growth or tissue regeneration when cells are rapidly dividing.

Biosynthesis of Purine Nucleotides

Three processes contribute to purine nucleotide biosynthesis (Fig. 9.1) in order of decreasing importance:

1. Synthesis from amphibolic intermediates (synthesis de novo).
2. Phosphoribosylation of purines.
3. Phosphorylation of purine nucleosides.

Salvage Reactions

Purines that result from the normal turnover of cellular nucleic acids or the small amount that is obtained from the diet and not degraded, can be converted to NTPs and used by the body. This is referred to as the 'salvage pathway' for purines.

Conversion of purine bases to nucleotides: Two enzymes are involved:

1. Adenine phosphoribosyltransferase (APRT).
2. Hypoxanthine-guanine phosphoribosyltransferase (HGPRT).

Both enzymes use phosphoribosyl pyrophosphate (PRPP) as the source of the ribose 5-phosphate group. The release of pyrophosphate and its subsequent hydrolysis by pyrophosphatase makes these reactions irreversible.

Clinical Correlation

Lesch-Nyhan syndrome:

1. This is an X linked, recessive, inherited disorder associated with a virtually complete deficiency of hypoxanthine-guanine phosphoribosyltransferase and therefore, the inability to salvage hypoxanthine or guanine.
2. The enzyme deficiency results in increased levels of PRPP and decreased levels of inosine monophosphate (IMP) and GMP, causing increased de novo purine synthesis.
3. This results in the excessive production of uric acid, plus characteristic neurologic features including self-mutilation and involuntary movements.

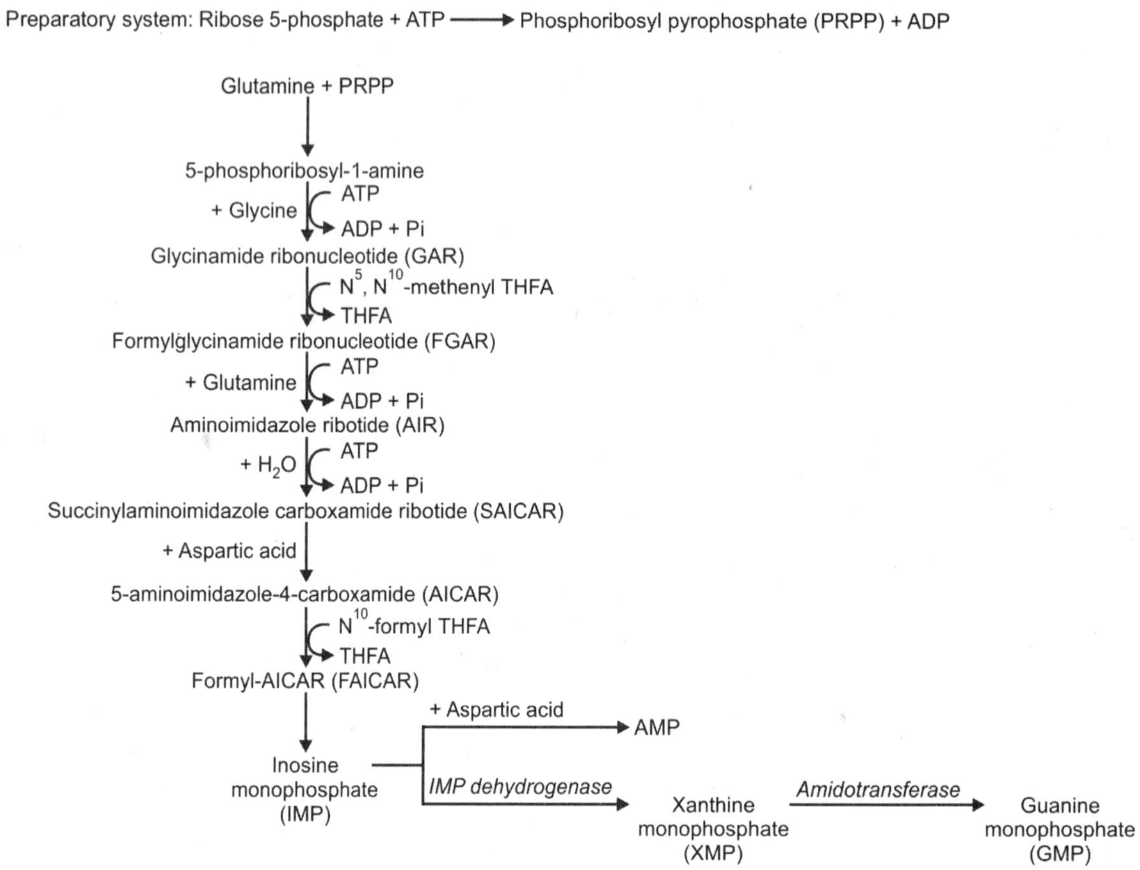

Fig. 9.1: De novo purine synthesis (AMP, adenosine monophosphate; ADP, adenosine diphosphate; ATP, adenosin triphosphate; GMP, guanosine monophosphate; THFA; tetrahydrofolate; pi, inorganic phosphate).

Biosynthesis of Pyrimidine Nucleotides

The precursors for the synthesis of pyrimidine ring are carbamoyl phosphate, which arises from glutamate and bicarbonate (HCO_3) and the amino acid aspartate. These two components are linked to N-carbamoyl aspartate and then converted into dihydroorotate. Dihydroorotate is oxidized to orotate by a flavin mononucleotide dependent dehydrogenase. Orotate is then linked with phosphoribosyl diphosphate (PRPP) to form the nucleotide orotidine 5-monophosphate (OMP). Finally, decarboxylation yields uridine 5-monophosphate (UMP) (Fig. 9.2).

Clinical Correlation

Orotic aciduria

The orotic aciduria that accompanies Reye's syndrome probably is a consequence of the inability of severely damaged mitochondria to utilize carbamoyl phosphate, which then becomes available for cytosolic overproduction of orotic acid.

Type I orotic aciduria reflects a deficiency of both orotate phosphoribosyltransferase and orotidylate decarboxylase and the rarer type II orotic aciduria is due to a deficiency of orotidylate decarboxylase only.

DNA STRUCTURE

The DNA is a polymer of deoxyribonucleoside monophosphates covalently linked by 3'5'-phosphodiester bonds. With the exception of a few viruses that contain single-stranded (ss) DNA. DNA exists as a double-stranded (ds) molecule in which the two strands wind around each other, forming a double helix. Each molecule is a strand of DNA a chemically linked chain of nucleotides. Each of which consists of a sugar, a phosphate and one of four kinds of aromatic hydrocarbon 'nitrogen bases'. The nitrogen bases can be adenine (A), thymine (T), cytosine (C), and guanine (G).

Watson and Crick Model of DNA Structure

The salient features are:

1. Right-handed double helix (Fig. 9.3): In double helix, the two chains are coiled around a common axis called

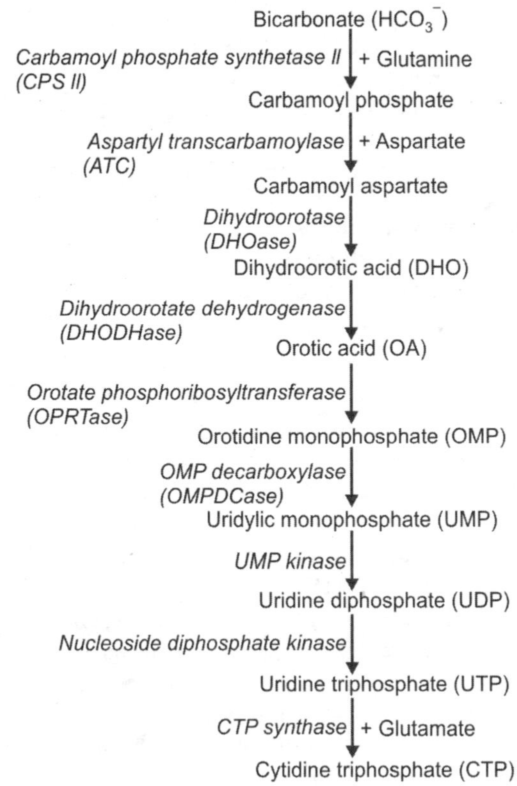

Fig. 9.2: Pyrimidine synthesis

axis of symmetry. The chains are paired in an anti parallel manner, 5'-end of one strand is paired with the 3'-end of the other strand (Fig. 9.3). In DNA helix, the hydrophilic deoxyribose-phosphate backbone of each chain is on outside of the molecule, whereas the hydrophobic bases are stacked inside. The overall structure resembles a twisted ladder.

2. Base pairing rule: The bases of one strand of DNA are paired with the bases of the second strand, so that an adenine is always paired with a thymine and a cytosine is always paired with a guanine. Given the sequence of bases on one chain, the sequence of bases on the complementary chain can be determined. The specific base pairing in DNA leads to the Chargaff rule—in any sample of dsDNA, the amount of adenine equals the amount of thymine, the amount of guanine equals the amount of cytosine, and the total amount of purines equals the total amount of pyrimidines.
3. Hydrogen bonding: The base pairs are held together by hydrogen bonds such as two between A and T and three between G and C. These hydrogen bonds, plus the hydrophobic interactions between the stacked bases, stabilize the structure of the double helix.
4. Antiparallel: Two strands run antiparallel, i.e. one strand runs in 5'-3' direction, while the other is in 3'-5' direction.
5. Other features: In each strands of DNA, the nitrogen bases are stacked at a distance of 0.34 nm almost at right angles to the axis of the helix. Each base is rotated relative to the preceding one by an angle of 35°. A complete turn of the double helix (360°), therefore contains around 10 base pairs, i.e. the pitch of the helix is 3.4 nm. Between the backbones of the two individual strands there are two grooves with different widths. DNA-binding proteins and transcription factors usually enter into interactions in the area of the major groove.

REPLICATION OF DNA

The DNA replication or DNA synthesis is the process of copying a double-stranded DNA strand, prior to cell division. The two resulting double strands are identical (if the replication goes well) and each of them consists of one original and one newly synthesized strand. This is called semiconservative replication (Fig. 9.4).

Origin of Replication

The origin of replication (also called replication origin or oriC) is a unique DNA sequence at which DNA replication is initiated and proceeds bidirectionally or unidirectionally.

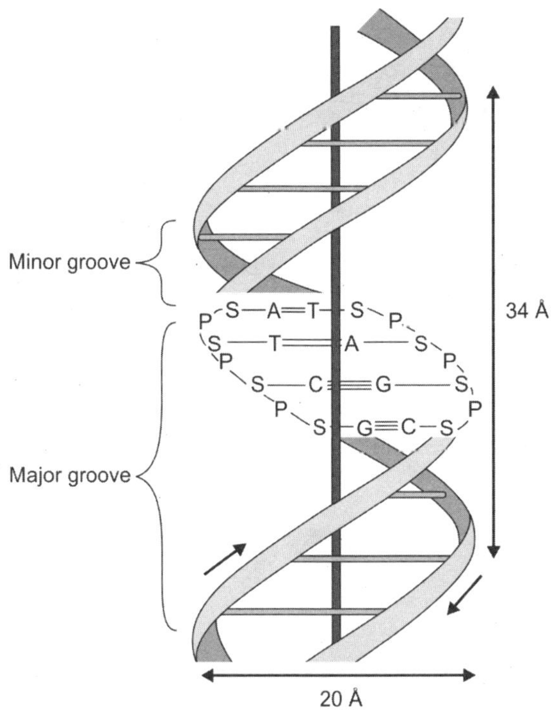

Fig. 9.3: Watson and Crick model of deoxyribonucleic acid (DNA)

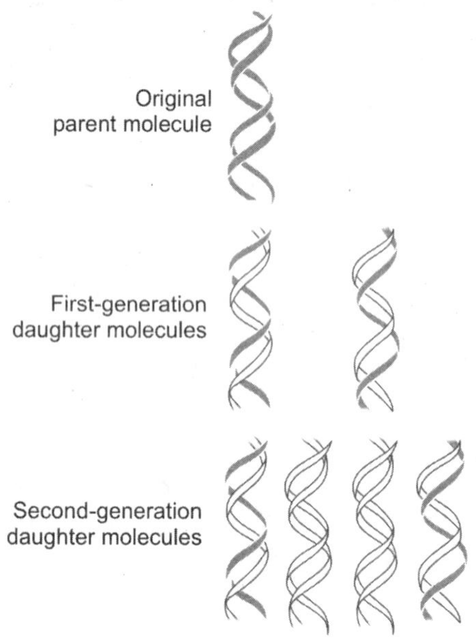

Fig. 9.4: Semiconservative mode of deoxyribonucleic acid (DNA) replication

Replication Fork

The replication fork is a structure, which forms when DNA is ready to replicate itself. It is created by topoisomerase, which breaks the hydrogen bonds holding the two DNA strands together. The resulting structure has two branching 'prongs', each one made up of a single strand of DNA. DNA polymerase then goes to work on creating new partners for the two strands by adding nucleotides (Fig. 9.5).

Basic Molecular Events at Replication Forks

Leading strand synthesis

Leading strand synthesis is the continuous synthesis of one of the daughter strands in a 5'–3' direction.

Lagging strand synthesis

1. Okazaki fragments: One of the newly synthesized daughter strands is made discontinuous. The resulting short fragments are called Okazaki fragments.

   These fragments are later joined by DNA ligase to make a continuous piece of DNA. This is called lagging strand synthesis. Discontinuous synthesis of lagging strands occur because DNA synthesis always occurs in a 5'–3' direction (Fig. 9.6).
2. Direction of new synthesis: As the replication fork moves forward, leading strand synthesis follows. A gap forms on opposite strand because it is in the wrong orientation to direct continuous synthesis of a new strand. After a lag period, the gap that forms is filled in by 5'–3' synthesis. This means that new DNA synthesis on the lagging strands is actually moving away from the replication fork.

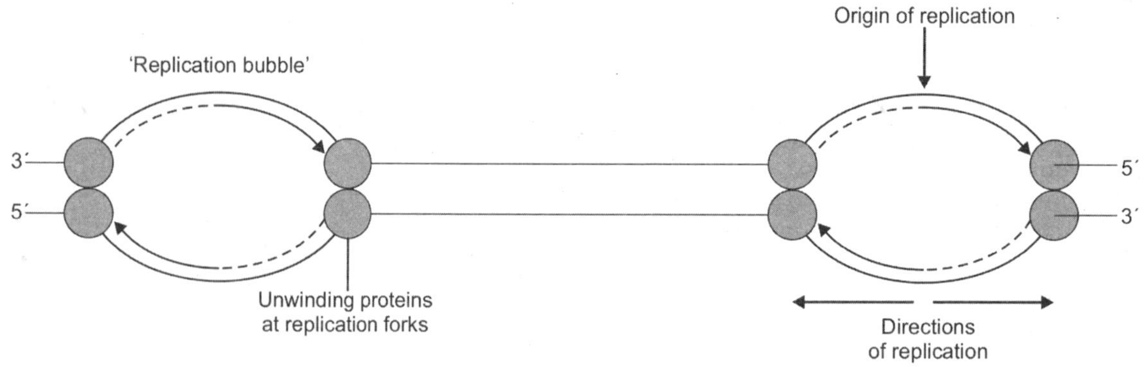

Fig. 9.5: Replication fork

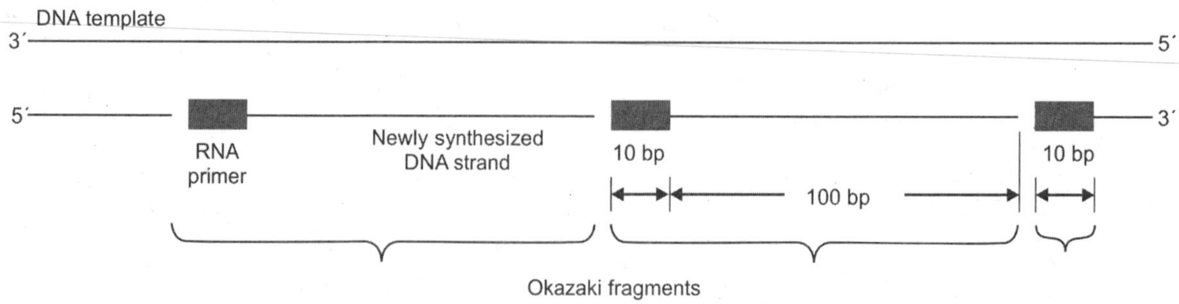

Fig. 9.6: Formation of Okazaki fragments (bp, base pairs; DNA, deoxyribonucleic acid; RNA, ribonucleic acid)

3. Priming of okazaki fragment synthesis:
   a. Enzyme: An enzyme called primase is the catalytic portion of a primosome that makes the RNA primer needed to initiate synthesis of Okazaki fragment. It also makes the primer that initiates leading strand synthesis at the origin.
   b. Primers provide a 3'-hydroxyl group that is needed to initiate DNA synthesis. The primers made by primase are small pieces of RNA (4–12 nucleotides) complementary to the template strand.
4. Joining of Okazaki fragments: After DNA polymerase (Table 9.1) has removed the RNA primer and replaced it with DNA, an enzyme called DNA ligase can catalyze the formation of a phosphodiester bond given an unattached, but adjacent 3'OH and 5'phosphate. This can fill in the unattached gap left when the RNA primer is removed and filled in. The DNA polymerase can organize the bond on the 5' end of the primer, but ligase is needed to make the bond on the 3' end.

Table 9.1: Multiple eukaryotic DNA polymerases

Mammalian DNA* polymerase	Function
α DNA polymerase	One of subunits carries the polymerase activity, responsible for the initiation of Okazaki fragments
β DNA polymerase	DNA repair
γ DNA polymerase	Mitochondrial DNA synthesis
δ DNA polymerase	Leading strand and lagging strand synthesis
ε DNA polymerase	Leading strand synthesis

*DNA, deoxyribonucleic acid

Other Factors Needed for Propagation of Replication Forks

1. Topoisomerase is responsible for initiation of the unwinding of the DNA.
2. Helicases are enzymes that catalyze the unwinding of the DNA helix.
3. Gyrase: Positive supercoils would build up in advance of a moving replication fork without the action of gyrase, which is a topomerase.
4. Single strand binding protein (ssBP):
   a. Function: SSBP enhances the activity of helicase and binds to a single strand template DNA until it can serve as a template. It may also serve to protect single strand DNA from degradation by nucleases.

Replisome

It is believed that all the replication enzymes and factors are part of a large macromolecular complex called replisome. It has been suggested that the replisome may be attached to the membrane and that instead of the replisome moving along the DNA during replication, DNA passed through the stationary replisome.

Termination of Replication

Replication sequences (e.g. ter protein) direct termination for replication. A specific protein [the termination utilization substance (TUS) protein] binds to these sequences and prevents the helicase DNAB protein from further unwinding DNA. This facilitates the termination of replication (Fig. 9.7).

DNA REPAIR MECHANISM

1. Base excision repair: A defective DNA in which cytosine is deaminated to uracil is acted upon by uracil DNA glycosylase. This results in removal of defective base uracil. Gap created is filled by the action of DNA polymerase and DNA ligase.
2. Nucleotide excision repair: The DNA damaged due to ultraviolet light or ionizing radiation is repaired by this mechanism. The DNA double helix is unwound to expose the damaged part. An excision nuclease cuts the DNA and the gap is filled by DNA polymerase. Xeroderma pigmentosum is due to a defect in this method.
3. Mismatch repair: It corrects a single mismatch base pair. For example, C to A instead of T to A. Hereditary non-polyposis colon cancer, an inherited cancer is linked with faulty mismatched repair.
4. Double strand break repair: This in DNA results in genetic recombination, which can lead to cell death. They can be repaired by homologous recombination or non-homologous end joining (Table 9.2).

Table 9.2: Deoxyribonucleic acid (DNA) repair mechanism

Mechanism	Defect	Repair
Mismatch repair	Copying error 1–5 bases unpaired	Strand cutting, exonuclease, digestion
Nucleotide excision repair (NER)	Chemical damage to a segment	30 bases removed, then correct bases added
Base excision repair	Chemical damage to single base	Base removed by N-glycosylase; new base added
Double strand break	Free radicals and radiation	Unwinding, alignment and ligation

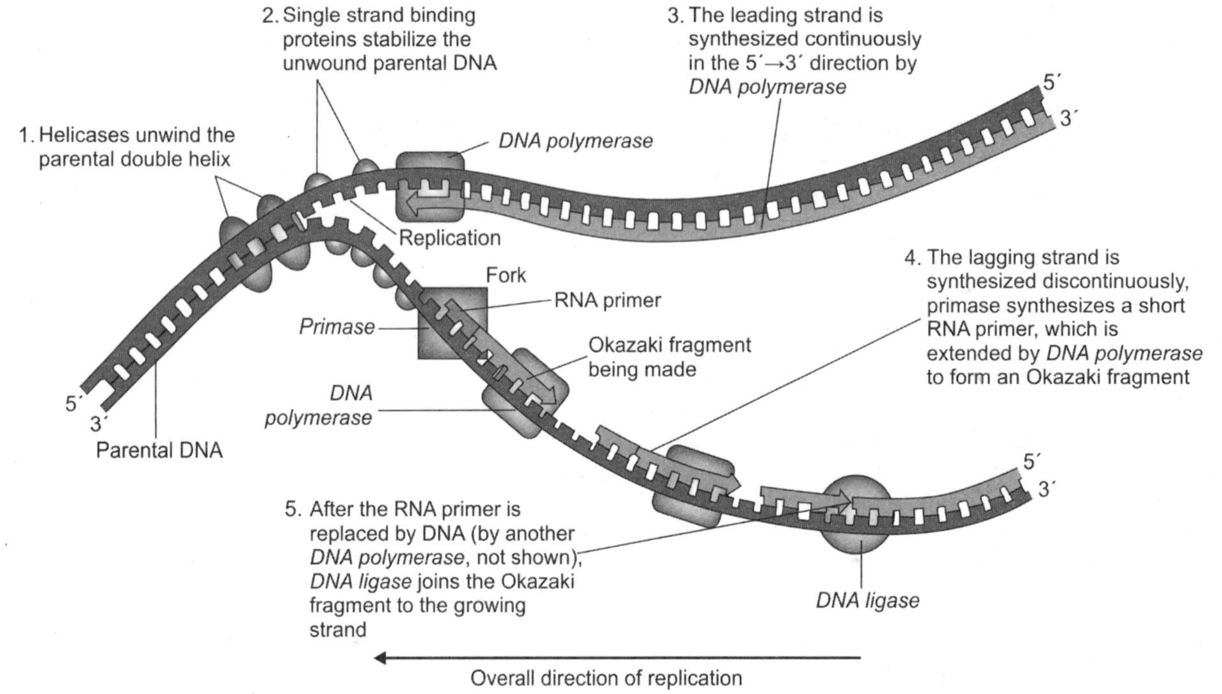

Fig. 9.7: Summary of DNA replication (DNA, deoxyribonucleic acid; RNA, ribonucleic acid)

Clinical Correlations

Diseases associated with DNA repair:

1. Defects in the repair mechanism of DNA can lead to cancer.
2. Xeroderma pigmentosum can result from a deficiency in the excinuclease, which removes pyrimidine dimers. Individuals with this disease frequently die from metastases of malignant skin tumors before the age of 30 years.
3. Defective mismatch repair can result in hereditary non-polyposis colorectal cancer. Mutations build up in the genome over time until eventually a gene controlling cell proliferation is altered, resulting in a cancerous tumor.

TRANSCRIPTION AND TRANSLATION

Transcription

The process of RNA synthesis directed by a DNA template is termed transcription and occurs in three phases such as initiation, elongation and termination.

In transcription, DNA is copied to RNA by an enzyme called RNA polymerase (Fig. 9.8).

Transcription to yield a messenger RNA (mRNA) is the first step of protein biosynthesis (Fig. 9.9).

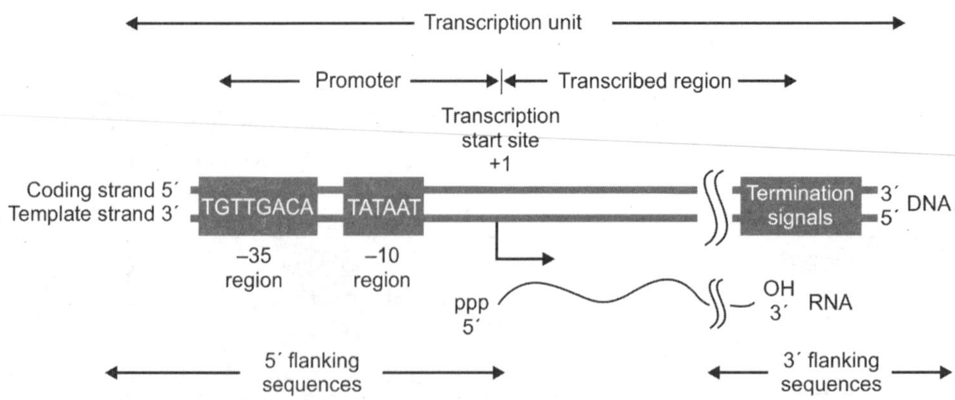

Fig. 9.8: Transcription unit (DNA, deoxyribonucleic acid; RNA, ribonucleic acid; OH, hydroxyl group; ppp, 5′-triphosphate)

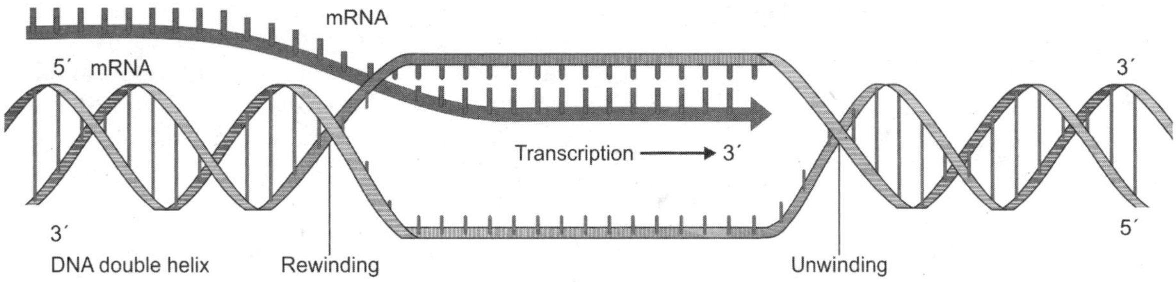

Fig. 9.9: Transcription (DNA, deoxyribonucleic acid; RNA, ribonucleic acid)

Initiation

Promoter sequences: Unlike the initiation of replication, transcriptional initiation does not require a primer. Promoter sequences are responsible for directing RNA polymerase to initiate transcription at a particular point.

Promoter sequences differ between prokaryotes and eukaryotes.

In genetics, a promoter is a DNA sequence that enables a gene to be transcribed.

The promoter is recognized by RNA polymerase (RNAP), which then initiates transcription.

Prokaryotic promoters

The promoters for most prokaryotic genes have three sequence elements:

1. Initiation site: Transcription for most genes alway-starts at the same base (position one). The initiation site is usually purine.
2. Pribnow box: Lies 9–18 base pairs upstream of the initiation site. It is either identical to or very similar to the sequence TATAAT. The pribnow box also called -10 sequences because it is usually found 10 base pair (bp) upstream of the initiation site.
3. The -35 sequence is a component of a typical prokaryotic promoter. It is a TTGAGA. Called -35 sequence because it is usually found 35bp upstream of the initiation site.

Eukaryotic promoters

Each type of eukaryotic RNA in polymerase uses different promoter. The promoters used by RNA polymerase I and II are similar to the prokaryotic promoter in that they are upstream of the initiation site. However, the promoters used by RNA polymerase III are unique because they are usually downstream of the initiation site. The initiation factors are as follows:

1. Prokaryotic σ factor is required for accurate initiation of transcription.
2. Eukaryotic initiation factors: The initiation of transcription in eukaryotes is considerably more complex than in prokaryotes, partly because of the increased complexity of eukaryotic RNA polymerases and partly because of the diversity of their promoters.

Elongation

The basic requirement and fundamental mechanism of the elongation phase of RNA synthesis is the same in prokaryotes and eukaryotes:

1. Template: A single strand of DNA acts as a template to direct the formation of complementary RNA during transcription.
2. Substrates: The four nucleosides triphosphates are needed as substrates for RNA synthesis.
3. Direction of synthesis: RNA chain growth proceeds in the 5′-3′ direction.
4. Enzyme:
   a. Prokaryotes have a single RNA polymerase responsible for all cellular synthesis. The structure of RNA polymerase is complex.
   b. Eukaryotes have one mitochondrial and three nuclear RNA polymerase. The latter are distinct enzymes that function to synthesize different RNAs.

Termination

In prokaryotes: There are two basic classes of termination event in prokaryotes:

1. Intrinsic termination (Rho-independent termination), which involves terminator sequences within the RNA as it is being made that signal the RNA polymerase to stop. The terminator sequence is usually a palindrome DNA sequence that forms a 'hairpin'.
2. Rho-dependent termination uses a termination factor called P factor to stop RNA synthesis at specific sites. When factor reaches the RNAP, it causes RNAP to dissociate from the DNA, terminating transcription.

In eukaryotes: Very little is known about how they terminate transcription.

Translation

Protein biosynthesis is the process in which cells build proteins. The term is sometimes used to refer only to protein translation, but more often it refers to a multistep process, beginning with transcription and ending with protein translation.

Ribosome

A ribosome is an organelle composed of rRNA (synthesized in the nucleolus) and ribosomal proteins. It translates mRNA into a polypeptide chain (e. g. a protein). It can be thought of as a factory that builds a protein from a set of genetic instructions.

Free ribosomes: It occurs in all cells and usually produce proteins that are used in the cytosol or in the organelle they occur in.

Membrane bound ribosomes: When certain proteins are synthesized by a ribosome, it can become 'membrane bound,' associated with the membrane of the nucleus and the rough endoplasmic reticulum (in eukaryotes only) for the time of synthesis.

Translation (also called protein biosynthesis or polypeptide synthesis) is the second process in gene expression. In translation, mRNA is used as a template to produce a specific polypeptide according to the rules specified by the genetic code.

Phases

Translation proceeds in three phases such as initiation, elongation and termination (Figs 9.10A to C) (all describing the growth of the amino acid chain or polypeptide that is the product of translation).

Initiation: The initiation of translation involves the small ribosomal subunit binding to the 'start' codon on the mRNA, which indicates where the mRNA starts coding for the protein. This codon is most commonly an AUG. In eukaryotes, amino acid encoded by the start codon is methionine. In bacteria, the protein starts instead with the modified amino acid N-formyl methionine (f-Met). In f-Met, the amino group has been blocked by a formyl group to form an amide, so this amino group cannot form a peptide bond. This is not a problem because the f-Met is at the amino terminus of the protein.

Elongation: The large subunit then forms a complex with the small subunit and elongation proceeds. A new activated tRNA enters the A site of the ribosome and base pairs with the mRNA. The enzyme peptidyl transferase forms a peptide bond between the adjacent amino acids. As this happens, the amino acid on the P site leaves its transfer RNA (tRNA) and joins the tRNA at the A site. The ribosome then moves in relation to the mRNA shifting the tRNA at the A site on to the P, while releasing the empty tRNA, this process is known as translocation.

Termination: This procedure repeats until the ribosome encounters one.

MUTATIONS

A mutation is defined as a change in nucleotide sequence of DNA. This may be either gross, so that large areas of chromosome are changed or may be subtle with a change in one or a few nucleotides.

Mutation may be defined as an abrupt spontaneous origin of new character.

Mutagenic Agents

Any agent, which will increase DNA damage or cell proliferation causing increased rate of mutations are called mutagens. X-ray, γ-ray, UV ray, acridine orange, etc. are well-known mutagens.

Classification

First Type

There are two types of mutations as given below:
1. Point mutation.
2. Multisite mutation.

Point mutation

A point mutation is defined as change in a single nucleotide. This may be subclassified as:

a. Substitution.
b. Deletion.
c. Insertion.

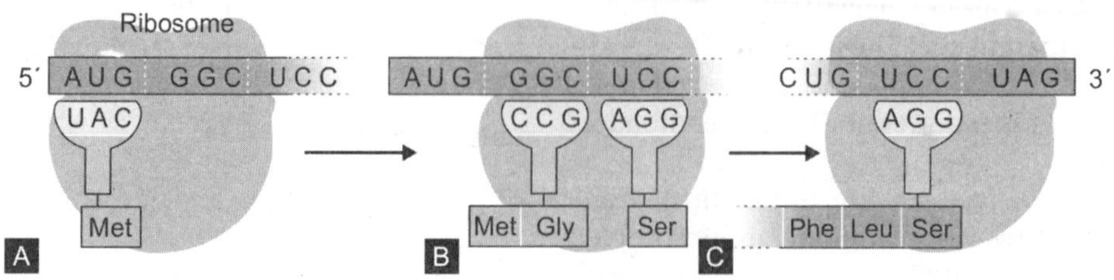

Figs 9.10A to C: Stages of translation. **A.** Initiation; **B.** Elongation; **C.** Termination. (A, adenine; C, cytosine; G, guanine; U, uracil; Gly, glycine; Leu, lerecine; Met, methionine; Phe, phenyl alanine; Ser, serine).

Substitution: One base is replaced by another and it falls into two categories:

1. Transitions: One purine is replaced by another (A → G or G → A) or one pyrimidine is replaced by another (C → T or T → C).
2. Transversions: A purine is replaced by a pyrimidine (A → C or T; G → C or T) or a pyrimidine is replaced by a purine (C → A or G; T → A or G).

Deletion: Remove one or more nucleotides from the DNA. These mutations can alter the reading frame of the gene. They are irreversible:

1. Large gene deletions, e.g. α-thalassemia (entire gene) or hemophilia (partial).
2. Deletion of a codon, e.g. cystic fibrosis [one amino acid, 508th phenyl alanine is missing in the cystic fibrosis transmembrane conductance regulator (CFTR) protein].
3. Deletion of a single base, which will give rise to frameshift effect.

Insertion: Add one or more extra nucleotides into the DNA:

1. Single base additions: Leading to frameshift effect.
2. Trinucleotide expansions: In Huntington's chorea, CAC trinucleotides are repeated 30–300 times. This leads to a polyglutamine repeat in the protein. The severity of the disease is increased as the numbers of repeats are more.
3. Duplications: In Duchenne muscular dystrophy (DMD), the gene is duplicated.

Second Type

Silent mutation: A point mutation may change the codon of one amino acid to a synonym for the same amino acid. Then the mutation is silent and has no effect on the phenotype. For example, CUA is mutated to CUC; both code for leucine and so this mutation has no effect.

Missense mutation: Both substitution and frameshift mutation give rise to an altered codon, which specifies a different amino acid from that normally located at a particular position in the protein. This is called missense mutation.

Frameshift mutation (insertion or deletion on one strand): Usually through a polymerase error when copying repeated sequences:

1. Deletions: One or more bases are removed. Unless this mutation results in the loss of a multiple of three bases, a frameshift will occur in coding sequences, drastically altering every codon downstream of the mutation and therefore the final amino acid composition of the protein.
2. Insertions: One or more bases are added. The effects are same as deletions, resulting in frameshift mutations.

Nonsense mutation: When a nonsense codon (UAA, UAG, UGA) is formed within a gene by mutation, the protein synthesis is terminated prematurely and a partial polypeptide is produced during translation. This is called nonsense mutation.

Manifestations of Mutation

Lethal Mutations

The alteration is incompatible with life of the cell or the organism. For example, mutation producing 4α globin genes is lethal and so the embryo dies.

The mutation may alter the regulatory mechanisms. Such a mutation in a somatic cell may result in uncontrolled cell division leading to cancer. Any substance causing increased rate of mutation can also increase the probability of cancer. Thus, all carcinogens are mutagens.

Silent Mutations

Alteration at an insignificant region of a protein may not have any functional effect.

Beneficial Mutations

Although rare, beneficial spontaneous mutations are the basis of evolution. Such beneficial mutants are artificially selected in agriculture. Normal maize is deficient in tryptophan. Tryptophan rich maize varieties are now available for cultivation.

Carcinogenic Effect

The mutation may alter the regulatory mechanisms. Such a mutation in a somatic cell may result in uncontrolled cell division leading to cancer. Any substance causing increased rate of mutation can also increase the probability of cancer. Thus, all carcinogens are mutagens.

REGULATION OF GENE EXPRESSION

Regulatory proteins (transcription factors) are involved in controlling gene expression in all cells. These regulatory proteins bind to specific DNA sequences and thereby activate or inhibit the transcription of genes (transcription control).

Depending on their mode of action, various terms are in use both for the proteins themselves and for the DNA sequences to which they bind. Control elements that bind activating factors are termed enhancers, while elements that bind inhibiting factors are known as silencers.

The expression of some genes is constitutive meaning that they are expressed at a reasonably constant rate and not known to be subject to regulation. These are often referred to as housekeeping genes. As a result of mutation, some inducible gene products become constitutively expressed. A mutation resulting in constitutive expression of what was formerly a regulated gene is called constitutive mutation.

If a factor operator blocks transcription, it is referred to as a repressor; otherwise, it is called an inducer. DNA sequences to which regulatory proteins bind are referred to as control elements. In prokaryotes, control elements that serve as binding sites for RNA polymerases are called promoters, whereas repressor-binding sequences are usually called operator site.

Lactose Operon

The well-investigated lactose operon of the bacterium *Escherichia coli* can be used here as an example of transcriptional control. The lac operon is a DNA sequence that is simultaneously subject to negative and positive control. The operon contains the structural genes for three proteins that are required for the utilization of lactose (one transporter and two enzymes) as well as control elements that serve to regulate the operon (Figs 9.11A and B).

Repression of lac operon: When lactose is absent repressor molecule bind to receptor cell, so RNAP cannot work and genes are in 'off' position.

Induction or derepression of lac operon: Lactose act as repressor; so repressor cannot bind to operator site, which is free; genes are in 'on' position; protein is synthesized.

RECOMBINANT DNA TECHNOLOGY

Recombinant DNA (Fig. 9.12) are the altered DNA that results from the insertion of a sequence of deoxynucleotides not previously present into an existing molecule of DNA by enzymatic or chemical means.

Applications

1. It offers a rational approach to understanding the molecular basis of a number of diseases (e.g. familial hypercholesterolemia, sickle cell disease, thalassemia, cystic fibrosis and muscular dystrophy).
2. Human proteins can be produced in abundance for therapy (e.g. insulin, growth hormone, tissue plasminogen activator).
3. Proteins for vaccines (e.g. hepatitis B) and for diagnostic testing (e.g. AIDS tests) can be obtained.
4. This technology is used to diagnose existing diseases and predict the risk of developing a given disease.
5. Special techniques have led to remarkable advances in forensic medicine.
6. Gene therapy for sickle cell disease, the thalassemias, adenosine deaminase deficiency and other diseases may be devised.

Vectors

A vector is a molecule of DNA to which the fragment of DNA to be cloned is joined. Essential properties of a vector include:

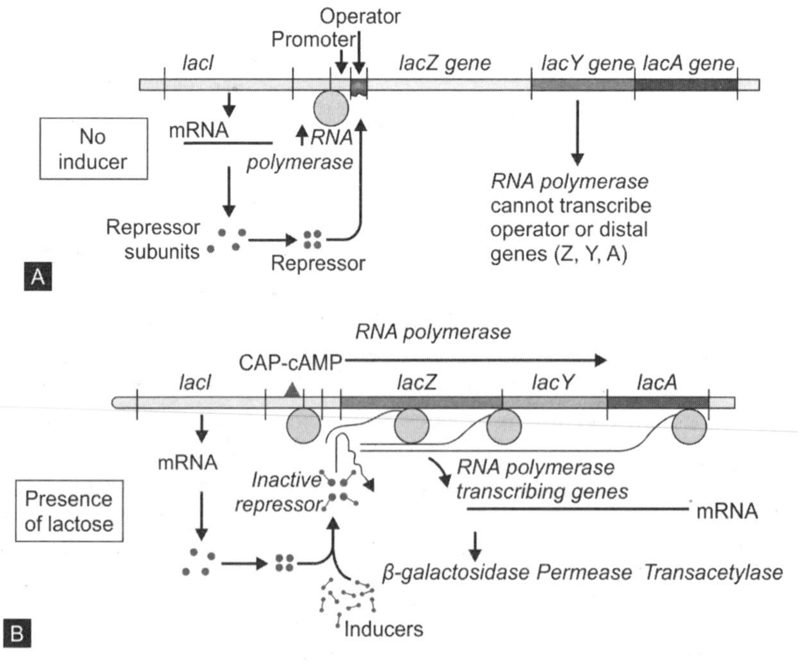

Figs 9.11A and B: Lactose operon. **A.** Transcription is blocked by repressor; **B.** Operator is not blocked, RNA polymerase can initiate transcription (cAMP, cyclic adenosine monophosphate; CAP, catabolic activator protein; mRNA, messenger ribonucleic acid).

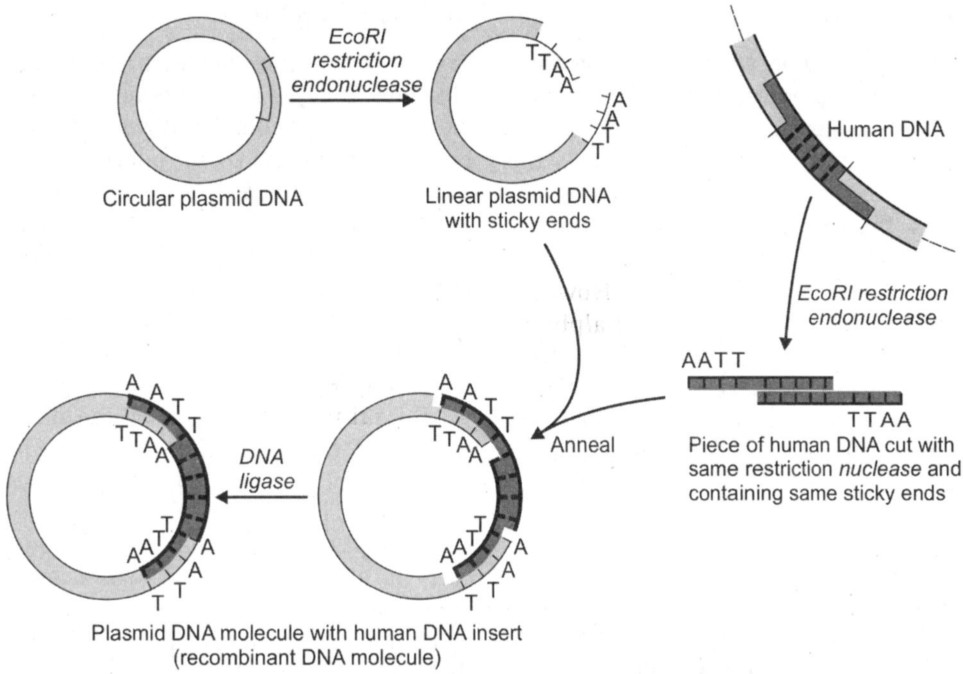

Fig. 9.12: Formation of recombinant DNA (A, adenine; DNA, deoxyribonucleic acid; T, thymine)

1. It must be capable of autonomous replication within a host cell.
2. It must contain at least one specific nucleotide sequence recognized by a restriction endonuclease.
3. It must carry at least one gene that confers the ability to select for the vector such as an antibiotic resistance gene.

Commonly used vectors include plasmids and viruses.

GENE THERAPY

Gene therapy is intracellular delivery of genes to generate a therapeutic effect by correcting an existing abnormality. Only somatic gene therapy by inserting the new gene into somatic cell of the patient is under trial. Germ cell gene therapy is considered as unethical.

Procedure

1. Isolate the healthy gene along with the sequence controlling its expression.
2. Incorporate this gene into a carrier or vector as an expression cassette.
3. Finally deliver the vector to the target cells.

Introducing Genes

1. In ex vivo strategy, where the patients' cells are cultured in the laboratory and the new genes are infused into the cells, and modified cells are administered back to the patient.
2. In situ strategy, when the expression cassette is injected to the patient either intravenously or directly to the tissue.
3. In vivo strategy, where the vector is administered directly to the cell, e.g. *cystic fibrosis (CF)* gene to the respiratory tract cells.

Retrovirus

1. Retroviruses are RNA viruses that replicate through a DNA intermediate. Moloney murine leukemia virus (MMLV) is commonly used. The *gag, pol, env* genes are deletcd from wild type retrovirus rendering it incapable of replication inside human body. Then the human gene is inserted into the virus.
2. This is introduced into a culture containing packaging cells having *gag, pol* and *env* genes. These cells provide the necessary proteins to pack the virus.
3. The replication is deficient, but infective retrovirus vector carrying the human gene, now comes out of the cultured cells. These are introduced into the patient. The virus enters into the target cell via specific receptor.
4. In the cytoplasm of the human cells, the reverse transcriptase carried by the vector converts the RNA to proviral cell DNA, which is integrated into the target cell DNA. The normal human gene can now express.

GENETIC CODE

Most of the genetic information stored in the genome codes for the amino acid sequences of proteins. For these proteins to be expressed, a text in 'nucleic acid language' therefore has to be translated into 'protein language'. This is the origin of the use of the term translation to describe protein biosynthesis. The dictionary used for the translation is the genetic code (Table 9.3).

There are 20 proteinogenic amino acids. However, there are only four letters in the nucleic acid alphabet (A, G, C, and U or T). To obtain 20 different words from these, each word has to be at least three letters long (with two letters, there would only be 42 = 16 possibilities). And in fact the codons do consist of three sequential bases (triplets).

Features

1. As the genetic code provides 43 = 64 codons for the 20 amino acids, there are several synonymous codons for most amino acids—the code is degenerate.
2. Three triplets, UAA, UAG, UGA do not code for amino acids, but instead signal the end of translation (stop codons).
3. Another special codon, the start codon (AUG) marks the start of translation. It codes for methionine.
4. The code shown here is almost universally applicable; only the mitochondria and a few microorganisms deviate from it slightly.

TRANSFER RNA

Transfer RNA molecules vary in length from 74 to 95 nucleotides. They are also generated by nuclear processing of a precursor molecule. The tRNA molecules serve as adapters for the translation of the information in the sequence of nucleotides of the mRNA into specific amino acids. There are at least 20 species of tRNA molecules in every cell, at least one (and often several) corresponding to each of the 20 amino acids required for protein synthesis.

Although each specific tRNA differs from the others in its sequence of nucleotides, the tRNA molecules as a class have many feature in common (Fig. 9.13).

The primary structure, e.g. the nucleotide sequence of all tRNA molecules allows extensive folding and intrastrand complementarity to generate a secondary structure that appears like a cloverleaf.

At the same time, at their 3' end (sequence CCA-3) they carry the amino acid that is assigned to the relevant mRNA codon according to the genetic code. All tRNA molecules contain four main arms. The acceptor arm terminates in the nucleotides CpCpAOH. These three nucleotides are added post-transcriptionally. The tRNA appropriate amino acid is attached to the 3CEOH group of the A moiety of the acceptor arm.

The molecule contains a high proportion of unusual and modified components.

These include pseudouridine (Ψ), dihydrouridine (D), thymidine (T), which otherwise only occurs in DNA. The D, T Ψ C and extra arms helps to define a specific tRNA.

Table 9.3: Genetic codes

Nucleotide base					
First	Second				Third
	Uracil (U)	Cytosine (C)	Adenine (A)	Guanine (G)	
Uracil (U)	F phenylalanine (phe)	S serine (ser)	Y tyrosine (tyr)	C cysteine (Cys)	U
	F phenylalanine (phe)	S serine (ser)	Y tyrosine (tyr)	C cysteine (Cys)	C
	L leucine (leu)	S serine (ser)	Stop codon	Stop codon	A
	L leucine (leu)	S serine (ser)	Stop codon	W tryptophan (Trp)	G
Cystosine (C)	L leucine (Leu)	P proline (Pro)	H histidine (His)	R arginine (Arg)	U
	L leucine (Leu)	P proline (Pro)	H histidine (His)	R arginine (Arg)	C
	L leucine (Leu)	P proline (Pro)	Q glutamine (Gin)	R arginine (Arg)	A
	L leucine (Leu)	P proline (Pro)	Q glutamine (Gin)	R arginine (Arg)	G
Adenine (A)	L isoleucine (iLE)	T threonine (Thr)	N asparagine (Asn)	**S serine (Ser)**	U
	L isoleucine (iLE)	T threonine (Thr)	N asparagine (Asn)	**S serine (Ser)**	C
	L isoleucine (iLE)	T threonine (Thr)	K lysine (Lys)	R arginine (Arg)	A
	Start (methionine)	T threonine (Thr)	K lysine (Lys)	R arginine (Arg)	G
Guanine (G)	V valine (Val)	A alanine (Ala)	D aspartic acid (Asp)	G glycine (Gly)	U
	V valine (Val)	A alanine (Ala)	D aspartic acid (Asp)	G glycine (Gly)	C
	V valine (Val)	A alanine (Ala)	E glutamic acid (Glu)	G glycine (Gly)	A
	V valine (Val)	A alanine (Ala)	E glutamic acid (Glu)	G glycine (Gly)	G

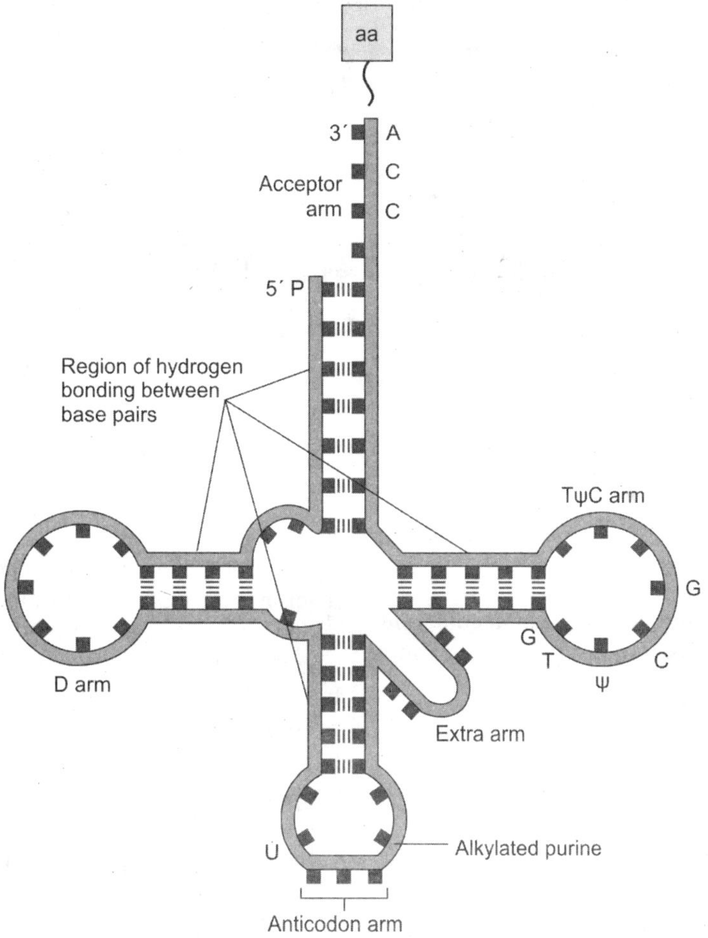

Fig. 9.13: Structure of transfer RNA (tRNA)

Although tRNAs are quite stable in prokaryotes, they are somewhat less stable in eukaryotes. The opposite is true for mRNAs, which are quite unstable in prokaryotes, but generally stable in eukaryotic organisms.

Chapter 10

Xenobiotics

FREE RADICALS

A free radical is defined as a molecule or a molecular species that contains one or more unpaired electrons and is capable of independent existence.

Types of Free Radicals

- Superoxide anion radical ($O_2^{\bullet}$)
- Hydroperoxyl radical ($HOO^{\bullet}$)
- Hydrogen peroxide ($H_2O_2^{\bullet}$)
- Hydroxyl radical ($OH^{\bullet}$)
- Lipid peroxide radical ($ROO^{\bullet}$)
- Singlet oxygen ($^1O_2$)
- Nitric oxide ($NO^{\bullet}$)
- Peroxynitrite ($NO_3^{\bullet}$).

Features of Free Radicals

The common characteristic features of free radicals are listed below:

1. Highly reactive.
2. Very short half-life.
3. Can generate new radicals by chain reaction.
4. Cause damage to biomolecules, cells and tissues.

Reactive Oxygen Species

The products of partial reduction of oxygen are highly reactive and create havoc in the living systems (Fig. 10.1). Hence, they are also called reactive oxygen species (ROS).

OXIDATIVE STRESS

Various ROS are formed continuously as by-products of aerobic metabolism, through reactions with drugs and environmental toxins. When their level is increased or the level of antioxidants is diminished, it creates a condition called oxidative stress. The ROS can cause serious chemical damage to deoxyribonucleic acid (DNA), proteins, carbohydrates and unsaturated lipids and can eventually lead to cell death. The ROS have also been implicated in a number of pathological processes including ischemia, cancer, diabetes, inflammatory disease, etc.

Generation of Free Radicals

1. The free radicals are constantly produced during the normal oxidation of foodstuffs, due to leaks in the electron transport chain in mitochondria.
2. Some enzymes such as xanthine oxidase and aldehyde oxidase form superoxide anion radical or hydrogen peroxide.
3. Nicotinamide adenine dinucleotide phosphate (NADPH) oxidase in the inflammatory cells (neutrophils, eosinophils, monocytes and macrophages) produces superoxide anion by a process of respiratory burst during phagocytosis. The superoxide is converted to hydrogen peroxide and then to hypochlorous acid (HClO) with the help of superoxide dismutase (SOD) and myeloperoxidase (MPO). Along with the activation of macrophages, the consumption of oxygen by the cell is increased drastically; this is called respiratory burst. In chronic granulomatous disease (CGD),

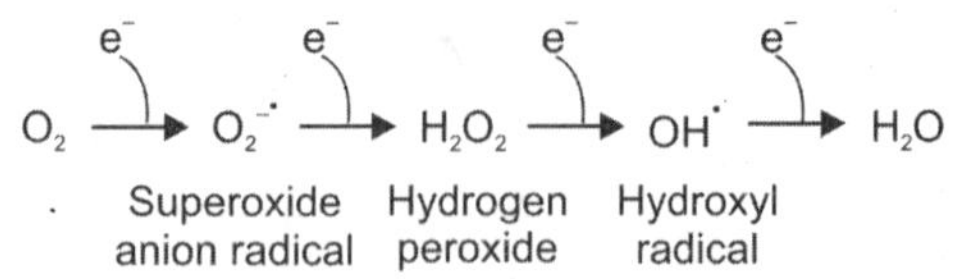

Fig. 10.1: Formation of reactive oxygen species from molecular oxygen (e, electron)

the NADPH oxidase is absent in macrophages and neutrophils.

4. Macrophages also produce NO from arginine by the enzyme nitric oxide synthase.
5. Light of appropriate wavelengths can cause photolysis of oxygen to produce singlet oxygen.
6. Peroxidation is catalyzed by lipoxygenase in platelets and leukocytes.

LIPID PEROXIDATION

Free radical-induced peroxidation of membrane lipids occurs in three stages—initiation, propagation and termination.

Initiation Phase

Initiation step involves the removal of hydrogen atom (H) from polyunsaturated fatty acids (RH), caused by hydroxyl radical.

$$RH + OH^{\bullet} \longrightarrow R^{\bullet} + H_2O$$

Propagation Phase

Under aerobic conditions, the fatty acid radical ($R^{\bullet}$) takes up oxygen to form peroxyl radical ($ROO^{\bullet}$). The latter, in turn, can remove H^- atom from another polyunsaturated fatty acid (PUFA) (RH) to form lipid hydroperoxide (ROOH).

$$R^{\bullet} + O_2 \longrightarrow ROO^{\bullet}$$

$$ROO^{\bullet} + RH \longrightarrow ROOH + R^{\bullet}$$

The hydroperoxides are capable of further stimulating lipid peroxidation, as they can form alkoxy ($RO^{\bullet}$) and peroxyl ($ROO^{\bullet}$) radicals.

Termination Phase

Lipid peroxidation proceeds as a chain reaction until the available PUFA gets oxidized (Fig. 10.2).

Role of Free Radicals in Diseases

They have been found to play significant role in diseases ranging from the diabetes mellitus to arthritis to acquired immunodeficiency syndrome (AIDS) and infertility:

1. Lipid peroxidation and oxidative process are said to be one of the important factors contributing to the pathogenesis of atherosclerosis.

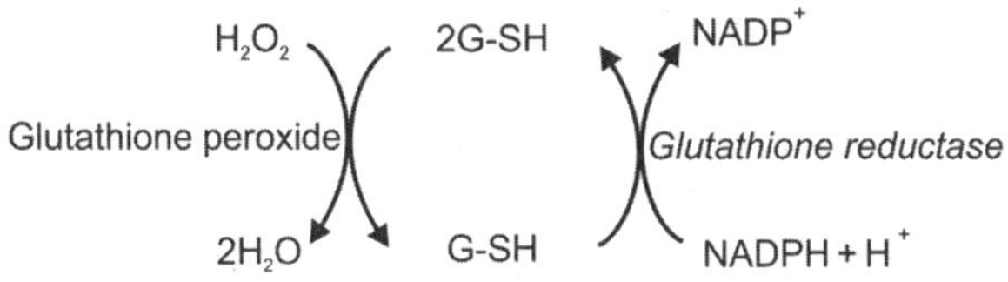

Fig. 10.2: Polyunsaturated fatty acid

2. Many substances including free radicals induce genomic damage that play important role in number of neoplastic diseases.
3. Diabetes has also been found to be associated with increased free radical damage. In diabetic patients, **serum thiobarbituric acid reactive material** (a well-known biomarker for assessing free radical mediated-tissue damage) is found to be elevated.
4. Increased lipid oxidation and oxidative stress has been attributed to the increased plasma glucose level.
5. Free radicals have been found to be associated with the aging phenomenon.
6. Accumulation of **lipofuscin** (the so-called age pigment) has been correlated with the aging.
7. **Inflammatory diseases:** Rheumatoid arthritis is a chronic inflammatory disease. The free radicals produced by neutrophils are the predominant causative agents.
8. **Respiratory diseases:** Direct exposure of lungs to 100% oxygen for a long period (more than 24 hours) is known to destroy endothelium and cause lung edema. This is mediated by free radicals. ROS are also responsible for adult respiratory distress syndrome (ARDS), a disorder characterized by pulmonary edema.
9. **Cataract:** Increased exposure to oxidative stress contributes to cataract formation.
10. **Retrolental fibroplasia** seen in premature infants is due to free radicals.
11. **Skin diseases** such as psoriasis and leukoderma may result.

Free Radical Scavenger Systems

Superoxide Dismutase

The mitochondrial SOD is manganese dependent; cytoplasmic enzyme is copper-zinc dependent. SOD is a nonheme protein.

Clinical correlation: A defect in *SOD* gene is seen in patients with amyotrophic lateral sclerosis (Lou Gehrig's disease).

$$O_2 + O_2 + 2H^+ \xrightarrow{SOD} H_2O_2 + O_2$$

$$2H_2O_2 \xrightarrow{Catalase} 2H_2O + O_2$$

Glutathione Peroxidase

In the next step, the H_2O_2 is removed by glutathioneperoxidase (POD). It is a self-dependent enzyme.

Glutathione Reductase

The oxidized glutathione, in turn, is reduced by glutathione reductase (GR), in presence of NADPH. This NADPH is generated with the help of glucose-6-phosphate dehydrogenase (GPD) in hexose monophosphate (HMP) shunt pathway.

Catalase

When H_2O_2 is generated in large quantities the enzyme catalase is also used for its removal.

$$2\,H_2O_2 \xrightarrow{\textit{Catalase}} O_2 + 2H_2O$$

Polyphenols

Consumption of polyphenol-rich fruits, vegetables and beverages is beneficial to human health.

Dietary polyphenols represent a wide variety of compounds that occur in fruits, vegetables, wine, tea and chocolate. They contain flavonoids, isoflavones, flavonols, catechins and phenolic acids.

They shows antioxidant, antiapoptosis, antiaging, anticarcinogenic, anti-inflammatory, antiatherosclerotic effects. They are protective against cardiovascular diseases. Grape polyphenols can prevent brain damage due to alcohol. Oral administration of grape polyphenol extract ameliorates cerebral ischemia-induced neuronal carnage. Grape-seed procyanidins prevent lower grade inflammation by modulating cytokine expression in rats.

ANTIOXIDANTS

A biological antioxidant may be defined as a substance (present in low-concentrations compared to an oxidizable substrate) that significantly delays or inhibits oxidation of a substrate. Antioxidants may be considered as the scavengers of free radicals.

Role of Antioxidants

Apart from the scavenging enzymes, there are two types of antioxidants.

Preventive Antioxidants

The antioxidants will inhibit the initial production of free radicals. They are catalase, glutathione peroxidase and ethylenediaminetetraacetate (EDTA).

Chain-breaking Antioxidants

The antioxidants can inhibit propagative phase. They include superoxide dismutase, uric acid and vitamin E. The α-tocopherol (T-OH) (vitamin E) would intercept the peroxyl free radical and inactivate it before a PUFA can be attacked.

$$\text{T-OH} + \text{ROO} \longrightarrow \text{TO}' + \text{ROOH}$$
$$\text{TO}' + \text{ROO} \longrightarrow \text{inactive products}$$

Vitamin E (α-tocopherol) acts as the most effective naturally occurring chain-breaking antioxidant in tissues.

Important Antioxidants

- **Vitamin E** is the lipid phase antioxidant
- **Vitamin C** is the aqueous phase antioxidant
- **Ceruloplasmin** can act as an antioxidant in extracellular fluid
- **Caffeine** is an effective antioxidant
- Cysteine, glutathione and **vitamin A** are minor antioxidants. **Beta carotene** can act as a chain-breaking antioxidant, but is less effective than α-tocopherol.

Antioxidants Used as Therapeutic Agents

1. Vitamin E.
2. Vitamin C.
3. Dimethylthiourea.
4. Dimethyl sulfoxide.
5. Allopurinol.

Commercial Use of Antioxidants

Antioxidants are regularly used in food industry to increase the shelf-life of products. Commercially used food preservatives are vitamin E, propyl gallate, butylated hydroxyanisole (BHA) and butylated hydroxytoluene. They prevent oxidative damage of oils, particularly those containing PUFA and prevent rancidity.

METABOLISM OF XENOBIOTICS OR DETOXIFICATION

Detoxification refers to the series of biochemical reactions occurring in the body to convert the foreign (often toxic) compounds to nontoxic or less toxic and more easily excretable forms.

Salient Features of Cytochrome P450

Multiple forms of cytochrome P450 are believed to exist, ranging from 20 to 200. They are all **heme proteins,** containing heme as the prosthetic group. Cytochrome P450 species are found in the highest concentration in the microsomes of liver. In the adrenal gland, they occur in mitochondria.

The mechanism of action of cytochrome P450 is complex and is dependent on NADPH. The phospholipid-phosphatidylcholine is a constituent of cytochrome P450 system, which is necessary for the action of this enzyme. Cytochrome P450 is an inducible enzyme. Its synthesis is increased by the administration of drugs such as phenobarbital.

Phases of Detoxification

1. Phase one reactions:
   - Oxidation
   - Reduction
   - Hydrolysis.
2. Phase two reactions is conjugation reactions.

Phase One Reactions

Oxidative reactions: It may be either aromatic or aliphatic hydroxylation. The reactions also include sulfoxidation, N-oxidation and epoxidation. For example, toluene is hydroxylated to benzyl alcohol by mixed function oxidase system. The oxidation and detoxification of alcohol is also an important function of the liver. Two enzymes are involved in this process; alcohol dehydrogenase oxidizes alcohol to aldehyde and aldehyde dehydrogenase oxidizes aldehyde to acid.

Oxidation of some compounds may result in production of substances, which are more toxic. For example:

Methanol ⟶ Formic acid

Ethylene glycol ⟶ Oxalic acid

Reduction reactions: The major group of compounds, which are reduced and detoxified by the liver are nitro compounds. These are reduced to their amines, while aldehydes or ketones are reduced to alcohols.

Nitrobenzene ⟶ Aniline

Picric acid ⟶ Picramic acid

Para-nitrophenol ⟶ Para-aminophenol

Hydrolysis: It is a chemical reaction in which the addition of water splits the toxicant into two fragments or smaller molecules. The hydroxyl group (OH^-) is incorporated into one fragment and the hydrogen atom is incorporated into the other.

Esters, amines, hydrazines, amides, glycosidic bonds and carbamates are generally biotransformed by hydrolysis, e.g. aspirin, acetanilide, procaine, xylocaine.

Aspirin, which has analgesics, antipyretic, actions is widely used in clinical practices. It undergoes hydrolysis during detoxification.

$$\text{Aspirin} \xrightarrow{+H_2O} \text{Salicylic acid + Acetic acid}$$

Phase Two Reactions (Conjugations)

Phase two reactions are conjugation reactions, i.e. a molecule normally present in the body is added to the reactive site of the phase one metabolite. In most cases, the conjugation will make the compounds non-toxic and easily excretable.

Glucuronic acid conjugation: In general, sulfation decreases the toxicity of xenobiotics. The highly polar sulfate conjugates are readily excreted through urine. Often glucuronidation or sulfation can conjugate the same xenobiotics.

Phenolic and alcoholic compounds are conjugated with sulfate. The enzyme is sulfotransferase and the sulfate group is transferred from [phosphoadenosine phosphosulfate (PAPS)].

R-OH + PAPS ⟶ $R\text{-}O\text{-}SO_3$ + PAP

Phenol + PAPS ⟶ Phenyl sulfate + PAP

Indole + PAPS ⟶ Indoxyl sulfate + PAP

Important compounds excreted as their sulfates include steroids and indole compounds.

Cysteine and glutathione: The cysteine is derived from glutathione, which is the active conjugating agent. Alkyl or aryl halides, epoxides and alkenes are detoxified in this manner.

Acetylation: Conjugation with acetic acid is taking place with drugs like sulfanilamide, isoniazid and para-amino salicylic acid (PAS).

Conjugation with glycine: Benzoic acid is conjugated with glycine to form hippuric acid (benzoyl glycine), which is excreted in urine.

Conjugation with glutamine: Phenyl acetic acid is conjugated with glutamine to form phenyl acetyl glutamine.

Methylation reactions: Amino, hydroxy or thiol groups are methylated. S-adenosyl methionine (SAM) is the methyl donor and the enzyme is usually O-methyl transferase.

Phase Three Reactions

Phase three reactions are not very common. Typical example is further conjugation with glutathione.

The xenobiotics that enter the body are mostly drugs and they are detoxified by the enzymes concerned with drug metabolism. Induction of cytochrome P450 system may even produce unwanted effects in some persons. For example, induction of aminolevulinic acid (ALA) synthase by barbiturates will precipitate attacks in acute intermittent porphyria.

Chapter 11

Cancer

Cancer is the **second largest killer disease** (the first being coronary heart disease) in the developed countries. It is characterized by the loss of control of cellular growth and development leading to excessive proliferation and spread of cells.

TUMORS

Uncontrolled growth of cells result in tumors. The tumors are of two types:

1. **Benign tumors:** They usually grow by expansion and remain encapsulated in a layer of connective tissue. Normally, benign tumors are not life-threatening, e.g. moles, warts.
2. **Malignant tumors or cancers:** They are characterized by uncontrolled proliferation and spread of cells to various parts of the body, a process referred to as **metastasis.** Malignant tumors are invariably life-threatening, e.g. lung cancer, leukemia.

CANCER

The word cancer is derived from Latin word cancrum meaning 'Crab'. The disease is so-called because of swollen vein around the area, which resembles crab limb.

Definition of Cancer

Indiana University Cancer Center (IUCC) defined cancer as a disturbance of growth characterized by excessive proliferation of cells without relation to the physiological demand of the organ involved.

Etiology of Cancer

Cancers are multifactorial in origin. The causative agents (also called carcinogens) can be grouped into:

1. **Chemical compounds:** Carcinogenesis may be caused by both organic and inorganic compounds (Table 11.1).

Table 11.1: Organic and inorganic compounds

Organic compounds	Inorganic compounds
Methylcholanthrene	Nickel
Benzpyrene	Chromium
Benzidine	Cadmium
2-naphthylamine	Beryllium

2. **Endocrine factors:** Hormones responsible for the onset of cancers include estrogen for premenopausal breast carcinoma and androgens for prostatic carcinoma.
3. **Oncogenic viruses:** The viruses causing malignancies in humans are:
   - Deoxyribonucleic acid (DNA) viruses, e.g. papovavirus group
   - Ribonucleic acid (RNA) viruses, e.g. leukoviruses.
4. **Ionizing radiations:** X-rays, γ rays and ultraviolet (UV) rays.

Molecular Basis of Cancer

Oncogenes

Oncogenes are cellular genes that can trigger uncontrolled cell proliferation, if their sequence is altered or their expression is incorrectly regulated. They were first discovered as viral (v-) oncogenes in retroviruses that cause tumors (tumor viruses). Viruses of this type sometimes incorporate genes from the host cell into their own genome. If these genes are reincorporated into the host DNA again during later infection, tumors can then be caused in rare cases.

Proto-oncogenes

The cellular form of oncogenes (known as c-oncogenes or **proto-oncogenes)** code for proteins involved in controlling growth and differentiation processes. They only become oncogenes, if their sequence has been altered by mutations, deletions and other processes or when excessive amounts of the gene products have been produced as a result of overexpression. The overexpression can occur when **amplification** leads to numerous functional copies of the respective gene or when the gene falls under the influence of a highly active promoter. If the control of oncogene expression by **tumor suppressor genes** is also disturbed, **transformation** and unregulated proliferation of the cells can occur.

A single activated oncogene does not usually lead to a loss of growth control. It only occurs when over the course of time, mutations and regulation defects accumulate in one and the same cell.

If the immune system does not succeed in eliminating the transformed cell over the course of months or years, it can grow into a macroscopically visible **tumor.**

Antioncogenes or Oncosuppressor Genes

A special category of gene called oncosuppressor genes or more commonly antioncogenes are identified (Table 11.2).

Table 11.2: Important oncosuppressor genes

Name of the oncosuppressors	Abbreviations
Retinoblastoma	RB
Wilms' tumor	WT
Familial adenomatous polyposis	FAP
Deleted in colorectal cancer	DCC
Gene for protein-53	*p53*

The products of these genes apply breaks and regulate cell proliferation.

The loss of these suppressor genes remove the growth control of cells and is believed to be a key factor in the development of several tumors.

TUMOR MARKERS

Tumor markers are substances, usually proteins that are produced by the body in response to cancer growth or by the cancer tissue itself (Fig. 11.1).

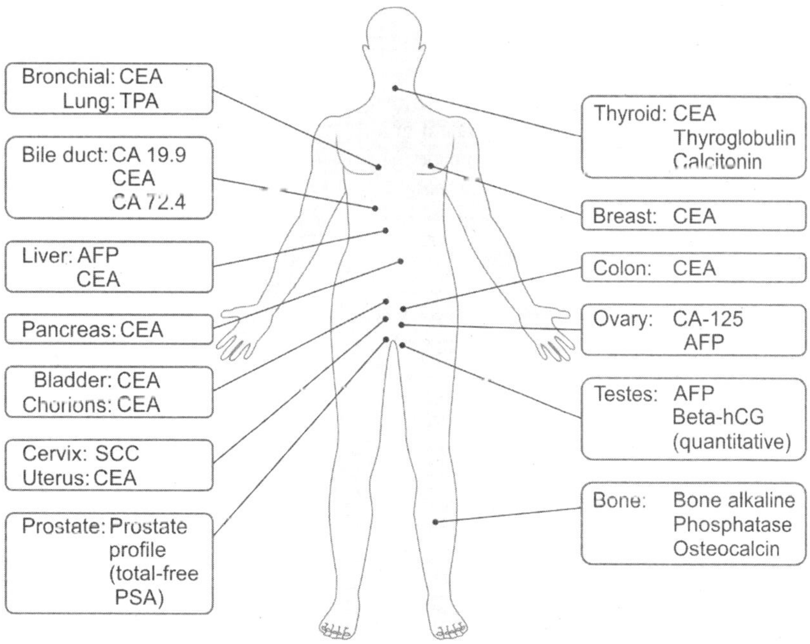

Fig. 11.1: Tumor markers (AFP, alpha-fetoprotein; CEA, carcinoembryonic antigen; CA, cancer antigen; hCG, human chorionic gonadotropin; SCC, squamous cell carcinoma; TPA, tissue polypeptide antigen).

Some tumor markers are specific, while others are seen in several cancer types. Many of the well-known markers are also seen in non-cancerous conditions. Consequently, these tumor markers are not diagnostic for cancer.

Importance

Tumor markers are not diagnostic in themselves. A definitive diagnosis of cancer is made by looking at the biopsy specimens (e.g. of tissue) under a microscope. However, tumor markers provide information that can be used to:

1. Screen: Most markers are not suited for general screening, but some may be used in those with a strong family history of a particular cancer. In the case of genetic markers, they may be used to help predict risk in family members [prostate-specific antigen (PSA) testing for prostate cancer is an example].
2. Help diagnose: In a patient who has symptoms, tumor markers may be used to help identify the source of the cancer (Table 11.3).
3. Stage: If a patient does have cancer, tumor marker elevations can be used to help determine how far the cancer has spread to other tissues and organs.
4. Determine prognosis.
5. Guide treatment.
6. Determine recurrence: Currently, one of the biggest uses for tumor markers is to monitor for cancer recurrence. If

Table 11.3: Important tumor markers

Tumor markers	Produced by	Elevated	Levels	Importance
		Cancer conditions	Non-cancer conditions	
Carcinoembryonic antigen (CEA)	Embryonic tissue of liver, gut and pancreas	Colorectal cancer	Alcoholic cirrhosis (70%), emphysema (57%) and diabetes mellitus (38%)	Indicator to detect the burden of tumor mass and monitoring the treatment
Alpha-fetoprotein (AFP)	Yolk sac in early fetal life	Cancers of liver and germ cells of testis and to some extent carcinomas of lung, pancreas and colon	Cirrhosis, hepatitis and pregnancy	A sensitive index for tumor therapy and detection of recurrence
Beta human chorionic gonadotropin (β-hCG)	Placenta	Testicular and ovarian cancers (germ cell tumors) and in gestational trophoblastic disease, mainly choriocarcinoma	A woman who still has a large uterus after pregnancy has ended and men with an enlarged testicle or anyone with a tumor in their chest	Detection of recurrence
Cancer antigen (CA-125)	Ovary	Epithelial ovarian cancer, lung, pancreatic, breast, liver and colon cancer	Uterine fibroids or endometriosis	Cancer antigen (CA)-125 has been studied as a screening test in women whose cancer has not spread outside the ovary
Prostate-specific antigen (PSA)	Cells of the prostate gland	Prostate cancer	Benign prostatic hyperplasia (BPH), infected or inflamed prostates	Very valuable in monitoring the response to treatment and in the follow-up of men with prostate cancer

Table 11.4: Commonly used anticancer drugs

Anticancer drugs	Chemical nature	Mode of action
Methotrexate	Folic acid analogue	Competitive inhibitor of dihydrofolate reductase (involved in THFA* synthesis); THFA is required for nucleotide synthesis
6-Mercaptopurine	Purine analogue	Inhibits the formation of AMP† from IMP‡
6-Thioguanine	Purine analogue	Inhibits the synthesis of purine nucleotide
Mitomycin C	Antibiotic	Formation of cross bridges between DNA§ base pairs
Vinblastine and vincristine	Alkaloids	Inhibit spindle movement and interfere with cytoskeleton formation

*THFA, tetrahydrofurfuryl alcohol; †AMP, adenosine 5′ monophosphate; ‡IMP, inosine monophosphate; §DNA, deoxyribonucleic acid.

If a tumor marker is elevated before treatment, low after treatment and then begins to rise over time, then it is likely that the cancer is returning.

ANTICANCER DRUGS

Synthetic analogs of purine and pyrimidine bases and their derivatives serve as anticancer drugs either by inhibiting an enzyme of nucleotide biosynthesis or by being incorporated into DNA or RNA (Table 11.4). For example, methotrexate, 6-mercaptopurine, 6-thioguanate, vincristine and vinblastine, etc.

APOPTOSIS

Apoptosis is also called programmed cell death. It refers to the removal of superfluous, aged and partially damaged cells.

Apoptosis is characterized by:

1. Nuclear shrinking.
2. Condensation of chromatin.
3. Membrane blobbing.
4. Shrinking of cells.
5. DNA fragmentation.
6. Disintegration.

Chapter 12

Biotechniques

Biochemistry is an experimental rather than a theoretical science. The understanding and developments of biochemistry are based on the laboratory tools employed for biochemical experimentation. Thus, the development of sensitive and sophisticated analytical techniques has contributed to the understanding of biochemistry.

ELECTROPHORESIS

The term refers to the movements of charged particles through an electrolyte when subjected to an electric field.

Factors Affecting Electrophoresis

- Net charge on the particles
- Mass and shape of the particles
- The pH of the medium
- Strength of electrical field
- Properties of the supporting medium.

Types of Electrophoresis

- Zone electrophoresis
  - Paper electrophoresis
  - Gel electrophoresis.
- Isoelectric focusing
- Immune electrophoresis.

Normal Pattern

In agar gel electrophoresis, normal serum is separated into five bands. Their relative concentrations are given below:

- Albumin: 55%–65%
- Alpha 1-globulin: 2%–3%
- Alpha 2-globulin: 6%–12%
- Beta-globulin: 8%–12%
- Gamma-globulin: 12%–22%.

Abnormal Patterns in Clinical Disease

1. Chronic infections.
2. Multiple myeloma: A sharp spike is noted and termed as **M band.** This is due to monoclonal origin of immunoglobulins in multiple myeloma.
3. Fibrinogen.
4. Primary immune deficiency.
5. Nephrotic syndrome.
6. Cirrhosis of liver.
7. Chronic lymphatic leukemia.
8. Alpha 1-antitrypsin deficiency.

POLYMERASE CHAIN REACTION

Principle

The purpose of polymerase chain reaction (PCR) is to make a huge number of copies of a gene. This is necessary to have enough starting template for sequencing.

Reaction Cycle

There are three major steps in PCR, which are repeated for 30–40 cycles. This is done on an automated cycler, which can heat and cool the tubes with the reaction mixture in a very short time.

Denaturation

During the denaturation at 95°C for 15 seconds to 2 minutes, the double strand melts open to single-stranded deoxyribonucleic acid (DNA), all enzymatic reactions stop. For example, the extension from a previous cycle.

Primer

Primers annealing at 50°C for 0.5 seconds to 2 minutes hybridize with their complementary single-stranded DNA produced in the first step (denaturation).

Extension

Extension at 72°C for 30 seconds is the ideal working temperature for the polymerase. PCR requires the use of a DNA polymerase, i.e. thermu saquaticus (Taq) polymerase derived from the bacterium *Thermus aquaticus* to make the copies of the complementary DNA sequence used as a template.

The bases (complementary to the template) are coupled to the primer on the 3′ side [the polymerase adds deoxynucleotide triphosphate (dNTP) from 5′ to 3′, reading the template from 3′ to 5′ side, bases are added complementary to the template].

Applications of Polymerase Chain Reaction

A PCR has become a very common tool for a large number of applications. These include:

1. Comparison of a normal cloned gene with an uncloned mutant form of the gene: PCR allows the synthesis of mutant DNA in sufficient quantities for a sequencing protocol without laboriously cloning the altered DNA.
2. Detection of low-abundance nucleic acid sequences. For example, viruses that have a long latency period, such as human immunodeficiency virus (HIV) are difficult to detect at the early stage of infection using conventional methods. PCR offers a rapid and sensitive method for detecting viral DNA sequences even when only a small proportion of cells are harboring the virus.
3. Forensic analysis of DNA samples: DNA fingerprinting by means of PCR has revolutionized the analysis of evidence from crime scenes. DNA isolated from a single human hair, a tiny spot of blood or a sample of semen is sufficient to determine whether the sample comes from a specific individual. The DNA markers analyzed for such fingerprinting are most commonly short tandem repeat polymorphisms.
4. Prenatal diagnosis of inherited disorders where cells obtained from fetus by amniocentesis are very few.
5. Detection of cancer.
6. Fossil studies: DNA can be isolated and PCR amplified from the fossils and is used to study evolution by comparing the sequences in the extinct and living organism.

RADIOIMMUNOASSAY

Radioimmunoassay (RIA) technique has revolutionized the estimation of several compounds in biological fluids that are found in exceedingly low concentrations (nanogram or picogram). RIA is a highly sensitive and specific analytical tool. It combines the principles of radioactivity of isotopes and immunological reactions of antigen and antibody, hence the name.

Suppose, blood level of thyroxine is to be assayed the thyroxine (T_4) hormone is the antigen (Ag) in this case. It is made to react with a specific antibody (Ab). A constant amount of isotope-labeled hormone, constant amount of antibody and variable quantities of unlabeled hormone are taken in different tubes.

In tube A, the labeled hormone molecules are combined with the antibody molecule; so there is no radioactivity in the supernatant. In tube B, equal quantity of unlabeled hormone is added, when labeled and unlabeled antigen molecules compete for the antibody. Thus, half of radioactivity is in the supernatant and half in the precipitate. The displacement of labeled antigen is proportional to the unlabeled antigen in the system.

A series of test tubes are taken in which constant quantity of antibody, constant quantity of labeled antigen and different, but known quantities of unlabeled antigen are added. After a few hours of incubation, a precipitating agent is added when antigen-antibody complex being high molecular weight substance is precipitated. The radioactivity in the precipitate is inversely related to the unlabeled antigen added (Fig. 12.1).

ENZYME-LINKED IMMUNOSORBENT ASSAY

Enzyme-linked immunosorbent assay (ELISA) is a nonisotopic immunoassay. An enzyme is used as a label in ELISA in place of radioactive isotope employed in RIA. ELISA is as sensitive as or even more sensitive than RIA. In addition, there is no risk of radiation hazards (as in case with RIA in ELISA.

A ELISA is based on the immunochemical principles of antigen-antibody reaction.

Indirect ELISA

Indirect ELISA is useful to detect small quantities of antibodies in the blood. A good example is the test for detection

$$Ag + Ag^{*} + Ab \longrightarrow \underset{\text{(bound radio-activity)}}{[Ag - Ab]} + [Ag^{*} - Ab] + Ag + \underset{\text{(free radio-activity)}}{Ag^{*}}$$

Fig. 12.1: Principle of radioimmunoasssy (*Ag, stands for radioactivity; Ag, antigen; Ab, antibody)

of HIV antibody. In patients with acquired immunodeficiency syndrome (AIDS), the human immunodeficiency virus (HIV) produces specific antibody. To detect the HIV antibody, the following method is used.

Antigen coated well $\xrightarrow{\text{wash}}$ antibody in patient's serum binds to antigen $\xrightarrow{\text{wash}}$ enzyme-linked antibody binds to specific antibody $\xrightarrow{\text{wash}}$ substrate added; color proportional to antibody in patient's serum.

Sandwich ELISA

Sandwich ELISA is useful to detect small quantities of antigens in the blood.

Antibody coated plate ⟶ add patient's serum containing antigen (T4) ⟶ add antibody (anti thyroxine raised in rabbit) ⟶ add horseradish peroxidase (HRP) conjugated second antibody (anti-rabbit IgG raised in goat) ⟶ add substrate ⟶ develop color; read on plate reader.

DNA FINGERPRINTING

There are tandem repeats (TR) in chromosomes. These are short sequences of DNA, located at scattered sites. The number of these repeat units varies person to person, but is unique for a particular person. Therefore, it serves as a molecular fingerprint. It is also known as DNA profile. Probability of similarity between two persons is only one in 3×10^{10} persons.

A DNA probes have been developed, so that at low stringency they hybridize to a number of these loci to produce individual specific fingerprints. The technique is used to pinpoint the culprit of the crime and also in disputes of parenthood. DNA can be isolated from stains on clothing made of blood or semen stained even several years before. Sperm nucleic acid can also be separated from vaginal swabs of rape victims.

Restriction Fragment Length Polymorphism

Human genome contains hundreds of variations in base sequences that do not affect the phenotype. The property of the molecules to exist in more than one form is known as polymorphism.

A polymorphic gene is one in which the variant alleles are common in more than 1% of the total population. The existence of two or more types of restriction fragment patterns is called restriction fragment length polymorphism (RFLP). This can be used as a genetic marker.

The DNA is treated with restriction enzymes, which cleave DNA into fragments of defined lengths. Then electrophoresis is done in agarose gels, when the fragments are separated. Finally, the DNA from the agarose gel is transferred onto nitrocellulose paper (Southern blotting) and hybridized with labeled probe sequences. Genotypic changes can be recognized by the altered restriction fragments.

Clinical Correlations

1. Useful in disputed parenthood: An individual, who is heterozygous for a polymorphism has a sequence variation in the DNA of one chromosome and not in the DNA of the companion chromosome. In such cases, each chromosome can be traced from parent to offspring by the presence or absence of this marker.
2. Useful in human population genetics: Geographical isolates and comparison of genetic make up of related species. Genetic diseases will produce alteration in size distribution of restriction endonuclease (RE) fragments and show RFLP.

TOOLS IN BIOCHEMISTRY BLOTTING TECHNIQUES

Blotting refers to the process of immobilization of sample nucleic acids on solid support (nitrocellulose or nylon membranes). The blotted nucleic acids are then used as targets in the hybridization experiments for their specific detection.

Types of Blotting Techniques

The most commonly used blotting techniques are listed below:

- Southern blotting (for DNA)
- Northern blotting (for RNA)
- Dot blotting (DNA/RNA)
- Western blotting involves the transfer of protein blots.

The Southern blotting is named after the scientist Edwin Southern (1975) who developed it. The other names Northern blotting and Western blotting are laboratory jargons, which are now accepted.

Southern Blotting

Southern blotting technique is based on DNA hybridization. This is used to detect a specific segment of DNA in the whole genome (Fig. 12.2).

Importance: Mutant genes such as hemoglobin S (HbS), cystic fibrosis, Duchenne's muscular dystrophy (DMD), phenylketonuria (PKU) as well as presence of viral DNA (hepatitis virus B and C) can be identified by this method).

DNA is isolated from the tissue

↓

Fragmented by restriction *endonucleases*

↓

Electrophoresed on agarose gel

↓

Treated with NaOH to denature the DNA

↓

DNA pieces become single stranded

↓

Blotted (adsorbed) over to a nitrocellulose membrane

↓

Adsorption of single-stranded DNA in the nitrocellulose membrane

↓

Exact replica of the pattern in the gel reproduced on the membrane

↓

Baked at 80°C

↓

DNA is fixed on the membrane

↓

Radioactive DNA probe is placed over the membrane

↓

Probe will detect the complementary nucleotide sequence in the host DNA

↓

Probe is hybridized to the particular pieces of host DNA

↓

Membrane is then thoroughly washed to remove excess probes

↓

An X-ray plate is placed over the membrane in the dark for a few days

↓

Radiation from the fixed probe will produce its mark on the X-ray plate. This is called autoradiography

Fig. 12.2: Southern blotting (DNA, deoxyribonucleic acid; NaOH, sodium hydroxide)

Total RNA isolated from the cell

↓

Electrophoresed

↓

Blotted onto a membrane

↓

Probed with radioactive cDNA

↓

RNA-DNA hybridization

Fig. 12.3: Northern blotting (DNA, deoxyribonucleic acid; RNA, ribonucleic acid)

Isolation of proteins from the tissue

↓

Electrophoresis is done

↓

Transfer of electrophoresed protein bands to nylon or nitrocellulose membrane

↓

Probed with radioactive antibody

↓

Autoradiographed

Fig. 12.4: Western blotting

Northern Blotting

Northern blotting is the technique for the specific identification of RNA molecules (Fig. 12.3).

Importance: This is used to detect the gene expression in a tissue.

Western Blotting

Western blotting involves the identification of proteins (Fig. 12.4).

Importance: It is very useful to understand the nucleic acid functions, particularly during the course of gene manipulations.

Chapter 13

Clinical Chemistry

Based on the functional capabilities of the organs, specific biochemical investigations have been developed in the laboratory to assess their function. Biochemical functions are done mainly to assess the functioning of liver, kidney, stomach and pancreas.

LIVER FUNCTION TESTS

Liver is an important organ, which weighs about 1.5 kg and performs a variety of functions related to the metabolism of macromolecules, synthesis of proteins, biotransformation, storage and endocrine functions. It is better known as the **chemical workshop of the body**.

Functions of Liver

1. Synthetic functions:
   a. Synthesis of plasma proteins: All plasma proteins except gamma globulins.
   b. Synthesis of coagulation factors: Preprothrombin (inactive form) is converted into prothrombin in liver in the presence of vitamin K. Other coagulation factors like factor V, VII and X are also synthesized in the liver.
   c. Synthesis of cholesterol: A substantial percentage of endogenous cholesterol synthesis from acetyl-CoA, takes place in the liver.
   d. Synthesis of triacylglycerol: When there is a good supply of nutrients in the resorptive (well-fed) state, the liver converts glucose via acetyl-CoA, into fatty acids.
   e. Lipoprotein synthesis.

2 Metabolic functions:
   a. Carbohydrates: Glycolysis, glycogen synthesis, glycogen breakdown, gluconeogenesis.
   The liver takes up glucose and other monosaccharides from the plasma. Glucose is then either stored in the form of the polysaccharide glycogen or converted into fatty acids. When there is a drop in the blood glucose level, the liver releases glucose again by breaking down the glycogen.
   b. Ketogenesis: Fatty acid synthesis and breakdown.
   c. Protein catabolism.
   d. Citric acid cycle, production of adenosine triphosphate (ATP).

3. Detoxification and excretion:
   a. Ammonia to urea.
   c. Bilirubin (bile pigment).
   d. Cholesterol.
   e. Drug metabolites.
4. Storage functions: Vitamin A, D, K, B_{12}.
5. Production of bile salts: Help in digestion.
6. Homeostasis: The liver's the functions primarily serve to cushion fluctuations in the concentration of all groups of metabolite substances in the blood, in order to ensure a constant supply to the peripheral tissues (homeostasis).

Classification of Liver Function Tests

For the assessment of liver functioning, one has to be aware with both its reserve capacity and the battery of function it performs.

Based on Laboratory Findings

Group I (tests of hepatic excretory function)

1. Serum: Bilirubin; total, conjugated and unconjugated. The normal serum bilirubin level varies from

0.2 to 0.8 mg/dL. The unconjugated bilirubin (bilirubin-albumin complex) (free albumin) varies from 0.2 to 0.7 mg/dL. The conjugated bilirubin (direct bilirubin) varies from 0.1 to 0.4 mg/dL.
2. Urine: Bile pigments, bile salts and urobilinogen (UBG). Normally, bile salts (sodium salts of taurocholic acid and glycocholic acid) are not present in the urine.
3. Bromsulphthalein test: This test is done to assess the excretory function of the liver. Bromsulphthalein (BSP) is a dye and is almost exclusively excreted by liver through bile. The BSP is administered intravenously (5 mg/body weight) and its serum concentration is measured at 45 minutes and at 2 hours. In normal individuals, less than 5% dye is retained at the end of 45 minutes. Any impairment in liver function test causes an increased retention of the dye.

Group II: liver enzyme panel (markers of liver injury/cholestasis)

1. Alanine aminotransferase (ALT) earlier known as serum glutamic pyruvic transaminase (SGPT). Normal serum ALT value is 5–40 IU/L.
2. Aspartate aminotransferase (AST) earlier known as serum glutamic-oxaloacetic transaminase (SGOT). Normal serum AST value is 5–45 IU/L.
3. Alkaline phosphatase (ALP). Normal serum ALP value is 3–13 KA units/dL.
4. Gamma glutamyltransferase (GGT). Normal GGT value is 5–40 mg/dL.

Group III: plasma proteins (tests for synthetic function of liver)

1. Total proteins.
2. Serum albumin, globulins, albumin/globulin (A/G ratio):
   a. Normal albumin level in blood is 3.5–5 g/dL.
   b. Normal globulin level in blood is 2.5–3.5 g/dL.
   c. Normal A/G ratio is 1.7–2, which is elevated due to cirrhosis, hypoalbuminemia and associated hypergammaglobulinemia.
3. Prothrombin time (PT): The half-life of prothrombin (clotting factor II) is only 6 hours and hence PT indicates the present function of the liver.

Group IV: special tests

1. Ceruloplasmin.
2. Ferritin.
3. Alpha -1-antitrypsin (AAT).
4. Alpha-fetoprotein (AFP).

Based on Clinical Aspects

Group I: markers of liver dysfunction

1. Serum: Bilirubin; total, conjugated.
2. Urine: Bile pigments, bile salts and UBG.
3. Total protein, serum albumin and A/G ratio.
4. Prothrombin time.
5. Blood ammonia, when indicated.

Group II: markers of hepatocellular injury

1. Alanine aminotransferase.
2. Aspartate aminotransferase.

Group III: markers of cholestasis

1. Alkaline phosphatase.
2. Gamma-glutamyltransferase.

Clinical Correlation

In various liver diseases, serum levels of several enzymes are elevated:

1. Alanine aminotransferase and aspartate aminotransferase:
   a. In viral hepatitis and other forms of the liver diseases associated with hepatic necrosis, ALT and ASP are elevated, even before symptoms appear.
   b. Increased levels are also seen in extrahepatic cholestasis and the increase is more in chronic obstruction.
   c. The 5- to 10-fold elevation of enzymes occur in patients with primary or metastatic carcinoma of liver.
2. Alkaline phosphatase:
   a. Elevation of ALP tends to be marked in extrahepatic obstruction.
   b. Increased ALP is marked in children due to ongoing bone growth.
3. Gamma-glutamyltransferase:
   Highly elevated GGT is noted in sera from people who are heavy drinkers. Hence, this enzyme has significance in detecting alcohol-induced liver diseases.

RENAL FUNCTION TESTS

Kidneys form a pair of organs, which perform many important functions.

Functions of Kidney

1. Excretion of urea and other wastes, such as acids, bases, toxins, drug metabolites, urea, creatinine.
2. Maintaining water balance.
3. Excretion of sodium (effect on blood pressure).
4. Excretion of potassium (effect on heart).
5. Excretion of hydrogen ions (maintenance of pH).
6. Activation of vitamin D (effect on bone).
7. Production of erythropoietin (effect on red blood cells).
8. Filtration: About 180 liters/day of water with all sodium, chloride, sugar and amino acids.
9. Reabsorption: About 178.5 liters reabsorbed; all glucose and amino acids reabsorbed; most of sodium and chloride reabsorbed.

Classification of Renal Function Tests

To Screen for Kidney Disease

1. Complete urine analysis.
2. Plasma urea and creatinine.
3. Plasma electrolytes.

To Assess Renal Function

To assess glomerular function: Following are to be done:

a. Glomerular filtration rate.
b. Clearance tests.
c. Glomerular permeability.
d. Proteinuria.

To assess tubular function:: Following are to be done:

a. Reabsorption studies.
b. Secretion tests.
c. Concentration and dilution tests.
d. Renal acidification.

Complete urine analysis: The complete urine analysis is given in Table 13.1.

Table 13.1: Urine analysis

Test and normal range	Interpretations
Specific gravity (1.015–1.025)	Low: Renal tubular acidosis, diabetes insipidus, polydipsia High: Excess water loss due to diarrhea, vomiting, diabetes mellitus (DM), glomerulonephritis
pH (4.5–8)	Low: Increased protein diet, acidosis High: Decreased protein diet
Blood	Glomerulonephritis, trauma of urinary tract stones, hemoglobinuria
Protein (< 150 mg/day)	Fever, exercise, proteinuria, glomerulonephritis, urinary tract infection (UTI), tubular diseases
Glucose	Diabetes mellitus, renal glycosuria, Fanconi's syndrome
Ketone bodies	Diabetes mellitus, starvation
Bilirubin	Hepatitis, obstructive jaundice
Urobilinogen	Concentrated urine, hepatitis, intravascular hemolysis
Bile salts	Obstructive jaundice

Plasma urea and creatinine: The estimation of urea is done by: the following:

1. Urease method.
2. Glutamate dehydrogenase (GLDH) method.
3. Diacetyl monoxime method (DAM).

Normal serum urea level: The normal value is 20–40 mg/dL.

Blood urea nitrogen: Sometimes used as a measurement of urea since 1½ molecular weight of urea contains nitrogen.

The normal range of blood urea nitrogen (BUN) is 5–25 mg/dL.

High BUN > 80 mg/dL, indicates impaired renal function.

Normal serum urea = BUN × 2.14.

Causes for increased blood urea

1. Prerenal conditions:
   a. Dehydration: Severe vomiting, intestinal obstruction, diarrhea.
   b. Diabetic coma and severe burns.
   c. Fever and severe infections.
2. Renal diseases:
   a. Acute glomerulonephritis.
   b. Nephrosis.
   c. Malignant hypertension.
   d. Chronic pyelonephritis.
3. Postrenal causes:
   a. Stones in the urinary tract.
   b. Enlarged prostate.
   c. Tumors of bladder.

Causes for decreased blood urea

a. During pregnancy.
b. Liver diseases.
c. Protein malnutrition.

Clinical Correlation

1. **Azotemia:** Increase in the blood levels of non-protein nitrogen (NPN) is referred to as azotemia and is the hallmark of kidney failure.
2. **Uremic syndrome:** Clinical syndrome that develops due to nitrogen retention due to renal failure.

Mnemonic:
Blood urea nitrogen (BUN): Creatinine elevation:
Causes **ABCD**:
- ***A***zotemia (prerenal)
- ***B***leeding [gastrointestinal (GI)]
- ***C***atabolic status
- ***D***iet (high protein parenteral nutrition)

Estimation of serum creatinine: Done by Jaffe's method.

1. Normal range (Table 13.2):
   a. Adult males: 0.7–1.4 mg/dL.
   b. Adult females: 0.6–1.3 mg/dL.
   c. Children: 0.4–1.2 mg/dL.

Plasma electrolytes: Are as given below:

1. Estimation of electrolytes (Na^+ and K^+):
   a. Flame photometry.
   b. By ion selective electrode method.

2. Normal range:
   a. Sodium: 135–150 mmol/L.
   b. Potassium: 3.5–5 mmol/L.

Table 13.2: Factors that increase and decrease serum creatinine

Factors reducing serum creatinine	Factors increasing serum creatinine
Low muscle mass	Old age
Females	Males
Malnutrition	Renal diseases: • Glomerulonephritis • Pyelonephritis • Renal failure • Urinary obstruction

Glomerular Function

When the blood is perfused through the Bowman's capsule, an ultrafiltrate of the blood is produced in glomerulus, while the cells and proteins are retained in the blood. The sieves of the glomeruli are such that hemoglobin is passed through to be excreted in urine, but albumin is retained in blood. Therefore, the earliest manifestation in the abnormal function of the glomeruli is appearance of albumin in urine.

Glomerular Filtration Rate

1. The renal blood flow is about 700 mL plasma or 1,200 mL of blood, which passes, kidney per minute.
2. The glomerular filtration rate (GFR) is 120–125 mL per minute in a person with 70 kg body weight.
3. Glomerular filtrate (GF) formed is about 170–180 liters per day, out of which only 1.5 liters are excreted as urine. Thus, 99% of GF is reabsorbed (Table 13.3).

Table 13.3: Glomerular filtration rate

Segment of nephron	Reabsorption	Secretion
Proximal convoluted tubule (PCT)	Sodium (85%), chloride (85%), bicarbonate (85%), glucose (100%), amino acids (100%), uric acid, water (obligatory)	H^+, acids and bases, NH_4^+, diodrast, hippuric acid
Loop of Henle	Na^+, Cl^-, Ca^{2+}, Mg^{2+}	-
Distal convoluted tubule (DCT)	Na^+, Cl^-, water (facultative)	H^+, K^+, NH_4^+, uric acid

Renal Threshold and Tubular Maximum

The renal threshold of a substance is the plasma level above which the compound is excreted in urine. The maximum reabsorptive capacity of the substances is known as the tubular maximum.

Markers of GFR

Clearance Tests: Measurement of GFR is a general index for assessment of renal damage. GFR is also affected by age, sex, body size, protein intake and pregnancy. Normal GFR for young adults is 120–130 mL/min/1.73 m^2.

Clearance is defined as the volume of blood or plasma completely cleared of a substance per unit time and is expressed as milliliter per minute. It is expressed as milliliter of plasma per minute (not as g or mg).

Clearance estimates the amount of plasma that must have passed through the glomeruli per minute. It is calculated by using the formula:

$$C = \frac{U \times V}{P}$$

where,

U = Concentration of the substance in urine;

P = Concentration of the substance in plasma or serum;

V = The mL of urine excreted per minute.

Creatinine clearance test

Volume of plasma (in mL) completely cleared off creatinine per minute.

Creatinine is a waste product, formed from creatine phosphate. This conversion is spontaneous, nonenzymatic and is dependent on total muscle mass of the body. Since the production is continuous, the serum level of creatinine level will not fluctuate much, making creatinine an ideal substance for clearance test.

Normal range of creatinine: As given below:
Adult males: 0.7–1.4 mg/dL.
Adult females: 0.6–1.3 mg/dL.
Children: 0.4–1.2 mg/dL.

Procedure: As follows:
Give about 500 mL of water to the patient, to promote good urine flow. After about 30 minutes, ask to empty the bladder and discard the urine. Exactly after 60 minutes, again void the bladder and collect the urine, and note the volume. Take one blood sample for serum creatinine estimation.

Since the value of creatinine level depends on total muscle mass, creatinine clearance corrected for surface area could be calculated as:

$$C = \frac{U \times V \times 1.73}{P \times A}$$

The value up to 75% of average normal range indicates adequate renal function.

Advantages: As follows:
1. Early detection of functional impairment of kidney without overt signs and symptoms.
2. Helpful in long-term monitoring of patients with renal insufficiency under a protein restricted diet.
3. Extrarenal factors will rarely interfere in the test.

4. Endogenous substances and a constant serum creatinine level are maintained, and hence blood may be collected at any time.

Disadvantages: As follows:

1. Value depends on total muscle mass. A person suffering from muscle wasting diseases, measurement of creatinine clearance is not a reliable indicator of GFR.
2. Very early stages of decreased GFR may not be identified by creatinine clearance.
3. Prerenal, renal and postrenal causes will influence creatinine clearance.

Creatinine coefficient: It is the urinary creatinine expressed in mg/kg body weight. The value is elevated in muscular dystrophy. Normal range is 20–28 mg/kg for males and 15–21 mg/kg for females.

Urea clearance test

Milliliter of plasma completely cleared or filtered off urea per minute. Urea is the end product of protein metabolism. Urea clearance is less than GFR, because urea is particularly reabsorbed.

Maximum urea clearance: The urea clearance is calculated by the formula:

$$C_M = \frac{U \times V}{P}$$

Where,
U = Milligram of urea per mL of urine;
P = Milligram of urea per mL of plasma
V = Milliliter of urine excreted per minute.
Normal value is found to be 75 mL/minute.

Standard urea clearance: If the clearance value is decreased when V, the volume of urine is less than 2 mL/minute, then it is called standard urea clearance.

Normal value is found to be 54 mL/minute and is calculated as:

$$Cs = \frac{U \times \sqrt{V}}{P}$$

Interpretation of urea clearance value: If the value is below 75% of the normal, it is considered to be abnormal, e.g. impaired renal function.

The clearance value may be abnormal even though the plasma urea values are within normal limits. The plasma urea values will start to rise only when the clearance value falls below 50% of the normal.

GASTRIC FUNCTION TESTS

The stomach is a major organ of digestion and performs the following functions:

1. Stomach is a reservoir of ingested foodstuffs.
2. Stomach produces HCl and some enzymes that are responsible for the initiation of digestive process.

Tests to Assess Gastric Function

Fractional Test Meal

Fractional test meal (FTM) involves collection of stomach contents by Ryle's tube in fasting. This is followed by gastric stimulation, giving a test meal. Stomach contents are aspirated by Ryle's tube at different intervals and the samples are analyzed.

Alcohol Test Meal

Test meal in the form of 100 mL of 7% alcohol is administered. The response is rapid and test time can be reduced to 1½ hour. Free-acidity levels are higher compared to FTM.

Pentagastrin Stimulation Test

Pentagastrin is a synthetic peptide, which stimulates gastric secretion. Stomach contents are aspirated by Ryle' s tube (residual juice). The basal secretion is collected and pentagastrin is introduced. Gastric juice is collected at 15 minute interval for 1 hour (represents maximum secretion). The end point is detected by titration.

Augmented Histamine Test Meal

Histamine is a powerful stimulant of gastric secretion. Basal gastric secretion is collected for 1 hour and histamine is administered subcutaneously. Gastric contents are aspirated and acid content is measured.

Insulin Test Meal (Hollander's Test)

Insulin test meal is done to assess the completeness of vagotomy. Insulin is given intravenously, which causes hypoglycemia usually within 30 minutes. If vagotomy operation is successful, insulin administration does not cause any increase in acid output.

Tubeless Gastric Analysis

Tubeless gastric analysis involves administration of cation-exchange resin that gets exchanged with H^+ ions of gastric juice. The resin is excreted in urine and measures for gastric acidity. Diagnex blue containing azure-A resin is employed in it.

Section 2

Practicals

Chapter

14

Qualitative Analysis

SCHEME FOR IDENTIFICATION OF IMPORTANT BIOLOGICAL PRODUCTS

Scheme for identification of important biological products is detailed in Figure 14.1.

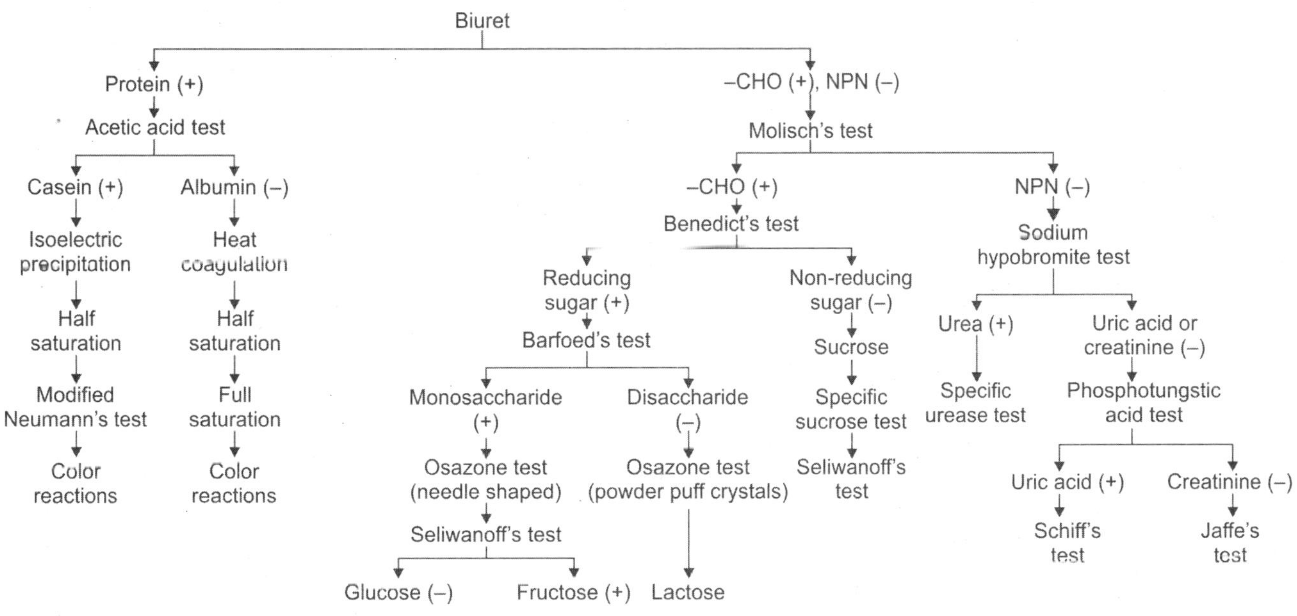

Fig. 14.1: Scheme for identification of important biological products (—CHO, carbohydrate; NPN, non-protein nitrogen)

REACTIONS OF CARBOHYDRATES (Table 14.1)

Table 14.1: Reactions of carbohydrates

Experiments	Observations	Inferences
1. Molisch's test To 1 mL of sugar solution, add 2–3 drops of Molisch reagent (1% α-naphthol in alcohol); add 2 mL of concentrated H_2SO_4 along the sides of it	Purple ring at the junction of two layers	Given solution is a carbohydrate; they form furfural derivatives when gets dehydrated by concentrated H_2SO_4; it condenses with α-naphthol forming purple product
2. Benedict's test To 5 mL Benedict's reagent (sodium citrate, sodium carbonate, copper sulfate) add eight drops of sugar solution and boil for 2 min	Red precipitate No red precipitate	Given solution is a reducing sugar; sugar solution in alkaline medium form enediols, which converts cupric ions to cuprous ions; $Cu(OH)_2$ formed during the process of heating is converted to red Cu_2O Given solution is a non-reducing sugar
3. Barfoed's test Mix equal volume of sugar solution and Barfoed reagent (copper acetate in glacial acetic acid) and keep in boiling water bath for 1 min; cool under tap water, add phosphomolybdic acid dropwise	Deep blue color No deep blue color	Given solution is a monosaccharide; they reduce cupric ions to cuprous ions in acidic medium, which converts phosphomolybdic acid to phosphomolybdous acid Given solution may be a disaccharide
4. Seliwanoff's test To 3 mL of Seliwanoff's reagent (resorcinol in HCl), add 1 mL of sugar solution; boil strongly for 30 s	Cherry red color	Given solution is a ketose sugar (fructose, sucrose); this on treating with HCl, dehydrated to furfural derivative, which condenses with resorcinol to form a cherry red color complex
	No cherry red color	Given solution is an aldose sugar (glucose, lactose); it will not answer this test Note: If boiled for longer duration, aldose will also give this test positive because of their conversion to ketose by HCl
5. Osazone formation Take one spatula of phenylhydrazine powder and add 2 mL of acetate buffer; heat to dissolve it; then add 2 mL of sugar solution to this test tube and keep it in boiling water bath for: • 20 min • 45 min Cool at room temperature; mount the crystals on a glass slide; cover with a cover slip and observe under a microscope	• Yellow long needle-shaped crystals (on heating with 20 min) • Hedgehog or powder puff-shaped crystals (on heating with 45 min)	Given solution may be glucose or fructose; glucoazone and fructoazone form yellow needle-shaped structures Given solution is lactose Reducing sugar is treated with phenylhydrazine to form phenylhydrazone, followed by the formation of characteristic crystalline-shaped osazones
6. Benedict's test after hydrolysis To 1 mL of sucrose solution, add few drops of concentrated HCl, boil for 2 min; cool and neutralize with 40% NaOH; the above solution is boiled with equal volume of Benedict's reagent for 2 min over a small flame	Red precipitate	Sucrose on hydrolysis by boiling with HCl, gives glucose and fructose will answer this test; reducing sugar under alkaline condition forms enediol, which reduces cupric ions to cuprous ions; the cuprous hydroxide formed during the process of heating is converted to red cuprous oxide

Related Test

Tests which are positive for:

1. Glucose: Molisch's test, Benedict's test, Barfoed's test, osazone formation.
2. Fructose: Molisch's test, Benedict's test, Barfoed's test, Seliwanoff's test, osazone formation.

3. Lactose: Molisch's test, Benedict's test, osazone formation.
4. Sucrose: Molisch's test, Benedict's test after hydrolysis.

COLOR REACTIONS OF PROTEINS (Table 14.2)

Table 14.2: Reactions of proteins

Experiments	Observations	Inferences
1. Biuret reaction To 2 mL of the test solution, add 1 mL of 5% NaOH mix; add two drops of 1% $CuSO_4$ solution	Violet color	Indicates the presence of proteins, compounds with two or more peptide bonds, gives a violet color with alkaline copper sulfate solution
2. Xanthoproteic reaction To 3 mL of the solution, add 1 mL of concentrated HNO_3; boil the contents till it turns yellow; cool and divide it into two parts; to one part add 40% NaOH	Yellow color deepens and changes to orange color in alkaline medium	This indicates presence of aromatic amino acids (Phenylalanine tryptophan tyrosine). On heating with concentrated HNO_3, benzene ring undergoes nitration to form yellow derivative; it is increased in strong alkaline medium
3. Aldehyde test (Hopkins-Cole test) To 1 mL of solution, add a drop of formalin and one drop of mercuric sulfate in H_2SO_4 mix and add 2 mL concentrated H_2SO_4 along the sides	Violet ring is formed at the junction	This indicates presence of indole ring containing amino acids (Phe); formaldehyde reacts with oxidized indole ring to give violet-colored complex
4. Sakaguchi reaction To 2 mL of the solution, add 1 mL of 40% NaOH solution and one drop of Molisch's reagent; after few min add few drops of alkaline hypobromide solution (bromine water)	Bright red color	Indicates the presence of arginine; the guanidine group of arginine reacts with α-naphthol to form a brightred-colored complex
5. Sulfur test To 2 mL of solution, add 2 mL of 40% NaOH and boil for 1 min; cool and add three drops of 2% lead acetate solution; boil for a min	Black precipitate	Indicates the presence of sulfur containing amino acids (cystine cysteine); the sulfur of the proteins in presence of NaOH is changed into Na_2S, which forms black lead sulfide when reacted with lead acetate
6. Millon's test To 1 mL of solution, add 1 mL of mercuric sulfate in H_2SO_4 and boil for 1 min; cool and add 1 mL of 1% sodium nitrate	Solution turns red color	Indicates the presence of phenol ring containing amino acid (Tyr); in the presence of H_2SO_4, phenol ring reacts with mercuric sulfate to form red mercuric phenolate
7. Pauly's test (Diazo reaction) To 0.5 mL sulfanilic acid, add 0.5 mL sodium nitrate, mix well and add 1 mL protein solution, mix and add 1 mL 10% sodium carbonate	A cherry-red color	Indicates the presence of tyrosine (Tyr) and histidine; the diazobenzene sulfanilic acid reacts with phenol group of tyrosine and imidazole group of histidine to form red-colored diazotized derivative

Reactions of Albumin (Table 14.3)

Table 14.3: Reactions of albumin

Experiments	Observations	Inferences
1. Half saturation test To 2 mL of protein solution is mixed with 2 mL of saturated ammonium sulfate solution and is allowed to stand for 5 min; with the filtrate, perform biuret test	Violet color	Egg albumin is not completely precipitated by half saturation; when an inorganic salt (ammonium sulfate) is added, the effective concentration of water or the protein is decreased and the protein gets precipitated
2. Full saturation test To 2 mL of protein solution, add ammonium sulfate till solution gets saturated; allow to stand for 5 min; perform biuret test with the filtrate	No violet color	Egg albumin is completely precipitated by full saturation

Contd...

Contd...

Experiments	Observations	Inferences
3. Heat coagulation test To 3 mL of solution, add two drops of chlorophenol red; if the solution is pink, add 1% acetic acid till it turns yellow; if it is yellow, add Na_2CO_3 till it turns pink and make it yellow by adding 1% acetic acid and boil it	A coagulum is formed	Indicates the presence of albumin; coagulation is irreversible when saturated at isoelectric point
4. Precipitation by heat and acetic acid Fill half of the test tube by albumin solution; boil the upper part of the solution by holding in a slanting position; add few drops of 1% acetic acid	A cloudy white precipitate in the upper part	Proteins are easily denatured when subjected to heat; they are coagulated and precipitated at their isoelectric point
5. Color reactions	-	-

Reactions of Casein (Table 14.4)

Table 14.4: Reactions of casein

Experiments	Observations	Inferences
1. Isoelectric precipitation test To two mL of protein solution, add 2 drops of bromocresol green; add 1% acetic acid drop by drop with mixing, until a green color is obtained	Initially, a deep blue color is formed, which turns to green with the formation of flocculent precipitate	Casein is precipitated at isoelectric pH 4.6; bromocresol green is used as an indicator; its pH ranges from 3.8 to 5.4 and color changes from yellow to blue
2. Acetic acid test To 3 mL of protein solution, add 1% acetic acid drop by drop	A white precipitate is formed that on further addition of acetic acid gets dissolved	The precipitate is formed at isoelectric pH and dissolves on further addition of acetic acid due to lowering of pH
3. Half saturation test To 3 mL of protein solution, add equal volume of saturated ammonium sulfate solution and filter; with 2 mL of filtrate, perform biuret test	No violet color	Casein gets completely precipitated at half saturation; when an inorganic salt like ammonium sulfate is added to a solution of protein, effective concentration of water or protein is decreased and the protein gets precipitated
4. Modified Neumann's test To 3 mL of casein solution, add 0.5 mL of 40% NaOH; boil strongly for few min; cool under tap water and add 0.5 mL concentrated HNO_3; add a pinch of ammonium molybdate and warm gently	Canary yellow precipitate is formed	This test detects the presence of organic phosphate; casein is a phosphoprotein and thus answer the test; organic phosphate when boiled with NaOH, is converted to inorganic phosphate; inorganic phosphate then reacts with ammonium molybdate to form ammonium phosphomolybdate
5. Color reactions	-	-

REACTIONS OF NON-PROTEIN NITROGENOUS SUBSTANCES

Non-protein nitrogenous (NPN) substance includes:

1. Urea.
2. Uric acid.
3. Creatinine.

Reactions of Urea (Table 14.5)

Table 14.5: Reactions of urea

Experiments	Observations	Inferences
1. Sodium hypobromite test To 2 mL urea solution, add 4–5 drops of freshly prepared sodium hypobromite NaOBr solution	Brisk effervescence	Hypobromite decomposes to nitrogen gas that appear as brisk effervescence $3NaOBr + NH_2\text{–}CO\text{-}NH_2 + 2NaOH \longrightarrow N_2 + Na_2CO_3 + 3NaBr + 3H_2O$
2. Specific urease test Take 3 mL of urea solution, add 2 mL of urease suspension; incubate for 30 min at room temperature; add two drops of phenolphthalein	Pink color	Urea is hydrolyzed by urease to form ammonium carbonate, which make the solution alkaline since the solution is alkaline. Phenolphthalein will give pink color $NH_2\text{-}CO\text{-}NH_2 + 2H_2O \longrightarrow 2NH_3 + H_2CO_3 \longrightarrow (NH_4)_2CO_3$

Reactions of Uric Acid (Table 14.6)

Table 14.6: Reactions of uric acid

Experiments	Observations	Inferences
1. Phosphotungstic acid reduction test To 2 mL of solution, add few drops of phosphotungstic acid reagent and 20% Na_2CO_3	Blue color	Uric acid under alkaline condition reduces phosphotungstic acid to tungsten blue
2. Schiff's test Wet a piece of filter paper with few drops of ammoniacal silver nitrate solution; dry and add two drops of uric acid solution on the filter paper	Black color	Uric acid reduces ammoniacal silver nitrate to black metallic silver

Reactions of Creatinine (Table 14.7)

Table 14.7: Reactions of creatinine

Experiments	Observations	Inferences
1. Jaffe's test Label two test tubes as 'test' and 'control' Into test, add 1 mL of creatinine solution; mix with 1 mL of saturated picric acid solution, add few drops of 5% NaOH	Orange color	Creatinine reacts with alkaline picrate solution to form orange-colored picrate
Into control, mix 1 mL of H_2O, 1 mL of picric acid and few drops of 5% NaOH	Yellow color	No creatinine

Chapter

15

Quantitative Analysis

INTRODUCTION TO CLINICAL BIOCHEMISTRY

Colorimetry

Measurement of concentration of colored substances in a solution is the basis of colorimetry. Colored solutions can absorb light rays of a particular wavelength called absorbants. This can be measured by photoelectric equipments.

Beer's law: The amount of light absorbed by a colored solution is proportional to the concentration of the solution.

Lambert`s law: The amount of light absorbed by a colored solution is proportional to the path length through which light passes in the solution.

Beer-lambert law is expressed as:

$$A_l = E_l \times C \times L$$

Where,

A_l = Absorbents of substances at a wavelength of l
E_l = Extension of coefficient at l
C = Concentration of colored substances in that solution
L = Length traveled by light in that solution.

Blood Glucose Estimation (Folin-WU Tube Method)

Alkaline copper (cupric ions) is reduced by glucose when boiled with protein-free filtrate to cuprous oxide. The cuprous oxide in turn reacts with phosphomolybdic acid to form blue-colored oxides of molybdenum. The intensity of color can be determined by measuring in a colorimeter at a wavelength of 680 nm.

Folin-Wu tube with constricted neck can be used to prevent the oxidation of cuprous ion, by atmospheric oxygen, during the period before adding phosphomolybdic acid.

Estimation of Serum Proteins (Biuret Method)

Proteins react with cupric ions in alkaline medium to form a purple-colored complex. The intensity of purple color is the concentration of total proteins present in the serum. Optical density measured at 540 nm. Serum albumin is determined by precipitating the globulin (G) with Na_2So_4. Albumin in globulin-free solution is estimated by biuret reagent. Differences between total proteins and albumin (A) can found out by A/G ratio.

Estimation of Serum Creatinine (Jaffe's Method)

Creatinine present in the protein-free filtrate of serum reacts with picric acid in alkaline medium to form an orange-colored complex. The intensity of color is proportional to the serum level. Optical density is measured at 540 nm.

Estimation of Urea in Blood

When urea is heated with substance containing two adjacent carboxyl groups like diacetyl monoxime, colored complexes are formed. On heating in acidic medium, diacetyl monoxime decomposes to give hydroxylamine and the diazine, which condenses with urea. Thiosemicarbazide and ferric ions are used as catalystsm, and pink color is produced. Intensity of the color is proportional to the amount of urea in the sample. Optical density is measured at 540 nm.

Chapter 16

Urine Analysis

PHYSICAL CHARACTERISTICS OF URINE

The physical characteristics of urine include observations and measurements of color, turbidity, odor, specific gravity, pH and volume. Visual observation of a urine sample can give important clues as evidence of pathology.

Color

The color of normal urine is usually light yellow to amber. Generally, the greater the solute volume, the deeper the color. The yellow color of urine is due to the presence of a yellow pigment, urochrome. Deviations from normal color can be caused by certain drugs and various vegetables, such as carrots, beets and rhubarb.

Odor

Slightly aromatic is the characteristic of freshly voided urine. Urine becomes more ammonia like, upon standing due to bacterial activity.

Turbidity

Normal urine is transparent or clear; becomes cloudy upon standing. Cloudy urine may be evidence of phosphates, urates, mucus, bacteria, epithelial cells or leukocytes.

pH

The pH ranges from 4.5 to 8.0 and average is 6.0, slightly acidic. High-protein diets and increase acidity, vegetarian diet and increase alkalinity. Bacterial infections also increase alkalinity.

Volume

Daily output of urine on an average is 1,500 mL/day. The volume of urine more than 2,500 mL/day is known as polyuria and urine output up to 500 mL/day is called oliguria.

Specific Gravity

The specific gravity of urine is a measurement of the density of urine; the relative proportions of dissolved solids in relationship to the total volume of the specimen. It reflects how concentrated or dilute a sample may be. Water has a specific gravity of 1.000. Urine will always have a value greater than 1.000, depending upon the amount of dissolved substances (salts, minerals, etc.) that may be present. Very dilute urine has a low specific gravity value and very concentrated urine has a high value. Specific gravity measures the ability of the kidney to concentrate or dilute urine depending on fluctuating conditions. Normal range is 1.005–1.035; average range is 1.010–1.025.

Low specific gravity is associated with conditions like diabetes insipidus, excessive water intake, diuretic use or chronic renal failure.

High specific gravity levels are associated with diabetes mellitus, adrenal abnormalities or excessive water loss due to vomiting, diarrhea or kidney inflammation. A specific gravity that never varies is indicative of severe renal failure.

Specific gravity can be determined by either of two methods using a refractometer or a urinometer.

Urinometer

urinometer is a weighted, bulb-shaped device that has a specific gravity scale on the stem end:

1. Fill the cylinder with enough urine so that the urinometer will float in the urine and not touch the bottom.
2. Be careful not to drop the urinometer in the cylinder. Gently release it in order, not to break or burst the cylinder. It should not touch the sides or bottom of the cylinder.
3. The specific gravity can be read on the scale on the stem of the urinometer at the meniscus.
4. The specific gravity of water is 1.000 with respect to temperature. The urinometer can be checked periodically against this standard, to ensure quality control at that temperature.

Note: For very precise and exact measurements of specific gravity, corrections should be made ± 0.001 for each 3°C above or below 25°C. Add 0.001, if above 25° C; subtract 0.001 if below 25°C.

CHEMICAL CONSTITUENTS OF URINE

The chemical constituents of urine are detailed in Table 16.1.

Table 16.1: Chemical constituents of urine

Name	Procedure	Observation
Urea	1 mL urine + 3 mL NaOCl (sodium hypochlorite)	Evolution of N_2 gas
Uric acid	1 mL urine + 0.5 mL 10% NaOH + 1 mL Folin's reagent	Blue color
Creatinine	1 mL urine + few drops of saturated picric acid + few drops of NaOH 10%	Deep red color of creatinine precipitate
Chloride	1 mL urine + few drops of dilute HNO_3 + 1 mL $AgNO_3$ $Cl^- + AgNO_3 \longrightarrow AgCl + NO_3$	White precipitate of AgCl
Phosphate	1 mL urine + 1 mL concentrated HNO_3 + 1 mL ammonium molybdate	Yellow color
Carbonate	1 mL urine + few drops of concentrated HCl + Na_2CO_3 + $2HCl \longrightarrow H_2O + 2NaCl + CO_2$	Effervescence
Ammonia	1 mL urine + 1 mL phenol + 1 mL NaBr	Blue color
Sulfates	1 mL urine + 2 drops of concentrated HCl + few drops of $BaCl_2 \longrightarrow SO_4 + BaCl_2$ $\longrightarrow BaSO_4 + 2Cl^-$	White precipitate of $BaSO_4$

Qualitative Analysis of Urine for Abnormal Constituents

Substances, which are not present in easily detectable amounts in urine of normal healthy individuals, but are present in the urine under certain diseased conditions are said to be abnormal constituents of urine.

Glucose

Benedict's test

Principle: Copper sulfate of Benedict's qualitative solution is reduced by reducing substances on boiling, to form the colored precipitate of cuprous oxide.

Test for glucose

To about 5 mL of Benedict's reagent, add 0.5 mL of urine and boil for 2 minute:

1. Blue color appearance indicates that sugar is absent.
2. If light green precipitate appears, 0.1%–0.5% of reducing sugar is present.
3. If green precipitate appears, 0.5%–1.0% of reducing sugar is present.
4. If yellow precipitate appears, 1%–2% reducing sugar is present.
5. If brick red precipitate appears, above 2% reducing sugar is present.

Normal urine also contains a trace of glucose and glucuronates, but their amount is too small to cause reduction in Benedict's test. In diabetes mellitus and in renal glycosuria, glucose is found in urine. This gives a Benedict's test, positive.

Albumin

Sulfosalicylic acid test

Principle: Albumin, the protein is denatured by sulfosalicylic acid coagulation.

Add a few drops of sulfosalicylic acid to 2 mL of urine. If turbidity appears, indicates the presence of albumin.

Heat coagulation test

Principle: The albumin is coagulated after being heated. Fill three fourth of the test tube by urine. Heat the upper one third of the test tube by a small flame. If turbidity appears on the heated portion of the tube, it indicates the presence of albumin.

Ketone bodies

Rothera's test

Principle: Acetoacetic acid forms a complex with nitroprusside in alkaline solution, developing a permanganate color.

Saturate 5 mL of urine with ammonium sulfate by shaking vigorously. Then add 2 drops of freshly prepared 5% solution of sodium nitroprusside and 1 mL of ammonium hydroxide. Allow it to stand in a rack for a while. If a permanganate color develops just above the layer of undissolved ammonium crystals it indicates the presence of ketone bodies.

Chapter

17

Biochemical Pathways

The Biochemical pathways are show in Figures 17.1 to 17.15.

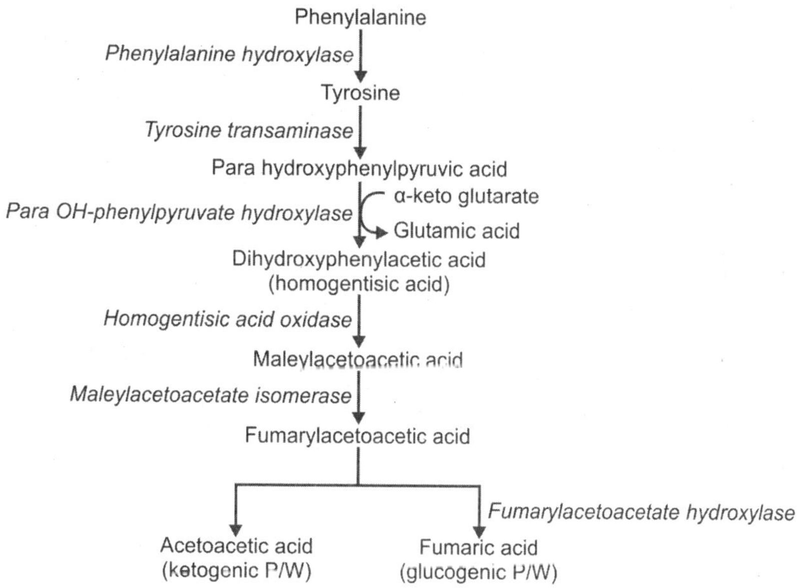

Fig. 17.1: Phenylalanine and tyrosine metabolism (P/W, pathway)

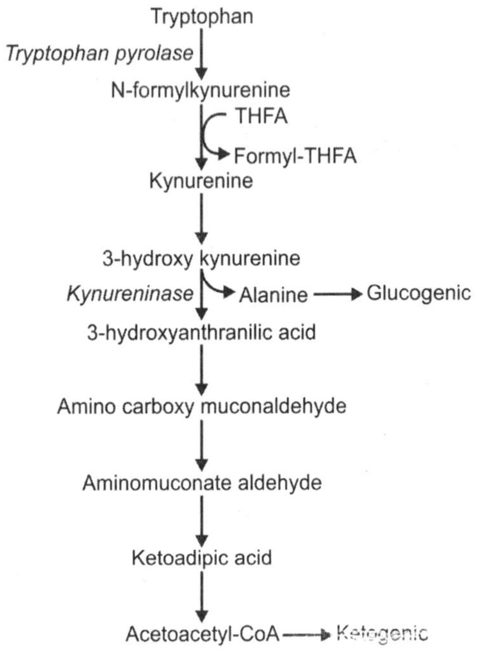

Fig. 17.2: Tryptophan metabolism

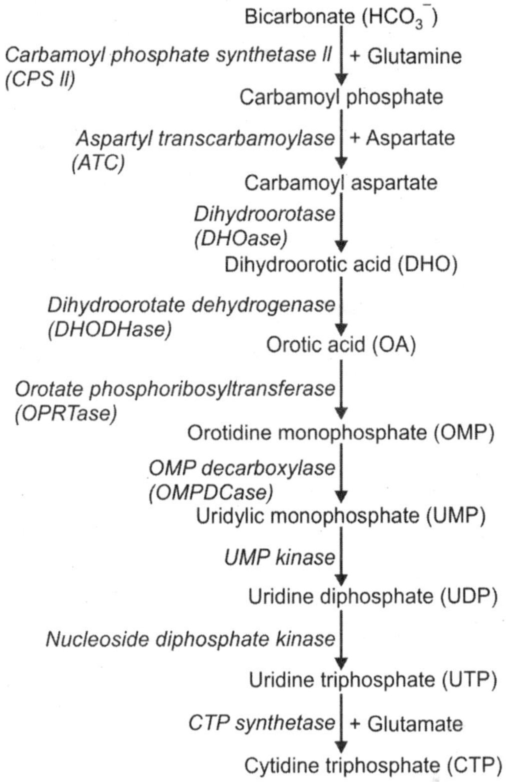

Fig. 17.3: Pyrimidine synthesis

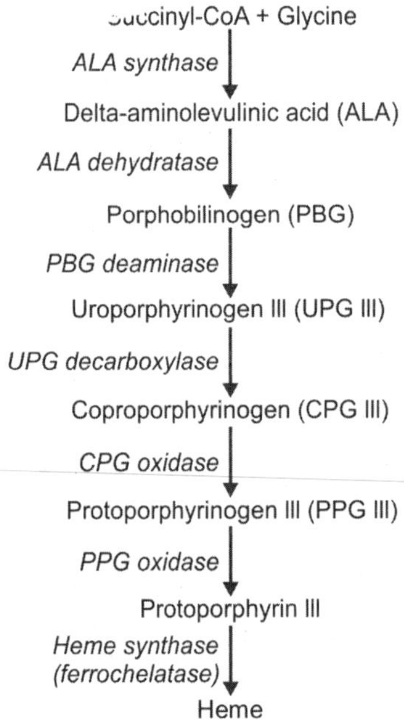

Fig. 17.4: Heme synthesis

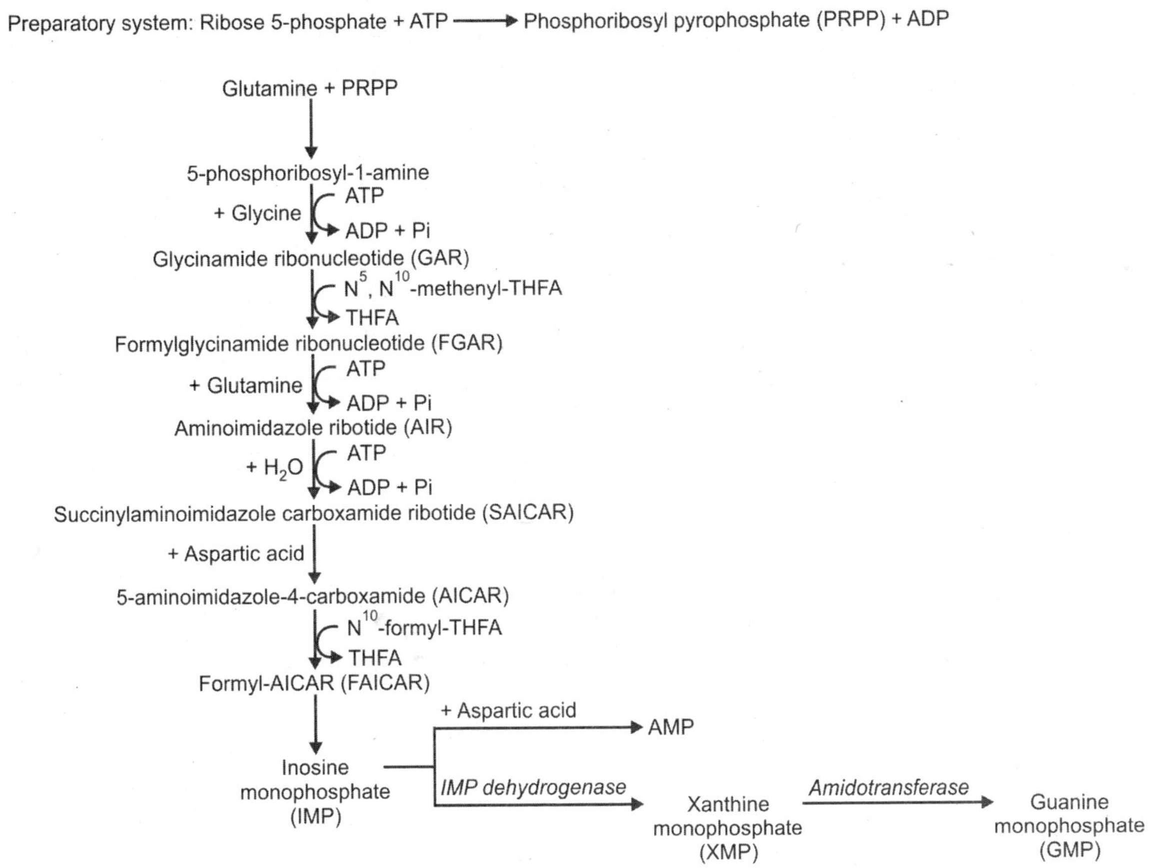

Fig. 17.5: De novo synthesis of purines

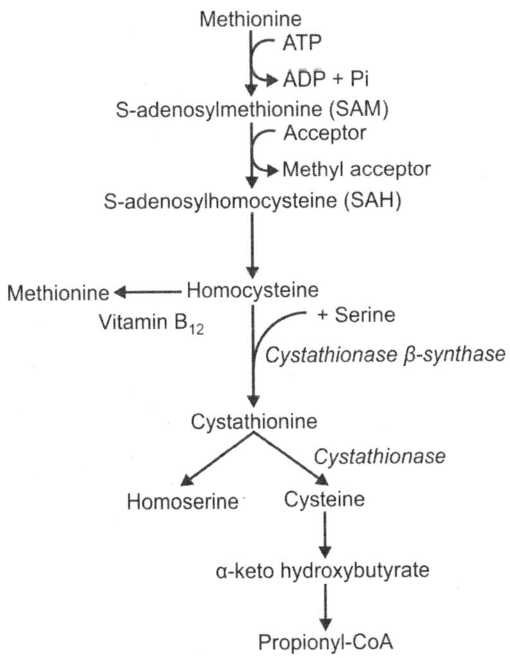

Fig. 17.6: Metabolism of sulfur containing amino acids
(ATP, adenosine triphosphate; ADP, adenosine diphosphate; Pi, inorganic phosphate)

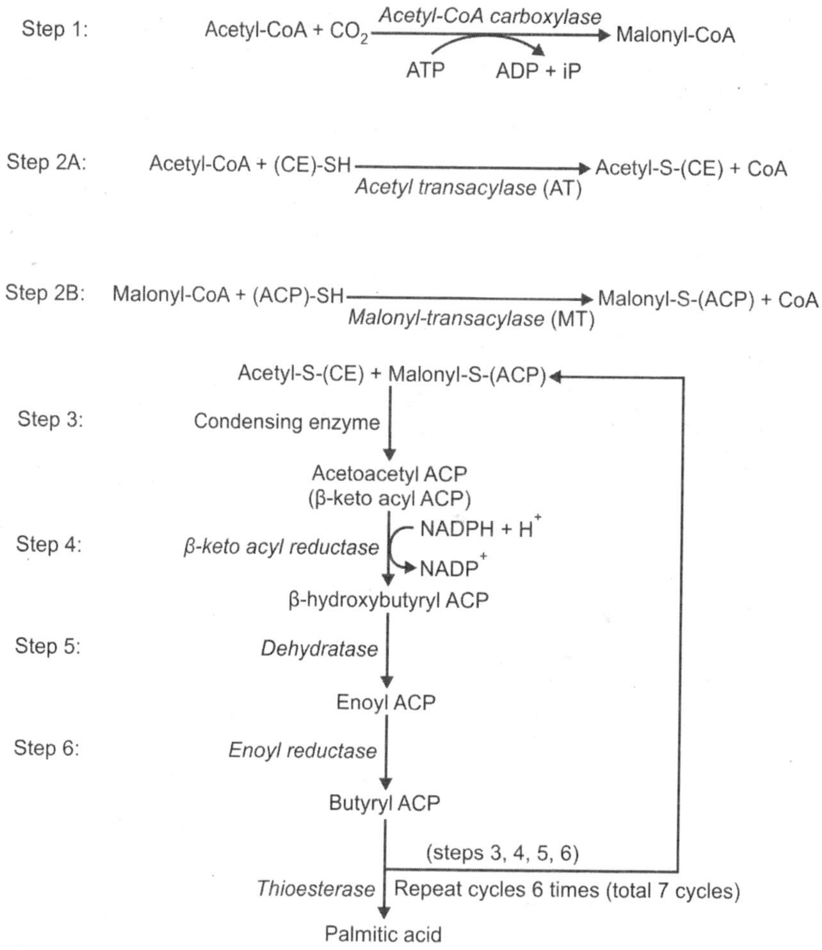

Fig. 17.7: De novo synthesis of fatty acids

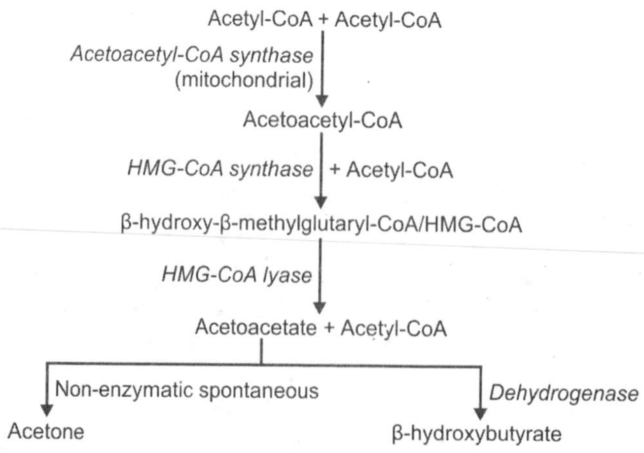

Fig. 17.8: Ketogenesis

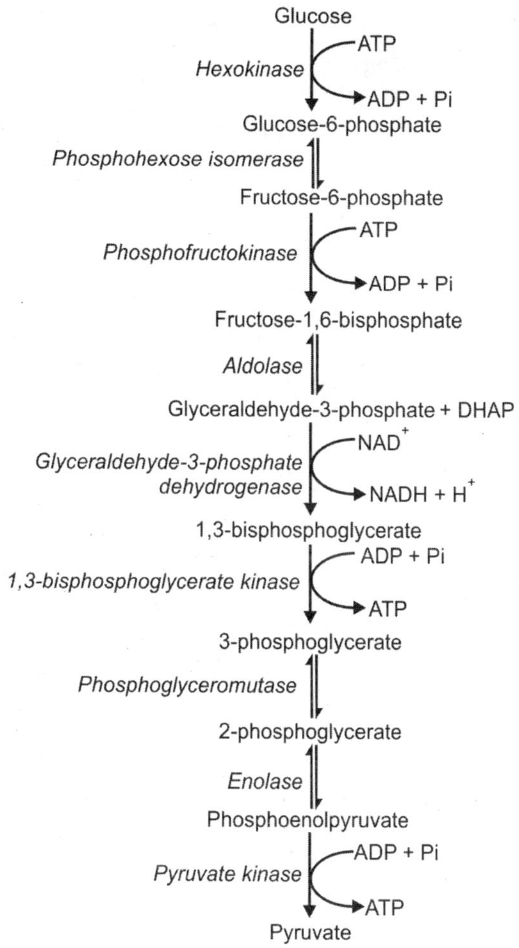

Fig. 17.9: Glycolysis

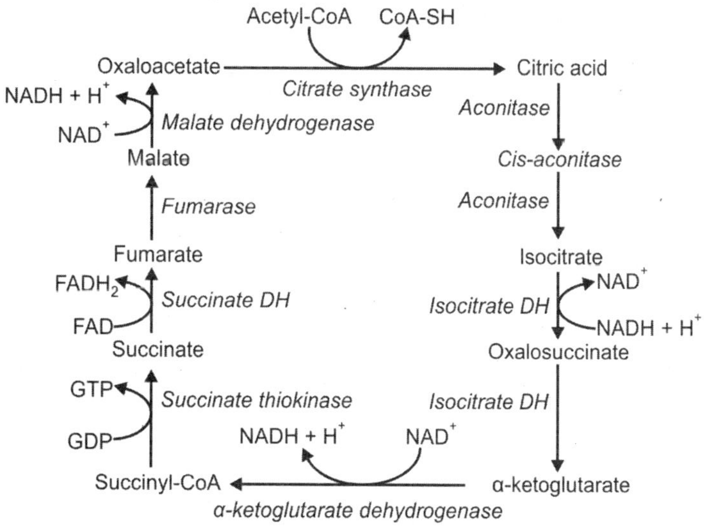

Fig. 17.10: Citric acid cycle

Acetyl-CoA + Acetyl-CoA

↓ *Acetoacetyl-CoA synthase (cytoplasmic)*

Acetoacetyl-CoA

↓ *HMG-CoA synthase* + Acetyl-CoA

HMG-CoA

(β-hydroxy β-methylglutaryl-CoA)

↓ *HMG-CoA reductase* 2NADPH + $2H^+$ → $2NADP^+$

Mevalonate (6C)

↓

5-phosphomevalonate (6C)

↓

5-pyrophosphomevalonate (6C)

↓

3-phospho-5-pyrophosphomevalonate (6C)

↓

Isopentenyl pyrophosphate (5C)

↓

Dimethylallyl pyrophosphate (5C)

↓

Geranyl pyrophosphate (10C)

↓

Farnesyl pyrophosphate (15C)

↓

Squalene (30C)

↓

Squalene epoxide

↓

Lanosterol (30C)

↓

Zymosterol (27C)

↓

Desmosterol (27C)

↓

Cholesterol (27C)

Fig. 17.11: Cholesterol biosynthesis

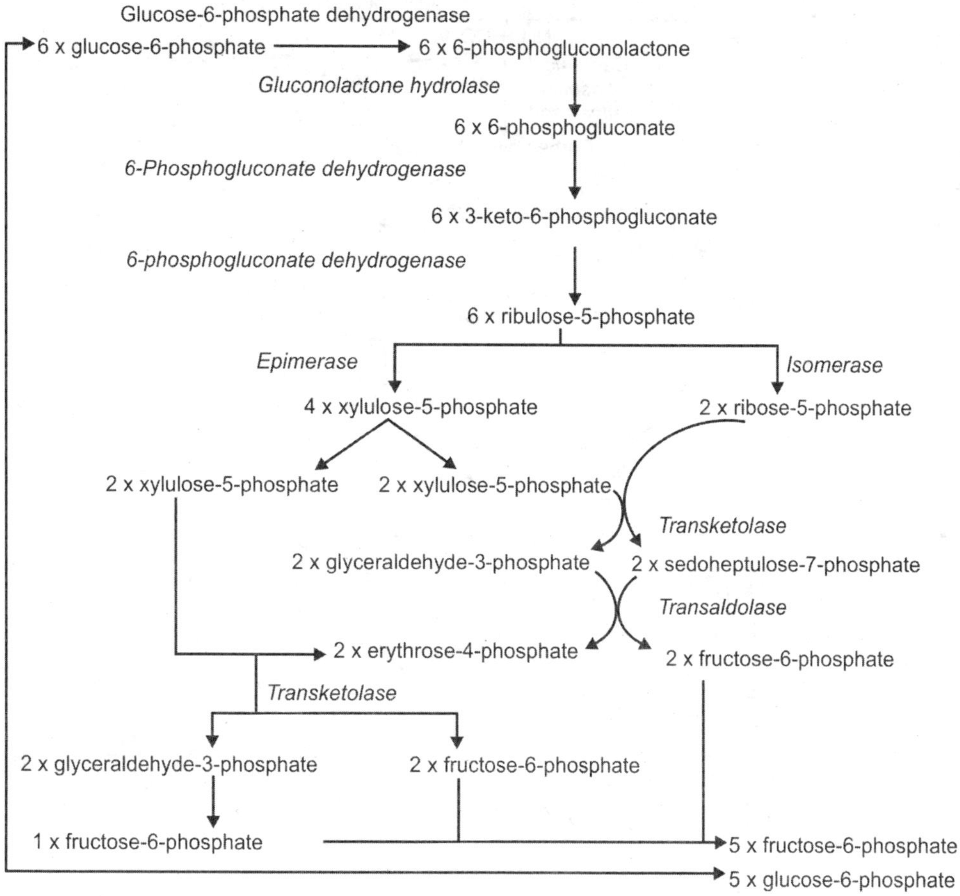

Fig. 17.12: HMP shunt pathway

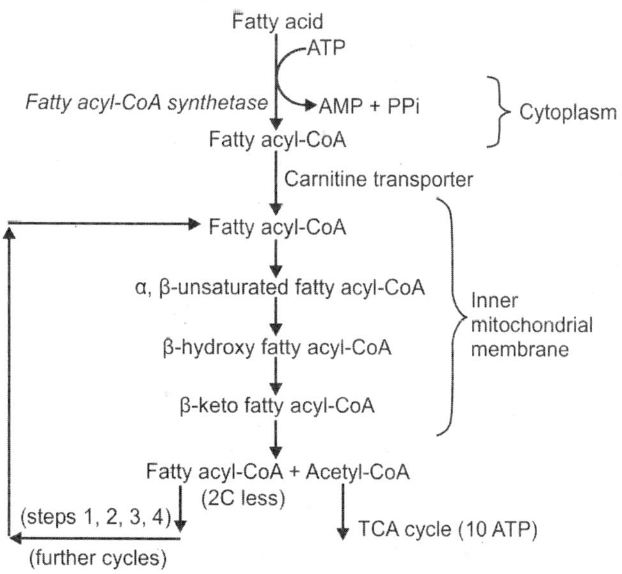

Fig. 17.13: Beta oxidation of fatty acids

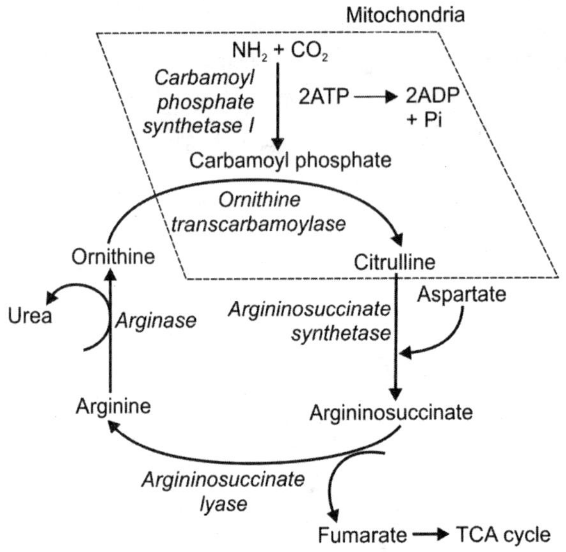

Fig. 17.14: Urea cycle/ornithine cycle/KREBS Henseleit cycle

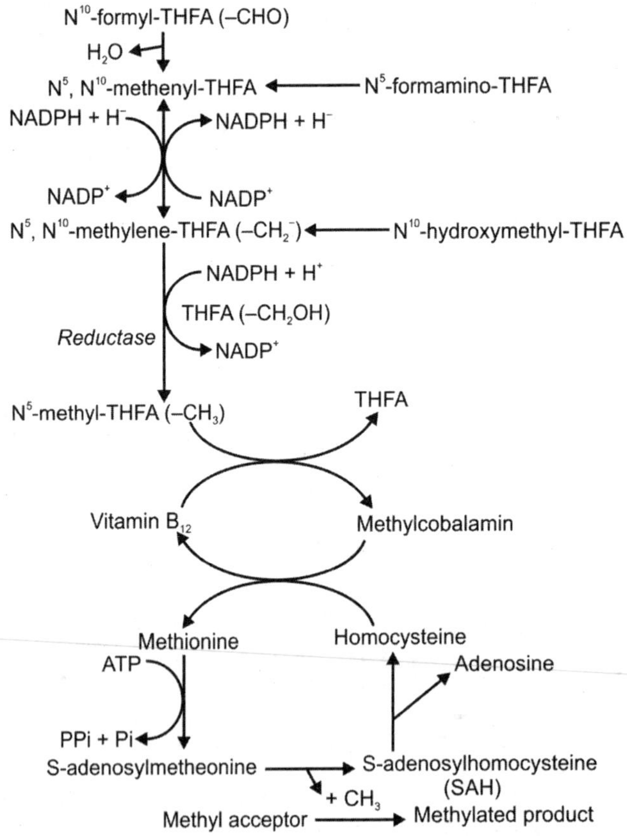

Fig. 17.15: One-carbon metabolism

Viva Voce

CELL AND SUBCELLULAR ORGANELLES

1. **What are the characteristics of fluid mosaic model?**
   Membrane is composed of lipid bilayer. Phospholipids are arranged in bilayers with a hydrophobic core.
2. **What are the components of membrane that alter the fluidity?**
   Cholesterol and unsaturated fatty acids.
3. **What are the functions of golgi complex?**
   Maturation and processing of nascent proteins:
   - Glycosylation of proteins
   - Secretion of newly synthesized proteins.
4. **What are the functions of endoplasmic reticulum?**
   Biosynthesis of proteins, drug metabolism, desaturation of fatty acids.
5. **What are cathepsins?**
   Cathepsins are intracellular proteolytic enzymes.
6. **What is the function of lysosomes?**
   Lysosomes are bags of hydrolytic enzymes that bring about degradation of macromolecules.
7. **What is lysozyme?**
   Lysosomes is an enzyme present in external secretions.

ENZYMOLOGY

1. **How are enzymes classified?**
   Enzymology are classified into six major classes—oxidoreductases, transferases, hydrolases, lyases, isomerases and ligases.
2. **Give an example of oxidoreductase.**
   Alcohol dehydrogenase.
3. **What is the function of transferases?**
   Transfer of groups other than hydrogen, e.g. hexokinase.
4. **What is the function of hydrolases?**
   Cleave the bond after adding water, e.g. acetylcholine esterase.
5. **What are coenzymes?**
   Coenzymes are non-protein part of enzyme. They are low- molecular weight organic substances without which the enzyme cannot exhibit any reaction. Coenzyme accepts one of the products of the reaction and acts as a cosubstrate.
6. **Give some examples of coenzymes involved in oxidoreductases.**
   Aldehyde dehydrogenase (NAD^+), nicotinamide adenine dinucleotide phosphate ($NADP^+$) and flavin adenine dinucleotide (FAD).
7. **What is the function of adenosine triphosphate (ATP)?**
   Adenosine triphosphate is the energy currency in the body. During the oxidation of foodstuffs, energy is released; a part of which is stored as chemical energy in the form of ATP.
8. **Name some enzymes containing copper.**
   Superoxide dismutase, tyrosinase and cytochrome oxidase.
9. **Which enzyme contains molybdenum?**
   Xanthine oxidase.
10. **Name some iron containing enzymes.**
    Cytochrome oxidase, catalase, peroxidase, etc.
11. **What is the active site of an enzyme?**
    The area of the enzyme where catalysis occurs is referred to as active site or active center.

12. What is meant by serine proteases?
Proteases (proteolytic enzymes) having a serine residue at its active center.

13. Give an example of a serine protease.
Trypsin, chymotrypsin, thrombin, etc.

14. What is the significance of 'Km' value?
'Km' is independent of enzyme concentration. Km value is thus a constant for an enzyme. It is the characteristic feature of a particular enzyme for a specific substrate.

15. What is the relation of Km value with the affinity?
Km denotes the affinity of enzyme to substrate. Thus, the lesser the numerical value of Km, the affinity of the enzyme for the substrate is more.

16. What are isoenzymes?
Isoenzymes are physically distinct forms of the same enzyme activity. They have identical catalytic properties, but differ in structure.

17. Glucose is absorbed at the luminal side of gastrointestinal cells by which mechanism?
Carrier-mediated cotransport with sodium is named as sodium-dependent glucose transporter (SGLT).

18. How glucose is released from intestinal cell into the bloodstream?
Glucose transporter type-2 (GluT2)

19. How glucose is taken up by cells?
In tissues helps in absorption of glucose from blood.

20. What is the importance of GluT4?
GluT4 is the glucose transporter present in muscle and adipose tissue.

CARBOHYDRATES

1. How carbohydrates are classified?
Based on the number of the sugar units available, they are classified as monosaccharides, disaccharides, oligosaccharides and polysaccharides.

2. Name some important monosaccharides.
Glucose, fructose, mannose, galactose.

3. Name a few pentoses.
Arabinose, xylose, ribose.

4. What is epimerism?
When sugars are different from one another, only in configuration with regard to a single carbon atom (other than the reference carbon atom), they are called epimers. For example, glucose and mannose are an epimeric pair, which differ only with respect to carbon atom 2. Similarly, galactose is the fourth epimer of glucose.

5. Anomerism is produced with reference to which carbon atom?
With reference to the first carbon atom in aldoses and second carbon atom in ketoses.

6. How polysaccharides are classified?
Homopolysaccharides (homoglycans) and heteropolysaccharides (heteroglycans).

7. What are homoglycans?
Homoglycans are composed of single kind of monosaccharides.

8. Give examples of homopolysaccharides.
Starch, glycogen.

9. Give examples of heteropolysaccharides.
Agar, hyaluronic acid, heparin, chondroitin sulfate.

10. What are mucopolysaccharides?
Mucopolysaccharides contain uronic acid and amino sugars.

11. Which heteropolysaccharide does not contain uronic acid?
Keratan sulfate.

12. What is the significance of glycolysis?
Anaerobic glycolysis forms the major source of energy in actively contracting muscles. Moreover, glycolysis is the only source of energy in red blood cells (RBCs).

13. Fluoride ions inhibit which enzyme?
Enolase.

14. What is the clinical significance of the fluoride ion inhibition?
Fluoride is used to prevent glycolysis, as preservative for blood before glucose estimation.

15. What are substrate-level phosphorylation steps in glycolysis?
1,3-bisphosphoglycerate (step 6) and pyruvate kinase (step 9).

16. What is Cori cycle (or lactic acid cycle)?
During exercise, lactate is produced in muscle. This lactate diffuses into the blood. Lactate then reaches liver, where it is oxidized to pyruvate. It is then becomes glucose. This glucose can enter into blood and then taken to muscle.

17. What is the energy yield from glycolysis during anaerobic conditions?
2 ATP.

18. In aerobic glycolysis, how much is the net yield from one glucose molecule?
7 ATP.

19. During complete oxidation, what is the net yield of ATP from one glucose molecule?
32 ATP.

20. How many ATPs are generated per one rotation of the citric acid cycle?
10 ATP.

21. What is function of 2,3-bisphosphoglycerate?
It reduces the affinity of hemoglobin toward oxygen.

22. What are the key gluconeogenic enzymes?
Pyruvate carboxylase, phosphoenolpyruvate carboxy kinase, fructose-1,6-bisphosphatase and glucose-6-phosphatase.

23. Gluconeogenesis is seen in which tissue?
Liver.

24. How many ATP molecules are required to convert two molecules of pyruvate into glucose?
6 ATP.

25. Which hormone will inhibit gluconeogenesis?
Insulin.

26. What is the significance of gluconeogenesis?
Gluconeogenesis is necessary to maintain blood glucose level, especially under conditions of starvation.

27. What is the key enzyme of glycogenolysis?
Glycogen phosphorylase.

28. Which hormones enhance glycogenolysis?
Adrenaline and glucagon causes glycogenolysis.

29. Which is the defective enzyme in von Gierke disease (glycogen storage disease type I)?
Glucose-6-phosphatase.

30. Which hormone controls hexase monophosphate (HMP) shunt pathway?
Insulin stimulates the pathway by activating the key enzyme.

31. What is the purpose of HMP shunt pathway?
HMP shunt pathway generates NADPH.

32. What is the clinical significance of transketolase?
The transketolase available in RBCs, is an index of the thiamine status of an individual.

33. Galactosemia is due the absence of which enzyme?
Galactose-1-phosphate uridyltransferase.

34. What is the treatment for galactosemia?
Lactose-free diet is given for first 5 years of life.

35. Why excess intake of alcohol produce hypoglycemia?
Because ethanol inhibits gluconeogenesis.

PROTEINS AND AMINO ACIDS

1. Benzene group is present in which amino acid?
Phenylalanine.

2. Phenol group is present in which amino acid?
Tyrosine.

3. Tryptophan contains what special group?
Indole group.

4. Which special group is present in histidine?
Imidazole group.

5. Name a purely ketogenic amino acid?
Leucine.

6. Name some glucogenic amino acids?
Glycine, serine, aspartic acid.

7. What are essential amino acids?
They cannot be synthesized in the body and so they are to be provided in the diet.

8. How many amino acids are essential?
Eight amino acids are essential; two are semiessential and the rest 10 are non-essential.

9. What is isoelectric point?
The pH at which the molecule carries no net charge is called isoelectric point.

10. What is produced when glutamic acid is decarboxylated?
Gamma-aminobutyric acid or GABA.

11. What is transamination?
The alpha amino group of amino acid can be transferred to alpha-keto acid to form the corresponding new amino acid and alpha-keto acid.

12. Give an example of transamination reaction?
Glutamic acid + pyruvic acid to alpha-ketoglutarate + alanine.

13. What force maintains the primary structure?
The primary structure is maintained by the covalent bonds of the peptide linkages.

14. What is a pseudopeptide?
The pseudopeptide is a peptide bond formed by carboxyl group, other than that of alpha position, e.g. glutathione (gamma-glutamyl-cysteinyl-glycine).

15. What are the forces that maintain the secondary, tertiary and quaternary structures of a protein?
Hydrogen bonds, electrostatic bonds, van der Waals forces and hydrophobic bonds.

16. Name the proteins having quaternary structure?
Hemoglobin, immunoglobulins.

17. What is the defect in maple syrup urine disease?
Deficient decarboxylation of branched-chain keto acids.

18. What is formiminoglutamic (FIGLU) acid excretion test?
In folic acid deficiency, there is a block in histidine metabolism and FIGLU is excreted in large quantities in urine.

19. What is FIGLU?
Formiminoglutamic acid, a product of histidine metabolism.

20. What is the defective enzyme in phenylketonuria?
Phenylalanine hydroxylase.

21. What is Hartnup disease?
Absorption of aromatic amino acids from intestine, as well as reabsorption from renal tubules are defective. So tryptophan deficiency and pellagra-like symptoms are seen. Tryptophan is excreted in large quantities.

LIPIDS

1. Classify fatty acids?
Depending on the total number of carbon atoms, they are classified as even chain and odd chain.

2. Name some saturated fatty acids?
Palmitic acid, stearic acid.

3. Name some unsaturated fatty acids?
Oleic, linoleic, linolenic and arachidonic acids.

4. Name some polyunsaturated fatty acids (PUFA)?
Linoleic, linolenic and arachidonic acids.

5. How many double bonds are there in arachidonic acid?
Four double bonds.

6. Which contains good quantity of PUFA?
Vegetable oils such as sunflower, groundnut oil.

7. Which contains very low level of PUFA?
Animal fats.

8. Which fatty acids are common in human fat?
Mainly oleic acid; then comes palmitic acid and lino leic acid.

9. What are the advantages of storing energy as triglycerides in the body?
a. Space requirement is less, as storage does not require water.
b. Can be mobilized whenever required.
c. Capacity for storage is unlimited.

10. What is lecithin?
Phosphatidylcholine.

11. What is phosphatidicacid?
It is made up of one glycerol, two fatty acid residues and a phosphoric acid.

12. What is cephalin?
Phosphatidylethanolamine.

13. What is cardiolipin?
Diphosphatidylglycerol.

14. What is sphingomyelin?
Sphingosine is attached to a fatty acid to form a ceramide. Ceramide with choline is sphingomyelin.

15. What are the coenzymes needed for fatty acid oxidation?
FAD and NAD.

16. What is the function of carnitine?
The long-chain fatty acyl-CoA cannot pass through the inner mitochondrial membrane. Therefore a transporter, carnitine is involved in transfer of fatty acids.

17. What is the net generation of ATP, when one molecule of palmitic acid (16 carbon) is oxidized completely?
106.

18. What is the product of beta oxidation of odd chain fatty acids?
Propionyl-CoA.

19. Refsum's disease is due to what?
Accumulation of phytanic acid, due to defective alpha oxidation.

20. What is the rate limiting enzyme of de novo synthesis of fatty acid?
Acetyl-CoA carboxylase.

21. What is the rate limiting step in ketone body formation?
3-hydroxy-3-methylglutary-CoA (HMG-CoA) synthase.

22. What is the ring structure present in cholesterol?
Perhydrocyclopentanophenanthrene ring.

23. What are the substances derived from cholesterol?
Glucocorticoids, mineralocorticoids, testosterone, estrogen, bile acids.

24. What is the normal level of total cholesterol?
140–200 mg/dL.

25. What is bad cholesterol?
Low-density lipoprotein (LDL) cholesterol.

26. What is LCAT?
Lecithin cholesterol acyltransferase.

27. What is good cholesterol?
High-density lipoprotein (HDL) cholesterol.

28. What is the key enzyme of urea synthesis?
Carbamoyl phosphate synthetase (CPS).

29. What are the two carbamoyl phosphate synthetases?
Carbamoyl phosphate synthetase-I (CPS-I) is involved in urea synthesis; CPS-II is required for pyrimidine synthesis. CPS-I is seen in mitochondria, while CPS-II is in cytosol.

30. What is the normal blood urea level?
20–40 mg/dL.

CELLULAR ENERGETICS

1. What are the steps in which carbon dioxide is liberated during oxidation of glucose?
Pyruvate dehydrogenase, isocitrate dehydrogenase, alpha-ketoglutarate dehydrogenase.

2. How many ATPs are generated per one rotation of the citric acid cycle?
10 ATP.

3. What is the net yield of ATP from one molecule of glucose in anaerobic glycolysis?
2 ATP.

4. What is the net yield of ATP from one molecule of glucose in aerobic glycolysis?
7 ATP.

5. During complete oxidation, what is the net yield of ATP from one glucose molecule?
32 ATP.

6. On hydrolysis of 1 mole of ATP to ADP, the release of energy will be approximately how much?
7 kcal.

NUTRITION

1. What is the reason for peripheral neuritis in pyridoxal deficiency?
Pyridoxal phosphate (PLP) is involved in the synthesis of sphingolipids. So, B_6 deficiency leads to demyelination of nerves and consequent peripheral neuritis.

2. What is the antagonist for biotin?
Avidin.

3. What is coenzyme form of pantothenic acid?
Coenzyme A.

4. What is the reason for anemia in pyridoxal deficiency?
Pyridoxal phosphate is required for aminolevulinic acid (ALA) synthase. So, hypochromic microcytic anemia may occur due to the inhibition of heme biosynthesis.

5. Lysine is deficient in which foodstuff?
Pulses.

6. Phenylalanine is deficient in which foodstuff?
Tapioca.

7. Methionine is deficient in which foodstuff?
Cereals.

8. What are the features of hemosiderosis?
Cirrhosis of liver diabetes mellitus, yellow, color of skin.

9. What is the major cause for hemosiderosis?
Repeated transfusion of whole blood.

10. What are the salient features of pellagra?
Dermatitis, diarrhea, dementia.

11. What is the precursor of niacin?
Tryptophan.

12. Tryptophan is deficient in which food stuff?
Maize and corn.

13. Transamination reaction requires, which vitamin?
Pyridoxal phosphate.

14. What is calcitriol?
1,25-dihydroxycholecalciferol or active vitamin D contains three hydroxyl groups at 1, 3 and 25 positions.

15. What is the complication of folic acid deficiency in pregnancy?
Folic acid deficiency during pregnancy may lead to neural tube defects (such as spina bifida) in the fetus.

16. What is folate trap?
The production of methyl tetrahydrofolate (THFA) is an irreversible step. Therefore, the only way for generation of free THFA is methyl THFA to THFA, by a vitamin B_{12} dependent step. When B_{12} is deficient, this reaction cannot take place.

TISSUE BIOCHEMISTRY

1. What is the normal serum albumin level?
3.5–5 mg/dL.

2. What is the normal value of total proteins in serum?
6–8 g/100 mL.

3. Name some transport proteins.
Retinol-binding protein, thyroxine-binding globulin, transcortin (cortisol) haptoglobin (hemoglobin), transferrin (iron), hemopexin (free heme).

4. What is the alkali reserve of the body?
Bicarbonate is the alkali reserve.

5. What is the normal ratio of bicarbonate to carbonic acid in blood?
Bicarbonate to carbonic acid ratio is 20.

6. What are the causes of metabolic alkalosis?
Prolonged vomiting, gastric aspirate and ingestion of antacids.

7. What are the causes of respiratory alkalosis?
Bronchial asthma.

8. What is the cause for respiratory alkalosis?
Hyperventilation, as in hysteria; salicylate poisoning.

MOLECULAR GENETICS

1. **What is base pairing rule (Chargaff's rule)?**
   Pairing (hydrogen bonding) of adenine with thymine and guanine with cytosine. Purine is paired with pyrimidine, i.e. A + T = G + C.
2. **What are histones?**
   Histones are nuclear proteins found in nucleus. They bind with deoxyribonucleic acid (DNA) and stabilizes DNA structure.
3. **What is nucleosome?**
   Deoxyribonucleic acid wrapped around histones.
4. **What are Okazaki fragments?**
   The small DNA molecules attached to its own primer RNA in the lagging strand are called Okazaki fragments.
5. **Xeroderma pigmentosum is due to deficiency of what process?**
   Defect in DNA repair mechanism (nucleotide excision repair).
6. **What is TATA box?**
   TATA box is a signal for initiation of transcription in prokaryotes. It is about 10 bp upstream of starting of mRNA synthesis.
7. **What are ribozymes?**
   Enzymes made up of ribonucleic acid (RNA) are called ribozymes.
8. **Give some examples of ribozymes?**
   Spliceosomes, RNase P (which generates the ends of tRNAs) and peptidyl transferase (present in ribosomes).
9. **Name the inhibitors of RNA synthesis?**
   Rifampicin, actinomycin, mitomycin and amanitin.
10. **Give examples for post-translational modifications.**
    Gamma carboxylation of prothrombin hydroxylation of proline in collagen, methylation of histones, glycosylation of proteins.
11. **Give examples of inhibitors of translation in eukaryotic cells?**
    Puromycin, cycloheximide diphtheria toxin, ricin.
12. **What are the vectors used for gene therapy?**
    Retrovirus, adenovirus plasmid, liposome complex.

CANCER

1. **Alpha-fetoprotein (AFP) level is used as a tumor marker for which cancer?**
   Hepatoma.
2. **What is the marker for colorectal cancers?**
   Carcinoembryonic antigen.
3. **What is the significance of beta chain of human chorionic gonadotropin?**
   It is a tumor marker for choriocarcinoma.
4. **What is the mechanism of action of methotrexate?**
   It is a folic acid antagonist.

BIOTECHNIQUES

1. **What is the advantage of radioimmunoassay (RIA)?**
   Very small quantities of substances could be accurately measured.
2. **What are the disadvantages of RIA, when compared to enzyme-linked immunosorbent assay (ELISA)?**
   a. Since radioisotopes are used, only approved laboratories could take up the assay.
   b. The shelf life of the reagent is short.
3. **What are the enzymes commonly used in ELISA technique?**
   Alkaline phosphatase (ALP) and horseradish peroxidase (HRP).
4. **What are the uses of Southern blotting?**
   a. To identify abnormal genes, to demonstrate virus integration. It is also used for prenatal diagnosis.
   b. Locating mutations in DNA.
5. **How are monoclonal antibodies produced in the laboratory?**
   By means of hybridoma technology.

CLINICAL CHEMISTRY

1. **What is the normal serum bilirubin level?**
   0.2–0.8 mg/dL.
2. **What is the normal level of unconjugated bilirubin?**
   0.2–0.6 mg/dL.
3. **What is the normal level of conjugated bilirubin?**
   Less than 0.2 mg/dL.
4. **What is alkaline tide?**
   When HCl is produced in stomach, bicarbonate level within the cell increases (formed from H_2CO_3), it is reabsorbed into bloodstream. This would account for the alkaline tide of plasma and urine, immediately after meals.
5. **Specific gravity of urine increased, when?**
   Diabetes mellitus and acute glomerulonephritis.
6. **Polyuria is seen in which conditions?**
   Diabetes mellitus; diabetes insipidus; chronic renal failure.
7. **What is the best method for assessing glomerular filtration rate?**
   Creatinine clearance test.
8. **What is the advantage of creatinine test?**
   Creatinine is formed spontaneously (non-enzymatic), so the blood level and excretion rate of creatinine are constant.
9. **What is the normal creatinine level in blood?**
   For adult males, 0.7–1.4 mg/dL; for adult females, 0.6–1.3 mg/dL.

Appendix 1

Important Topics

CELL AND SUBCELLULAR ORGANELLES

Essay

1. Explain the different types of transport mechanism with suitable examples. What is phagocytosis and pinocytosis?

Short Notes

1. Structure of cell membrane.
2. Lysosomes—functions and clinical applications.
3. Ionophores.

ENZYMOLOGY

Essay

1. What are the different types of enzyme inhibition? Explain with suitable examples.

Short Notes

1. Classify enzymes with examples.
2. Active site.
3. Define K_m. What is its significance?
4. Factors influencing enzyme reactions.
5. Allosteric inhibition.
6. Competitive inhibition and its clinical significance.
7. Covalent modification of enzymes.
8. Difference between competitive and non-competitive inhibition. Give two examples for each.
9. Specificity of enzymes.
10. Isoenzymes of myocardial infarction.

CARBOHYDRATES

Essays

1. Define glycolysis. Write down the steps of glycolysis. How many ATP is formed from anaerobic glycolysis? How is it regulated?
2. Metabolism of glycogen. Explain glycogen storage diseases.

Short Notes

1. Mutarotation.
2. Structure of sucrose.
3. Heteropolysaccharides.
4. Substrate-level phosphorylation.
5. Significance of HMP shunt pathway.
6. Galactosemia.
7. Key enzymes of gluconeogenesis.
8. Polyol pathway.
9. Essential pentosuria.
10. Write down the reactions of oxidative phase of HMP shunt pathway.
11. Glucose tolerance test.
12. Glycated Hb and its significance.
13. von Gierke disease.
14. Cori cycle.
15. Alcohol metabolism.
16. Complications of diabetes mellitus.
17. Metabolic derangements in diabetes mellitus.
18. Anomers and epimers.
19. Hereditary fructose intolerance.

PROTEINS AND AMINO ACIDS

Essays

1. Classify amino acids with examples.
2. Classify proteins with examples.
3. Give a brief account of structural organization of proteins.
4. What is the normal blood urea level? Describe urea cycle. Explain disorders of urea cycle.
5. Explain glycine metabolism. What are the important substances derived from glycine?
6. Describe the steps of catabolism of phenylalanine and tyrosine. Indicate the inborn errors of metabolism associated with this pathway.

Short Notes

1. Essential amino acids.
2. Peptide bond formation.
3. Examples of tripeptide.
4. Primary structure of proteins.
5. Secondary structure of proteins.
6. Transamination.
7. Transdeamination.
8. Transmethylation.
9. One-carbon metabolism.
10. Homocystinuria.
11. Phenylketonuria.
12. Alkaptonuria.
13. Hartnup diseases.
14. Tryptophan metabolism.
15. Maple syrup urine diseases
16. Folate trap.
17. Meister's cycle.
18. Vanillylmandelic acid.
19. Garrod's tetrad.
20. Tryptophan metabolism.
21. Gamma-aminobutyric acid.
22. Decarboxylation of amino acids.

LIPIDS

Essays

1. Explain β-oxidation of the palmitic acid by the following:
   a. Activation.
   b. Proper β-oxidation reaction.
   c. Energetics of β-oxidation.
2. Describe the reactions of de novo synthesis of fatty acids. How it is regulated?
3. Name the ketone bodies. How ketone bodies are formed and utilized in the body? Mention the causes and consequences of ketosis.
4. What is the normal serum cholesterol level? Write down major steps of cholesterol synthesis. How it is regulated? Which are the important compound drivatives of cholesterol?
5. Classify lipoproteins. Mention the functions of lipoproteins.
6. Classify lipids with examples. Mention the functions of phospholipids.
7. Metabolic alterations in well fed and starvation.

Short Notes

1. Rothera's test.
2. Refsum's disease.
3. Fatty liver.
4. Lipotropic factors.
5. Polyunsaturated fatty acid.
6. Prostaglandins and functions.
7. Lipid storage disease.
8. Inhibitors of ETC.
9. Bile acid formation.
10. Digestion and absorption of lipids.
11. Glucose transportes.
12. Leukotrienes.

CELLULAR ENERGETICS

Essays

1. Write down the reaction steps of TCA cycle. What is its significance? Mention the amphibolic role of TCA.
2. Depict the ETC indicating the sites of ATP synthesis. Explain chemiosmotic theory.

Short Notes

1. Uncouplers of oxidative phosphorylation.
2. Inhibitors of ETC.
3. High-energy compounds.

NUTRITION

Essays

1. Write down the sources, recommended daily allowance, biochemical functions and deficiency manifestations of vitamin A.
2. How vitamin D is synthesized in the body? Write down the recommended daily allowance, biochemical functions and deficiency manifestations of vitamin D.
3. Write down the sources, recommended daily allowance. Biochemical functions and deficiency manifestations of vitamin C.

4. What is normal serum calcium level? Enumerate the functions of calcium. How serum calcium level is maintained?

Short Notes

1. Vitamin K.
2. Vitamin E.
3. Thiamine pyrophosphate.
4. Pellagra.
5. Pyridoxal phosphate.
6. Folate trap.
7. Vitamin B_{12}.
8. Scurvy.
9. Iron metabolism and iron overdose diseases.
10. Metabolic role of selenium.
11. Fluorosis.
12. Name two copper containing enzymes.
13. Normal range of serum sodium and potassium.
14. Protein energy malnutrition.

TISSUE BIOCHEMISTRY

Essays

1. How heme is metabolized and catabolized in the body? Write down the rate-limiting step of heme synthesis.
2. Classify porphyria. Write down the Clinical features of different types of porphyria?
3. Classify jaundice. How do you investigate the different type of jaundice?
4. Classify immunoglobulin. Mention the functions of each. Draw the structure of IgG.
5. What is the normal pH of the blood? How blood pH is maintained?

Short Notes

1. van den Bergh's reaction.
2. Crigler-Najjar syndrome.
3. Hemoglobin S.
4. Thalassemia.
5. Acute phase proteins.
6. C-reactive proteins.
7. Normal range of serum sodium and potassium.
8. Anion gap.
9. Metabolic acidosis and metabolic alkalosis.
10. Respiratory acidosis and respiratory alkalosis.
11. Hemoglobinopathies.
12. Albumin: Globulin ratio.
13. Cyclic adenosine monophosphate.
14. Alkali reserve.
15. Plasma proteins.

MOLECULAR BIOLOGY

Essays

1. What is the normal serum uric acid level? Explain the purine catabolism.
2. De novo synthesis of pyrimidine.
3. Describe the process of DNA replication. Name two inhibitors of DNA replication.
4. Define transcription. Describe the steps of transcription. What are the post-transcriptional modifications? Name two inhibitors of transcription.
5. Define translation. Describe the steps of translation. What are the post-translational modifications? Name two inhibitors of translation.
6. What is mutation? What are mutagens? Describe point mutation and frameshift mutation.

Short Notes

1. Gout.
2. Purine salvage pathway.
3. Structure of purine.
4. Structure of pyrimidine.
5. Lesch-Nyhan syndrome.
6. Orotic aciduria.
7. Different types of DNA repair mechanism.
8. Difference between DNA and RNA.
9. Operon concept.
10. Induction.
11. Repression.
12. Recombinant DNA technology and its application.
13. Gene therapy.
14. Genetic code.
15. RNA polymer.
16. Structure and functions of tRNA.
17. Retrovirus.

XENOBIOTICS

Essay

1. Detoxification.

Short Notes

1. Free radicals.
2. Polyphenols.
3. Antioxidants.

CANCER

Short Notes

1. Oncogenes and proto-oncogenes.
2. Tumor markers.

BIOTECHNIQUES

Essay

1. Types of blotting techniques

Short Notes

1. Southern blotting.
2. Western blotting.
3. Restriction fragment length polymorphism.
4. Polymerase chain reaction.
5. Enzyme-linked immunosorbent assay.
6. Principle and applications of RIA.
7. Electrophoresis.

CLINICAL CHEMISTRY

Essay

1. Enumerate liver function test.

Short Note

1. Clearance test.

Appendix

2

Multiple Choice Questions

CELL AND SUBCELLULAR ORGANELLES

1. Blood is not a newtonian fluid because
   a. Density changes with velocity
   b. Viscosity changes with velocity
   c. Density does not changes with velocity
   d. Viscosity does not changes with velocity
2. About newtonian force, true is
   a. Viscosity is directly proportional to velocity
   b. Viscosity is inversely proportional to velocity
   c. Viscosity is equal to the velocity
   d. There is no relation between these two

Answers

1. a   2. b

ENZYMOLOGY

1. Which force does not act in an enzyme substrate complex?
   a. Covalent   b. Hydrogen
   c. Electrostatic   d. van der Waals
2. Which hormone uses an enzyme receptor for its action?
   a. Tyrosine   b. Insulin
   c. Estrogen   d. Steroid
3. Best enzyme marker for chronic alcoholism is
   a. Aldolase
   b. Serum glutamic oxaloacetate transaminase (SGOT)
   c. Serum glutamic pyruvic transaminase (SGPT)
   d. Gamma-glutamyltransferase (GGT)

Answers

1. d   2. b   3. d

CARBOHYDRATES

1. In glycolysis, rate-limiting enzyme is
   a. Pyruvate kinase
   b. Phosphofructokinase
   c. Glucokinase
   d. Glucose-6-dehydrogenase
2. Insulin does not facilitate glucose uptake in all of the following except
   a. Kidney   b. Liver
   c. Red blood cell   d. Heart
3. Pyruvate can be converted directly into all of the following except
   a. Lactate
   b. Acetyl-CoA
   c. Alanine
   d. Phosphoenol pyruvate
4. Glucose can be synthesized from all of the following except
   a. Glycerol   b. Amino acid
   c. Lactic acid   d. Acetoacetate
5. Glucose may be synthesized from
   a. Guanine   b. Glycosol
   c. Palmitic acid   d. Adenine
6. Malate shuttle is seen in
   a. Gluconeogenesis   b. HMP shunt
   c. Glycogenolysis   d. Glycolysis
7. The major fate of glucose-6-phosphate in tissue in a well-fed state is
   a. Isomerization to fructose-6-phosphate
   b. Hydrolysis to glucose
   c. Conversion to glycogen
   d. Conversion to ribulose-5-phosphate

8. Which of the following is not affected by gluconeogenesis?
   a. Glycerol b. Lactate
   c. Alanin d. Growth hormone
9. Cyclic GMP acts on
   a. Insulin b. Thyroxine
   c. AMP d. Growth hormone
10. Common enzyme in gluconeogenesis and glycolysis pathway is
   a. Hexokinase
   b. Fructose 2, 6-bisphosphat
   c. Phosphofructokinase
   d. Glucose-6-phosphate
11. All of the following are aldoses except
   a. Erythrose b. Ribose
   b. Ribulose d. Glucose
12. All of the following are ketoses except
   a. Ribulose b. Fructose
   c. Erythrose d. Sedoheptulose
13. The following monosaccharides contain six carbons except
   a. Glucose b. Mannose
   c. Galactose d. Xylulose
14. The number of asymmetric carbons present in glucose
   a. 2 b. 4
   c. 6 d. 8
15. The fasting blood glucose level in normal individuals
   a. 20–60 mg/dL b. 60–100 mg/dL
   c. 100–140 mg/dL d. 140–200 mg/dL
16. Insulin is required for glucose uptake in the following organ/tissue
   a. Brain b. Liver
   c. Muscle d. Erythrocytes
17. Under anaerobic conditions, the number of ATP synthesized in glycolysis
   a. 1 b. 2
   c. 4 d. 8
18. The enzyme glycerokinase is absent in
   a. Liver b. Kidney
   c. Adipose tissue d. None of the above
19. The amino acid that is predominantly transported from skeletal muscle to liver for gluconeogenesis
   a. Glycine b. Alanine
   c. Aspartate d. Tryptophan
20. The largest quantity of glycogen is present in
   a. Liver b. Muscle
   c. Brain d. Kidney
21. Hereditary fructose intolerance is due to the deficiency of enzyme
   a. Hexokinase b. Aldolase
   c. Fructokinase d. Triokinase
22. The preferred carbohydrate source of energy by sperms
   a. Glucose b. Galactose
   c. Ribose d. Fructose
23. Plants and microorganisms can convert fat to glucose via
   a. Gluconeogenesis b. Glyoxylate cycle
   c. Krebs cycle d. Glycolysis
24. In glyoxylate cycle, the enzyme that cleaves isocitrate to glyoxylate and succinate
   a. Isocitrate lyase b. Isocitrate synthase
   c. Citrate synthase d. Aconitase
25. Which of the following statements best describes glucose?
   a. It is a ketose and usually exists as a furanose ring in solution
   b. It is a C-4 epimer of galactose
   c. It is utilized in biological systems only in the L-isomeric form
   d. It is produced from dietary starch by the action of α-amylase
26. Which one of the following statements concerning glycolysis is correct?
   a. The conversion of glucose to lactate requires the presence of oxygen
   b. Hexokinase is important in hepatic glucose metabolism only in the absorptive period following consumption of a carbohydrate-containing meal
   c. Fructose 2, 6-bisphosphate is a potent inhibitor of phosphofructokinase
   d. The regulated reactions are also the irreversible reactions
27. The reaction catalyzed by phosphofructokinase-1
   a. Is activated by high concentrations of ATP and citrate
   b. Uses fructose 1-phosphate as substrate
   c. Is the rate-limiting reaction of the glycolytic pathway
   d. Is near equilibrium in most tissues
28. Compared with the resting state, vigorously contracting skeletal muscle shows
   a. An increased conversion of pyruvate to lactate
   b. Decreased oxidation of pyruvate to CO_2 and water
   c. A decreased $NADH/NAD^+$ ratio
   d. A decreased concentration of AMP

29. The conversion of pyruvate to acetyl-CoA and CO_2
    a. Is reversible
    b. Involves the participation of lipoic acid
    c. Is activated when pyruvate dehydrogenase (PDH, E1) of the pyruvate dehydrogenase complex is phosphorylated by PDH kinase in the presence of ATP
    d. Occurs in the cytosol
30. Which one of the following conditions decreases the oxidation of acetyl-CoA by the citric acid cycle?
    a. A low ATP/ADP ratio
    b. A low NADH concentration due to rapid oxidation to NAD^+ through the respiratory chain
    c. A low NAD^+/NADH ratio
    d. A high concentration of AMP
31. The synthesis of glucose from pyruvate by gluconeogenesis
    a. Occurs exclusively in the cytosol
    b. Is inhibited by an elevated level of glucagon
    c. Requires the participation of biotin
    d. Involves lactate as an intermediate
32. Which one of the following statements concerning gluconeogenesis is correct?
    a. It occurs in muscle
    b. It is stimulated by fructose 2, 6-bisphosphate
    c. It is inhibited by elevated levels of acetyl-CoA
    d. It is important in maintaining blood glucose during the normal overnight fast
33. Which one of the following reactions is unique to gluconeogenesis?
    a. Lactate ⟶ pyruvate
    b. Phosphoenol ⟶ pyruvate
    c. Oxaloacetate ⟶ phosphoenolpyruvate
    d. Glucose-6-phosphate ⟶ fructose-6-phosphate
34. The hormones, epinephrine and glucagon have which one of the following effects on glycogen metabolism in the liver?
    a. The net synthesis of glycogen is increased
    b. Glycogen phosphorylase is phosphorylated and active, whereas glycogen synthase is phosphorylated and inactive
    c. Both glycogen phosphorylase and glycogen synthase are activated by phosphorylation but at significantly different rates
    d. Glycogen phosphorylase is inactivated by a rise in Ca^2, whereas glycogen synthase is activated
35. In contracting skeletal muscle, a sudden elevation of the cytosolic Ca^2 concentration will result in
    a. Activation of cAMP-dependent protein kinase A
    b. Dissociation of cAMP-dependent protein kinase A into catalytic and regulatory subunits
    c. Inactivation of phosphorylase kinase caused by the action of protein phosphatase 1
    d. Direct activation of phosphorylase kinase b

Answers

1. b	2. d	3. d	4. d
5. b	6. a	7. c	8. b
9. c	10. c	11. c	12. c
13. d	14. b	15. b	16. c
17. b	18. c	19. b	20. b
21. b	22. d	23. b	24. a
25. b	26. d	27. c	28. a
29. b	30. c	31. c	32. d
33. c	34. b	35. d	

PROTEINS AND AMINO ACIDS

1. Amino acid with dissociation constant closest to physiological pH is
   a. Proline b. Serine
   c. Histidine d. Threonine
2. Basic amino acids are
   a. Lysine and arginine
   b. Serine and glycine
   c. Aspartate and glutamate
   d. None of the above
3. Sources of nitrogen in urea cycle is/are
   a. Uric acid
   b. Arginine and ammonia
   c. Glutamate and ammonia
   d. Aspartate and ammonia
4. Non-polar amino acid is
   a. Glycine b. Lysine
   c. Arginine d. Leucine
5. A destitute woman is admitted to the hospital with altered sensorium and dehydration. Urine analysis shows mild proteinuria and no sugar. What other test should be done?
   a. Hay's b. Fouchet's
   c. Rothera d. Benedicts'
6. If urine sample darkens on standing the most likely condition is
   a. Tyrosinemia b. Alkaptonuria
   c. Phenylketonuria d. Maple syrup disease
7. Which of the following is optically inactive amino acid?
   a. Glycine b. Proline
   c. Leucine d. Lysine

8. In brain, ammonia is detoxified to
   a. Uric acid b. Urea
   c. GAB d. Glutamine
9. Which of the following amino acid is excreted in urine in maple syrup urine disease?
   a. Arginine b. Phenylalanine
   c. Leucine d. Tryptophan
10. Most basic amino acid is?
    a. Alanine b. Histidine
    c. Lysine d. Arginine
11. Transamination of pyruvate with glutamate produces
    a. Oxaloacetate and aspartate
    b. Alanine and α-ketoglutarate
    c. Oxaloacetate and α-ketoglutarate
    d. Alanine and aspartate
12. If chymotrypsin molecule undergoes a ser-195-ala mutation then
    a. No affect will be observed
    b. Chymotrypsin will not bind the substrate
    c. Chymotrypsin will bind the substrate as well as cause cleavage
    d. Chymotrypsin will bind substrate, but does not cause cleavage
13. Property of photochromism is seen in which of following amino acid
    a. Unsaturated amino acid
    b. Aromatic amino acid
    c. Monocarboxylic acid
    d. Dicarboxylic acid
14. True statement regarding covalent bonds is
    a. They are weak bond
    b. Electrons have opposite spin
    c. Electrons have same spin
    d. None of the above
15. All of the following are required for hydroxylation of proline in collagen synthesis except
    a. Pyridoxal phosphate
    b. Vitamin C
    c. Oxygen (O_2)
    d. Dioxygenases
16. The cellular component for protein synthesis is
    a. Smooth endoplasmic reticulum
    b. Rough endoplasmic reticulum
    c. Ribosomes
    d. Mitochondria
17. All of the following are basic amino acids except
    a. Lysine b. Arginine
    c. Histidine d. Glutamate
18. One of the following is an aromatic non-essential amino acid
    a. Histidine
    b. Phenylalanine
    c. Tyrosine
    d. Tryptophan
19. The secondary structure of a protein is stabilized by
    a. Peptide bonds
    b. Hydrogen bonds
    c. Disulfide bonds
    d. Hydrophobic bonds
20. The minimum number of peptide bonds needed to answer biuret test
    a. 1 b. 2
    c. 3 d. 4
21. One of the following amino acids answers biuret test
    a. Tryptophan b. Tyrosine
    c. Phenylalanine d. Histidine
22. All of the following are structural proteins except
    a. Keratin b. Glutelin
    c. Elastin d. Collagen
23. One of the following amino acid cannot undergo transamination
    a. Glycine b. Alanine
    c. Lysine d. Glutamate
24. The 8th amino group of the following amino acid can be transaminated
    a. Lysine b. Arginine
    c. Ornithine d. Histidine
25. The amino acid predominantly involved in transdeamination reaction
    a. Alanine b. Glutamate
    c. Aspartate d. Glutamine
26. The number of ATP consumed in urea synthesis
    a. 1 b. 2
    c. 3 d. 4
27. The non-protein amino acid found in urea cycle
    a. Ornithine b. Citrulline
    c. Argininosuccinate d. All the above
28. The non-essential amino acid synthesized in urea cycle is
    a. Arginine b. Aspartate
    c. Glutamate d. Ornithine
29. A peptide bond
    a. Has a partial double-bond character
    b. Is ionized at physiologic pH
    c. Is cleaved by agents that denature proteins, such as organic solvents and high concentrations of urea
    d. Is stable to heating in strong acids

30. Which one of the following statements is correct?
    a. The α-helix can be composed of more than one polypeptide chain
    b. ß-sheets exist only in the antiparallel form.
    c. ß-bends often contain proline
    d. Domains are a type of secondary structure
31. Which one of the following statements about protein structure is correct?
    a. Proteins consisting of one polypeptide can have quaternary structure
    b. The formation of a disulfide bond in a protein requires that the two participating cysteine residues be adjacent to each other in the primary sequence of the protein
    c. The stability of quaternary structure in proteins is mainly a result of covalent bonds among the subunits
    d. The information required for the correct folding of a protein is contained in the specific sequence of amino acids along the polypeptide chain

Answers

1. c	2. a	3. d	4. d
5. c	6. b	7. a	8. d
9. c	10. d	11. b	12. b
13. b	14. b	15. a	16. c
17. d	18. c	19. b	20. b
21. d	22. b	23. c	24. c
25. b	26. d	27. d	28. d
29. a	30. c	31. d	

LIPIDS

1. Which of the following fatty acid is found exclusively in breast milk?
    a. Palmitic b. Linoleic
    c. Linolenic d. d-Hexanoic
2. Gaucher's disease is due to deficiency of
    a. Sphingomyelinase
    b. ß-galactosidase
    c. ß-glucosidase
    d. Hexosaminidase A
3. All of the following statements are correct about metabolism in brain except
    a. Ketone bodies are used in starvation
    b. Has no stored energy
    c. Fatty acids are utilized in starvation
    d. About 60% of total energy is utilized during resting stage
4. NADPH is required for
    a. Fatty acid synthesis
    b. Gluconeogenesis
    c. Glycogenolysis
    d. Glycolysis
5. Apoprotein A is found in
    a. Chylomicrons b. VLDL
    c. HDL d. LDL
6. Endogenous triglycerides in plasma are maximally transported by
    a. LDL b. HDL
    c. Chylomicron d. VLDL
7. The most important carrier of cholesterol in plasma is
    a. LDL b. Chylomicrons
    c. VLDL d. HDL
8. The number of carbon atoms present in stearic acid
    a. 1 b. 16
    c. 1 d. 20
9. The number of double bonds present in linoleic acid is
    a. 1 b. 2
    c. 3 d. 4
10. Phospholipids may be regarded as the derivatives of
    a. Lecithin b. Cephalin
    c. Phosphatidic acid d. Plasmalogen
11. The nitrogenous base present in chitin
    a. Choline b. Ethanolamine
    c. Serine d. Inositol
12. One of the following is a plant sterol
    a. Cholesterol b. Ergosterol
    c. Cortisol d. Lanosterol
13. All of the following are intracellular enzymes except
    a. Trypsin b. Fumarase
    c. Hexokinase d. Alcohol dehydrogenase
14. One of the following classes of enzymes is mostly involved in biosynthetic reactions
    a. Lyases b. Ligases
    c. Transferases d. Hydrolases
15. Besides the proteins, one of the following has been shown to act as enzymes
    a. DNA b. Carbohydrates
    c. RNA d. Lipids
16. The graphic representation of Lineweaver-Burk reciprocal plot is
    a. Bell shaped b. Hyperbola
    c. Straight line d. Sigmoid shaped
17. The optimum pH for urease activity
    a. 40°C b. 50°C
    c. 60°C d. 80°C

18. The following cation/anion is required by amylase
    a. Mg^{2+} b. Cl^-
    c. Na^+ d. SO_4^{2-}
19. The specificity of the enzyme is mostly dependent on the
    a. Apoenzyme b. Coenzyme
    c. Prosthetic group d. Cofactor
20. The major vehicles for intestinal absorption of lipids
    a. Chylomicron b. Liposomes
    c. Emulsions d. Micelles
21. The packed cell volume of human blood is around
    a. 35 b. 45%
    c. 55 d. 65%
22. The ketone body not metabolized
    a. Acetone b. Acetoacetic acid
    c. ß-hydroxybutyrate d. None of the above
23. The synthesis of ketone bodies occurs in
    a. Muscle b. Liver
    c. Brain d. Kidney
24. The precursor for the synthesis of ketone bodies (ketogenesis)
    a. Acetyl-CoA b. Malonyl-CoA
    c. Propionyl-CoA d. Acetate
25. The ketone bodies can be utilized by the following tissues/organ except
    a. Brain b. Liver
    c. Skeletal muscle d. Cardiac muscle
26. During prolonged starvation ketone bodies are the major energy sources for
    a. Skeletal muscle b. Cardiac muscle
    c. Brain d. Kidney
27. Ketoacidosis is commonly observed in
    a. Diabetes mellitus b. Starvation
    c. Atherosclerosis d. Fatty liver
28. Which one of the following statements about the digestion of lipids is correct?
    a. Lipid digestion begins with acid-stable lipases that primarily use TAG with long to very long-chain fatty acids as substrates
    b. Large lipid droplets are emulsified (have their surface area increased) in the mouth through the act of chewing (mastication)
    c. Colipase facilitates the binding of bile salts to mixed micelles, maximizing the activity of pancreatic lipase
    d. Patients with cystic fibrosis have difficulties with digestion because their thickened pancreatic secretions are less able to reach the small intestine, the primary site of lipid digestion
29. Which one of the following statements about the absorption of lipids from the intestine is correct?
    a. Dietary triacylglycerol must be completely hydrolyzed to free fatty acids and glycerol before absorption
    b. The TAG carried by chylomicrons is degraded to free fatty acids and glycerol by lipoprotein lipase on the endothelial surface of capillaries in muscle and adipose primarily
    c. Fatty acids that contain 10 carbons or less are absorbed and enter the circulation primarily via the lymphatic system
    d. Deficiencies in the ability to absorb fat result in excessive amounts of chylomicrons in the blood
30. Triacylglycerol molecules stored in adipose tissue represent the major reserve of substrate providing energy during a prolonged fast. During fast
    a. The stored fatty acids are released from adipose tissue into the plasma as components of the serum lipoprotein particle, VLDL
    b. Free fatty acids are produced at a high rate in the plasma by the action of lipoprotein lipase on chylomicrons
    c. Glycerol produced by the degradation of triacylglycerol is an important direct source of energy for adipocytes and fibroblasts
    d. Hormone-sensitive lipase is phosphorylated and activated by a cAMP-activated protein kinase
31. A 25-year-old woman with a history that included hepatosplenomegaly with eventual removal of the spleen, bone and joint pain with several fractures of the femur, and a liver biopsy that showed wrinkled looking cells with accumulations of glucosylceramides was presented at grand rounds. The likely diagnosis for this patient is
    a. Fabry's disease
    b. Farber's disease
    c. Gaucher's disease
    d. Krabbe's disease
32. A 20-year-old anemic man is found to have an abnormal form of ß-globin that is 172 amino acids long, rather than the 141 found in the normal protein. Which of the following point mutations is consistent with this abnormality?
    a. UAA ⟶ CAA b. UAA ⟶ UAG
    c. CGA ⟶ UGA d. GAU ⟶ GAC

Answers

1. b	2. c	3. c	4. a
5. c	6. d	7. a	8. c
9. b	10. c	11. a	12. b

13. a	14. b	15. c	16. c
17. c	18. b	19. a	20. d
21. b	22. a	23. b	24. a
25. b	26. c	27. a	28. d
29. b	30. d	31. c	32. a

CELLULAR ENERGETICS

1. The number of NADH + H^+ produced in citric acid cycle
   a. 1 b. 2
   c. 3 d. 4
2. When a molecule of glucose is completely oxidized, the number of ATP generated
   a. 2 b. 8
   c. 3. d. 129

Answers

1. c 2. d

NUTRITION

1. Similarity between vitamin C and vitamin K is
   a. Both helps in conversion of proline to hydroxyproline
   b. Both undergo post-translational modification
   c. Both have anti-infective activity
   d. Both are involved in coagulation cascade
2. Thiamine acts as a cofactor in
   a. Oxidation in respiratory chain
   b. Conversion of pyridoxal to pyridoxal phosphate
   c. Conversion of pyruvate to acetyl-CoA
   d. Transamination reactions
3. All of the following constitute dietary fibers except
   a. Pectin b. Riboflavin
   c. Hemicellulose d. Cellulose
4. Which vitamin is required for post-translational modifications of coagulants?
   a. Vitamin E b. Vitamin A
   c. Vitamin C d. Vitamin K
5. Protein binding to DNA is regulated by
   a. Copper b. Zinc
   c. Selenium d. Nickel
6. The number of isoprenoid units present in retinol is
   a. 1 b. 2
   c. 3 d. 4
7. Vitamin D in its structure resembles one of the following compounds
   a. Retinol b. Vitamin K
   c. Sterol d. Tocopherol
8. High consumption of one of the following vitamins protects against the development of heart diseases
   a. Vitamin A b. Vitamin D
   c. Vitamin E d. Biotin
9. One of the following is the least toxic among the fat-soluble vitamins
   a. Vitamin A b. Vitamin B
   c. Vitamin E d. Vitamin K
10. One of the following amino acids in certain clotting factors gets modified through the coenzyme function of vitamin K
    a. Aspartate b. Glutamate
    c. Glutamine d. Tyrosine
11. Ascorbic acid (vitamin C) resembles one of the following compounds in structure
    a. Monosaccharides b. Nucleotides
    c. Sterols d. Amino acid
12. The following vitamins/provitamins prevent several diseases (like cancer, heart attacks) by acting as antioxidants except
    a. Vitamin A b. Bicarbonate
    c. Vitamin E d. Vitamin C
13. One of the following is a poor source of folic acid
    a. Milk b. Leafy vegetables
    c. Liver d. Cereals
14. One of the following enzymes is absent is adults
    a. Renin b. Rennin
    c. Pepsin d. Chymotrypsin

Answers

1. b	2. c	3. b	4. b
5. b	6. b	7. c	8. c
9. c	10. b	11. a	12. a
13. a	14. b		

TISSUE BIOCHEMISTRY

1. One of the following is an example of the transport proteins
   a. Keratin b. Pepsin
   c. Actin d. Albumin
2. One of the following is an example of phosphoprotein
   a. Histone b. Casein
   c. Ceruloplasmin d. Albumin
3. One of the following proteins is not synthesized in the liver
   a. Albumin b. Transferrin
   c. Fibrinogen d. Immunoglobulin

4. Immunoglobulins are synthesized by
   a. T lymphocyte b. Liver
   c. Kidney d. B lymphocytes
5. The following immunoglobulin is elevated in allergic reactions
   a. IgA b. IgM
   c. IgD d. IgE
6. One of the following has been deleted from the list of blood clotting factors
   a. I b. VI
   c. I d. X
7. The extrinsic and intrinsic pathways of blood clotting result in the activation of the factor
   a. IX b. X
   c. XI d. XII
8. Hemophilia is caused due to the defect of factors
   a. V b. VI
   c. VII d. VIII
9. Christmas disease is due to deficiency of
   a. VIII b. IX
   c. X d. XI
10. Which one of the following statements concerning the hemoglobins is correct?
    a. Fetal blood has a higher affinity for oxygen than does adult blood because HbF has a decreased affinity for 2,3-BPG
    b. Purified HbF (stripped of 2,3-BPG) has a higher affinity for oxygen than does purified HbA
    c. The globin chain composition of HbF is $\alpha 2\gamma 2$
    d. HbA1c differs from HbA by a single, genetically determined amino acid substitution
11. Which one of the following statements concerning the ability of acidosis to precipitate a crisis in sickle cell anemia is correct?
    a. Acidosis decreases the solubility of HbS.
    b. Acidosis increases the affinity of hemoglobin for oxygen
    c. Acidosis favors the conversion of hemoglobin from the taut to the relaxed conformation
    d. Acidosis shifts the oxygen dissociation curve to the left
12. Which one of the following statements concerning the binding of oxygen by hemoglobin is correct?
    a. The Bohr effect results in a lower affinity for oxygen at higher pH values
    b. Carbon dioxide increases the oxygen affinity of hemoglobin by binding to the C-terminal groups of the polypeptide chains
    c. The oxygen affinity of hemoglobin increases as the percentage saturation increases
    d. The hemoglobin tetramer binds four molecules of 2,3-BPG
13. A 30-year-old woman presented with progressive shortness of breath. She denied the use of cigarettes. A family history revealed that her sister had suffered from unexplained lung disease. Which one of the following etiologies most likely explains this patient's pulmonary symptoms?
    a. Deficiency of proline hydroxylase
    b. Deficiency of α-1-antitrypsin
    c. Deficiency in dietary vitamin C
    d. Decreased elastase activity

Answers

1. d	2. b	3. d	4. d
5. d	6. b	7. b	8. d
9. b	10. a	11. a	12. c
13. b			

MOLECULAR BIOLOGY

1. Which RNA has abnormal purine bases?
   a. 16sRNA b. tRNA
   c. mRNA d. rDNA
2. False regarding gout is
   a. Has a predilection for the great toe
   b. Uric acid levels may not be elevated
   c. Due to increased metabolism of purines
   d. Due to increased metabolism of pyrimidines
3. Triple bonds are found between which of the following base pairs?
   a. C T b. A T
   c. C G d. A G
4. In xeroderma pigmentosa, primary defect is
   a. Formation of adenine dimers
   b. Defective exonuclease
   c. Formation of thymine dimers
   d. Defective poly ADP ribose polymerase
5. Translation occurs in
   a. Ribosomes
   b. Cytoplasm
   c. Nucleus
   d. Mitochondria
6. Gout is a disorder of
   a. Protein metabolism
   b. Oxalate metabolism
   c. Purine metabolism
   d. Pyrimidine metabolism
7. Enzyme involved in translation often referred to as fidelity enzyme is
   a. Amino acyl-reductase
   b. DNA polymerase

c. RNA polymerase
d. Aminoacyl-tRNA synthetase

8. Which of the following molecular phenomenon in Ig genes is responsible for affinity maturation of antibody response?
a. Somatic hypermutation
b. Altered RNA splicing
c. Junctional diversity
d. Chain shuffling

9. Okazaki segments are required in
a. Protein synthesis b. DNA synthesis
c. RNA synthesis d. None of the above

10. Strongest bond is
a. Hydrophobic b. van der Waals
c. Electrostatic d. Hydrogen

11. DNA restriction is done by which method?
a. Spectrophotometer
b. Spectrometry
c. Paper chromatograph
d. Gel electrophoresis

12. Restriction endonuclease
a. Breaks RNA
b. Breaks double-stranded DNA
c. Breaks single-stranded DNA
d. Breaks peptide chain

13. The mitochondrial DNA (mtDNA) is
a. Circular double stranded
b. Circular single stranded
c. Linear double helix
d. None of the above

14. DNA is found in all of the following except
a. Nucleus b. Mitochondria
c. Golgi apparatus d. Chloroplasts

15. One of the following is not a purine
a. Adenine b. Uric acid
c. Thymine d. Guanine

16. All of the following are pyrimidines except
a. Cytosine b. Thymine
c. Uracil d. Xanthine

17. Deoxyribose has one oxygen less than ribose at carbon
a. 2 b. 3
c. 4 d. 5

18. Thymine and uracil differ in their structure by the presence in thymine or absence in uracil of a/an
a. Amino group b. Methyl group
c. Hydroxyl group d. Phosphate group

19. One of the following is a major purine base found in tea
a. Caffeine b. Theobromine
c. Theophylline d. Hypoxanthine

20. All of the following bases exhibit tautomerism except
a. Adenine b. Guanine
c. Cytosine d. Thymine

21. Chemically uric acid is
a. 6-oxypurine
b. 2, 6 dioxypurine
c. 2, 6, 8 trioxypurine
d. 6-aminopurine

22. One of the following is regarded as the reserve bank of genetic information in higher organisms
a. Deoxyribonucleotide
b. Deoxyribonucleic acid
c. Protein
d. Ribonucleic acid

23. DNA is found in all of the following except
a. Nucleus b. Mitochondria
c. Golgi apparatus d. Chloroplasts

24. A 10-year-old girl is brought to the dermatologist by her parents. She has many freckles on her face, neck, arms and hands, and the parents report that she is unusually sensitive to sunlight. Two basal cell carcinomas are identified on her face. Which of the following processes is most likely to be defective in this patient?
a. Repair of double-strand breaks
b. Removal of mismatched bases from the 3'-end of Okazaki fragments
c. Removal of pyrimidine dimers from DNA
d. Removal of uracil from DNA

25. Telomeres are complexes of DNA and protein that protect the ends of linear chromosomes. In most normal human somatic cells, telomeres shorten with each division. In stem cells and in cancer cells, however, telomeric length is maintained. In the synthesis of telomeres
a. Telomerase, a ribonucleoprotein, provides both the RNA and the polymerase needed for synthesis
b. The RNA of telomerase serves as a primer
c. The polymerase of telomerase is a DNA-directed DNA polymerase
d. The shorter, 3' ⟶ 5' strand gets extended

26. The extent of DNA synthesis in a cell could most specifically be determined by measuring the incorporation of radiolabeled
a. Leucine b. Phosphate
c. Ribose d. Thymidine

Answers

1. b	2. d	3. c	4. c
5. a	6. c	7. d	8. a
9. b	10. c	11. d	12. b
13. a	14. c	15. c	16. d
17. a	18. b	19. c	20. a
21. c	22. b	23. c	24. c
25. a	26. d		

XENOBIOTICS

1. Mechanism of action of nitric oxide is through
   a. cGMP b. cAMP
   c. Tyrosine d. Ca^{2+}
2. Correct statement regarding nitric oxide is
   a. NO is released from mitochondria
   b. NO is synthesized from arginine
   c. NO causes vasoconstriction
   d. NO is spontaneously produced from NO_2
3. In cytochrome P450, P stands for
   a. Structural protein b. Polymer
   c. Substrate protein d. Pigment
4. Selenium is cofactor for
   a. Glutathione dehydrogenase
   b. Glutathione synthetase
   c. Glutathione reductase
   d. Glutathione peroxidase

Answers

1. a 2. b
3. d 4. d

CANCER

1. The following form of ionizing radiation is associated with highest risk of cancer
   a. α rays b. β rays
   c. γ rays d. X-rays
2. Important examples of tumor suppressor gene indicated in human cancer include the following except
   a. *RB gene* b. *TP53*
   c. *APC* d. *ERB-B*
3. An example of tumor associated antigen is
   a. Tests specific antigen
   b. Alpha-fetoprotein
   c. Carcinoembryonic antigen
   d. Prostate-specific antigen

Answer

1. a 2. d 3. d

CLINICAL CHEMISTRY

1. All are liver function tests except
   a. Alanine aminotransferase
   b. Aspartate aminotransferase (ALT)
   c. Gamma-glutamyl transferase (GGT)
   d. Lactic acid dehydrogenase (LDH)
2. Normal serum urea level is
   a. 20–40 mg/dL b. 40–45 mg/dL
   c. 5–10 mg/dL d. 10–15 mg/dL
3. Serum creatinine is estimated by
   a. Jaffe's method
   b. Schiff's method
   c. Modified Neumann test
   d. Millon's test

Answer

1. d 2. a 3. a

BIOTECHNIQUES

1. DNA fragments formed by the action of restriction endonucleases are separated by
   a. High pressure liquid chromatography
   b. Paper chromatography
   c. Gel electrophoresis
   d. Agarose gel electrophoresis
2. True about polymerase chain reaction is
   a. Enzyme DNA amplification
   b. Separation of protein fragments in serum
   c. Recombinant DNA amplification
   d. None of the above
3. Dietary cholesterol is transported to (PCR) is
   a. Enzymatic DNA amplification
   b. Separation of protein fragments in serum
   c. Recombinant DNA amplification
   d. None of the above

Answers

1. c 2. a 3. c

Index

Page numbers followed by *t* refer to table and *f* refer to figure

H

I

J

K

R

S

T

U

V

W

X

Z